Low Vision

Low Vision

What It's Like to Live with Vision Loss

Gordon E. Legge

OXFORD
UNIVERSITY PRESS

OXFORD
UNIVERSITY PRESS

Great Clarendon Street, Oxford, OX2 6DP,
United Kingdom

Oxford University Press is a department of the University of Oxford.
It furthers the University's objective of excellence in research, scholarship,
and education by publishing worldwide. Oxford is a registered trade mark of
Oxford University Press in the UK and in certain other countries.

Published in the United States of America by Oxford University Press
198 Madison Avenue, New York, NY 10016, United States of America

British Library Cataloguing in Publication Data

Data available

Library of Congress Control Number: 2025945839

ISBN 9780198946939

DOI: 10.1093/9780198946960.001.0001

The manufacturer's authorized representative in the EU for product safety is
Oxford University Press España S.A. of Parque Empresarial San Fernando de Henares,
Avenida de Castilla, 2 – 28830 Madrid (www.oup.es/en or product.safety@oup.com).
OUP España S.A. also acts as importer into Spain of products made by the manufacturer.

To Wend and Alex with love, and to all my academic children.

—Gordon E. Legge

January 2025

Acknowledgments

My wife Wendy Willson Legge is my source of inspiration and encouragement. She is also my best editor, advisor, and critic. It is a joy for me to thank her for help with this book.

Enormous thanks to Rachel Gage, my lab manager, who has played a critical role in putting this book together. The book would not have happened without Rachel's countless hours of care and attention.

I am grateful to my many academic children—former PhD students and postdocs—who have worked with me over many years to understand how both normal and low vision function. I am specifically grateful to those who helped review text and prepare figures for this book: Yingzi Xiong, Yingchen He, Walter Wu, Miyoung Kwon, Susana Chung, Quan Lei, Andrew Freedman, Siyun Liu, and Nilsu Atilgan.

I am so grateful to many research colleagues and friends who have reviewed drafts and answered questions. Aries Arditi encouraged me from the start and convinced me that this book would be worthwhile. He also reviewed several chapters, some more than once. It's a pleasure to acknowledge with thanks the generous advice and reviews I've received from Ian Bailey, Michael Beyeler, Chuck Bigelow, Peter Borden, Alex Bowers, Angela Brown, Sarah Creem-Regehr, Michael Crossland, Gislin Dagnelie, Dawn DeCarlo, Greg Goodrich, Chris Johnson, Rong Liu, Bob Massof, Sandra Montezuma, Eli Peli, Rob Shakespeare, Dennis Siemsen, Pawan Sinha, and Susanne Trauzettel-Klosinski.

I'm indebted to many people with low vision who have shared their personal experiences and insights with me over the years. I owe special thanks for help with this book to Bob Blyth, Christina Devine, Ross Doerr, Mary Ellen Kavanaugh, Luka Krmpotich, Mike May, the late Ken Mills, Kevin Moldenhauer, Lucas Nadolskis, Michael O'Day, and Walter Wu.

Thanks also to friends who helped me find the right publisher for this book—Catherine Alexander, Aries Arditi, Chuck Bigelow, and Denis Pelli. I am grateful to editors at Oxford University Press, Martin Baum, and Phoebe Aldridge, for recognizing merit in this project and for publishing this book. I also appreciate the excellent copy-editing and production work of Kanimozhi Ramamurthy, and Poornima I.

Finally, I'm grateful to colleagues at the University of Minnesota who have provided me with a friendly and supportive environment to teach and do research on low vision. I also want to acknowledge the research funding I've received for many years from the National Institutes of Health.

Contents

Introduction

Do you have low vision? Do you know someone with low vision? One out of every five people who live into their eighties will encounter vision loss. Some may grow up with normal, healthy vision and then experience vision loss from macular degeneration, glaucoma, or another eye disease later in life. Others may be born with an inherited or congenital condition that results in low vision such as albinism or retinopathy of prematurity. Most people with vision loss have useful remaining vision; we call it *low vision*. But what can they see? What is the impact of low vision on their daily lives? Put it simply, what's it like to live with low vision?

Low vision is not blindness. Rather, it is the broad spectrum between blindness and normal vision. Low vision is any kind of visual impairment that can't be corrected with glasses or contact lenses. It affects millions of people in the United States and hundreds of millions of people worldwide. The most common causes are disorders that occur as we grow older, so low vision will become more prevalent as our population ages.

Eye doctors diagnose and treat eye disorders and prescribe eyeglasses. Rehabilitation professionals and special educators provide advice on daily living skills to people with low vision. These experts play crucial roles in helping those of us with low vision to succeed in our daily lives. But, even these experts find it difficult to explain what the visual experience of living with low vision is like.

I am a vision scientist. My students, colleagues, and I have devoted more than 40 years to understanding the perceptual experience of people with low vision, and how the different forms of low vision affect everyday life. In this book, I describe the different visual experiences of people with low vision. By understanding the science behind these experiences, we will better understand the challenges and possibilities of life with low vision.

Low vision can result from deficits in three major aspects of vision—visual acuity (the ability to see fine details), contrast sensitivity (the ability to distinguish small differences in color or shades of gray between an object and its background), and the overall field of view (which can be disrupted by central vision loss or peripheral vision loss). These deficits have surprisingly

Low Vision. Gordon E. Legge, Oxford University Press. © Oxford University Press (2026).
DOI: 10.1093/9780198946960.003.0001

diverse effects on visual capabilities. In this book, I explain how these aspects of vision are measured and what the measurements mean. More importantly, I explore how these different forms of vision impairment affect what we see and don't see.

I have a personal as well as a professional interest in low vision. I've had low vision myself since childhood. Although most of this book deals with how low vision works and the science behind it, I include illustrative anecdotes from my own experience with low vision. I'll tell you a little about my history now. I grew up in Toronto, Canada. When I was six years old, I experienced a life-threatening disorder called Stevens–Johnson Syndrome. My temperature rose to 107 degrees. My skin erupted with blisters all over my body. My life was at stake. I spent nearly five months in the hospital recovering. I don't recall how or when it became clear that my eyes were affected, but I do recall eventually getting out of bed, looking out the window and not being able to see the people and cars on the street below. At the time, it didn't seem like such a big deal. What I cared about then was feeling better, being able to eat a chicken sandwich and have ice cream, hugging my teddy bears, and yearning to go home. Each day, I waited eagerly, listening for my mother's footsteps coming along the hospital corridor; she visited every day, often twice. As a six-year old in the hospital, I wasn't thinking about the impact of my decreased vision on my future life. My eyesight would get better, wouldn't it? For many adults who acquire low vision, the consequences—being no longer able to drive or read—are frightening and psychologically debilitating.

My corneas were damaged as were the tear glands that produce necessary moisture and metabolic support for the cornea. Although I didn't realize it at the time, my life had taken a huge turn. I was transformed from a child with normal vision to one with severe low vision.

I spent the next six months recovering at home. A home teacher came and drew very large letters on paper so that I could begin to learn my alphabet. In the following years, I was in and out of hospital for eye treatments and surgeries. I attended a residential school for the blind in Brantford, Ontario, where I learned to read braille. I then transferred to a mainstream high school in Toronto. With the benefit of parental support and dedicated teachers, I excelled in high school and was accepted to the Massachusetts Institute of Technology (MIT) to study science and engineering. I graduated with a Bachelor of Science degree in physics and went on to graduate studies at Harvard. I received a PhD in Psychology, specializing in vision science. Soon after, I was hired as a faculty member at the University of Minnesota where I've taught and done research ever since. Throughout these years, I have confronted many challenges, both professional and personal, related to my low vision.

Low vision is puzzling for normally sighted people to understand and difficult for those of us with low vision to explain. Sometimes people ask me, often hesitating for fear of offending me: “How well can you see?” This is a hard question to answer. I will sometimes turn the table on my normally sighted interrogator and ask, “Well, first tell me how well do you see?” This question usually stumps them and makes clear why it’s hard to verbalize one’s visual capability. If I’m talking to an eye doctor or vision expert, I can tell them about my acuity and visual field: “I have very low acuity, less than 20/1000 on a good day, but I have a full visual field. I have vascularized corneas, which result in very low contrast sensitivity. I experience a lot of problems with glare.” This answer is not very helpful for people outside the vision community. For them, I answer by example: “I can read the largest newspaper headlines or highly magnified letters on a computer screen, but I can’t recognize faces, no matter how close I get. I often have trouble with depth perception (is it a small thing nearby or a large thing far away) and the shapes of things (they often look like formless blobs). My vision is ‘better’ in familiar places. Yes, that bright orange thing is the cat dish on our kitchen counter. In an unfamiliar hotel room or friend’s home, it’s just an unidentified orange blob.”

If you are a normally sighted person, I hope this book makes low vision less puzzling for you. If you are a person with low vision, this book will help you explain your visual world to family and friends.

Textbooks for optometrists and ophthalmologists address the diagnosis and treatment of eye disease and the prescription of low-vision aids. This book is different. It is about the visual experience of living with low vision and the implications for everyday life. I am writing from the unusual perspective of someone who has studied low vision in its many forms and who has experienced low vision personally. My goal for this book is to describe what it’s like to live with low vision, in all its different forms and degrees.

In Part I of the book—*Measuring and Understanding What People See*—I’ll begin by explaining in more detail what low vision is and why it is misunderstood. Then, I’ll explain how acuity, contrast sensitivity, and visual fields are measured and how the resulting numbers can be interpreted. What are the implications of the deficits revealed by these measurements for seeing things around us?

Part II—*The Impact of Low Vision on Daily Life*—describes how low vision affects reading and mobility. Almost everyone with low vision has reading difficulty. What are the limitations and what can be done to help? Mobility can also be daunting: how do people with low vision get around on foot or by car? Yes, there are people with low vision who drive legally and safely!

Part III—*Recovery of Sight?*—addresses the hope of sight recovery from two perspectives. Chapter 9 deals with low vision in childhood. There have been remarkable recent advances in our understanding of inherited and other forms of low vision with onset in early life. Chapter 10 discusses the dreams and realities of vision restoration for those of us living our lives with low vision.

I conclude the book with a brief epilogue, looking ahead to future research relevant to low vision.

I have included an appendix with an overview of the major structures of the eye for quick reference. I do include some technical details of a few research studies for readers who are interested and some boxes with extra information. Feel free to skim and skip according to your interest. For the most part, the chapters are self-contained.

Low vision is a topic of worldwide importance. As an author living and working in the United States, I acknowledge my U.S.-centric perspective. One particular example is my frequent use of acuity measures using Snellen ratios in the 20/xx format, such as 20/20 and 20/200. In Chapter 2 on acuity, I explain the relationship to metric notation for acuity such as 6/6 or 6/60. In some cases throughout the book, I have included metric equivalents when I refer to acuities with the 20/xx notation.

I also note that my source citations are intended to provide pointers to relevant research literature and are not intended to be exhaustive. My choice of citations may sometimes be affected by my American viewpoint. I do admire and celebrate the growing interest in low vision throughout the world.

This is not a medical text, and I will not attempt to cover the details of the vast number of eye conditions that result in low vision. There are many online sources of valuable medical information on eye and vision disorders. Instead, by explaining how low vision works and the science behind it, I hope readers will achieve a better understanding of the nature, value, and limitations of low vision.

My goal is to talk to a broad readership, including people with low vision, their families and friends, and the professionals who interact with them—ophthalmologists, optometrists, occupational therapists, rehabilitation specialists, and special educators. This book should also be useful to the tech industry, policymakers, and others interested in inclusive design for visual accessibility. I hope that this book will introduce many students to the marvelous nature of human vision in its diversity. I also dare to hope that anyone who contemplates the wonder of human vision will enjoy reading these pages.

PART I

MEASURING AND UNDERSTANDING WHAT PEOPLE SEE

1
What Is Low Vision?

The concept of low vision is unfamiliar to many people. What is it? Who has it? What causes it? How is it related to legal blindness? Why is so little known about it? Let's begin this book by answering these questions. In later chapters, I'll describe the varieties of low vision and how they are measured and the impact of low vision on everyday activities such as reading, mobility, driving, and social interaction. A major purpose of this chapter, and the book as a whole, is to enhance the understanding and awareness of low vision among the public and among students and professionals with an interest in eye care and rehabilitation. Let's get started!

• • • • •

Ken was driving at night in a strange city. He narrowly missed hitting a pedestrian who was crossing the street. Ken was shaken. He confronted his own denial and admitted to himself for the first time that he had a serious vision problem. He spent the evening in his hotel room browsing the internet for information about vision impairment. He discovered the term "low vision" and realized it applied to him. It was a revelation. Ken was a highly educated man with a career in national media, and yet, he was unfamiliar with the concept and the term "low vision." He became an active advocate and educator on behalf of people with vision disabilities.

Like Ken, many people do not recognize or acknowledge the onset of low vision. They may bump into something, fail to recognize a friend at a restaurant, or miss seeing a pedestrian at a street crossing. "Why did that happen? … I better get my glasses checked." Then, a visit to the doctor or an accident due to vision loss brings home the stark reality of vision impairment. Even with this realization, the concept of low vision is alien to most people.

The reality of low vision may be hard to accept. But, once accepted, there is much to be understood and much to be done.

Low Vision. Gordon E. Legge, Oxford University Press. © Oxford University Press (2026).
DOI: 10.1093/9780198946960.003.0002

Defining low vision

Low vision refers to any permanent or long-standing form of vision impairment that adversely affects everyday function. In developed countries, the term "low vision" does not describe people who can achieve normal vision with the aid of glasses or contacts, nor does it refer to people who have normal vision in one eye and reduced vision in the other eye. The World Health Organization (WHO) and other international organizations do count people who lack access to glasses as having visual impairment. Later in this chapter, we'll consider more detailed clinical definitions of low vision based on reduced visual acuity and restricted visual field.

The term low vision was first used in the early 1950s by the ophthalmologists Eleanor Faye and Gerald Fonda to refer to vision lying between blindness and normal sight. They were seeing patients in their eye clinic at the New York Association for the Blind, also known as The Lighthouse. They preferred *low vision* to earlier terms for the same category of sight such as subnormal vision, defective vision, partial vision, partial blindness, and vision impairment. Faye and Fonda were among the first eye doctors to focus specifically on maximizing the usefulness of remaining vision. They believed that low vision was a more positive description than the earlier terms. A timeline of important events in the history of developments concerning low vision[1] is available at the website of the American Printing House for the Blind (APH).

Interest in low vision, though not yet named, was already in the air by the early 1950s. In 1932, the optometrist William Feinbloom initiated his pioneering work on optical aids for low vision by designing telescopic spectacles. The first regular production of large-print books was undertaken by the APH in 1947.

Prior to the mid-20th century, the category of low vision, by any name, was not widely recognized. This neglect was due in part to the erroneous belief that using vision in the presence of an eye disorder would accelerate vision loss. The sight-saving philosophy of the early 20th century promoted this view. People with low vision were told that they should refrain from using their eyes in order to preserve their dwindling vision. This concern was especially common among older adults with late-onset low vision from age-related eye diseases such as macular degeneration, glaucoma, and cataract. No wonder there was little demand for rehabilitation programs or assistive technology.

[1] https://aphconnectcenter.org/wp-content/uploads/sites/5/2023-Low-Vision-History-Timeline.pdf.

During the first 60 years of the 20th century, children with low vision were typically educated in residential schools for the blind. Children with low vision would sometimes leave school unable to read print. I attended a school for the blind in Ontario, Canada, in the late 1950s and early 1960s. I learned to read Braille. There was no instruction in print reading, even for children with moderate low vision. Use of optical aids and glasses was discouraged. The curriculum was comprehensive, but delivered entirely with a blindness focus. Fortunately, I had been taught to read print, and very large print it was, by a home teacher during the year before my enrollment at the school for the blind. During my childhood, I would practice my print reading by finding and reading newspaper headlines, which also stimulated my interest in current affairs.

Although the curriculum at the Ontario School for the Blind assumed no vision, the students were certainly aware of differences in vision status. As Canadians, we played hockey, dividing into kids who were totally blind and those with low vision. The kids who were blind used a crumpled tin can rather than a puck because of its rattling sound. A teammate would stand behind the opposing goal and yell "over here" to guide the blind players in directing the "puck." The "sighted" kids (those with adequate low vision) played with a regular hockey puck and could usually see the opposing goal. I played with the blind group and wore a blindfold so that I could not use my very low vision. Try closing your eyes and imagine hearing the scrape of skate blades on ice, the crack of wooden hockey sticks against each other, and the rattle of a tin can on ice. Sharp hockey skates, blind players wildly swinging hockey sticks, and a crumpled tin can with sharp edges made for a very rough game! Despite a few bruises, we had fun and the competition was intense.

The idea of sight-saving classes for children with low vision originated in England. In a book chapter, Michael Crossland (2024) tells us that the first class for children with progressive myopia and other forms of low vision (such as albinism and congenital cataract) was held in 1908 at the Boundary Lane School in London. The special class was intended to reduce the progression of myopia by reducing eye strain and by limiting physical activity that might lead to retinal detachment. Crossland reports that parents were advised, "... for the protection of your children's eyes ... do not let them read or write," and children were told that reading for pleasure is a vice until fully grown. The concept of sight-saving or "conservation" classes soon spread to other European countries and was imported to the United States by Edward Allen, Director of the Perkins School for the Blind in Massachusetts.

In 1964, Natalie Barraga, a teacher of the visually impaired, completed a PhD at Vanderbilt University addressing the feasibility of children with low vision using visual skills in school. Subsequently, as a faculty member at the University of Texas at Austin, she promoted the view that children with low vision would benefit from using their remaining vision and would not do harm to their eyesight by doing so. Those with adequate vision could learn to read print with the aid of glasses and magnifiers in addition to or instead of learning Braille.

Today, most children in the United States with vision impairment are integrated into mainstream schools. U.S. federal law now mandates that a free, appropriate public education be available to all disabled children. Typically, visually impaired children in mainstream classrooms, whether blind or low vision, are provided with supplementary services from their school districts, including help from specially trained teachers of the visually impaired.

Barraga's influential work in special education, following the awakening interest in low vision among eye-care clinicians (ophthalmologists and optometrists), raised the profile of low vision among clinicians, educators, and rehabilitation specialists and eventually brought the concept of low vision to the general public. But, even today, low vision remains poorly understood. One purpose of this book is to enhance awareness of low vision among the public, educators, and rehabilitation professionals.

Terminology for impaired vision abounds. Low vision is one of the three broad categories of sight, the other two being normal vision and blindness. Some people prefer the term "typical vision" to "normal vision" when referring to vision with no impairment. Dictionary synonyms for "normal" include "usual," "ordinary," "typical," and others. In this book, I will frequently use "normal vision" to refer to unimpaired vision. I will use the term "blindness" to refer to the lack of any useful pattern vision. As we will see below, "blindness" is sometimes used for statutory or demographic purposes to refer to people with low vision below some criterion level of visual acuity. Sometimes, people with low vision or blindness are referred to collectively as "visually impaired" (VI), "blind and visually impaired" (BVI), or "visually impaired people" (VIP). This plethora of terminology can be confusing.

In 2002, the eminent ophthalmologist August Colenbrander prepared a report for the International Council of Ophthalmology distinguishing among four different aspects of low vision—visual disorder, visual impairment, visual disability, and visual handicap. Table 1.1 defines these four terms.

The four terms in this table are often used interchangeably in everyday conversation but have subtly different meanings. The first two terms refer to the status of the eyes or visual system. The third and fourth terms refer to consequences in daily life for a person with visual impairment. It is wise to keep these distinctions in mind when discussing topics related to low vision.

Table 1.1 Additional terminology associated with low vision

Term	Definition	Examples
Visual disorder	Any deviation from normal in the status of the eyes, including diseases or chronic conditions.	Glaucoma, eye injury, droopy eyelid, dry eye, detached retina, lazy eye.
Visual impairment	Consequences of an eye disease or disorder on a measure of visual function.	Reduced acuity, contrast sensitivity, size of the visual field.
Visual disability	Restrictions on normal activities of daily life resulting from visual impairment.	Difficulties with reading, mobility, face recognition.
Visual handicap	A cultural, economic, or social disadvantage for a person resulting from visual impairment.	Reduced access to education, employment, commerce, social life.

People are often hesitant or embarrassed about how to refer to another person's vision status. Whether the person self identifies as "blind," "low vision," "visually impaired," "visually disabled," "visually handicapped," "visually challenged," or something else, depends on personal preference. When in doubt, my advice is to ask the person what they prefer. In my own case, I have very low vision. I am legally blind in the United States and would be classified as "blind" by the WHO. But, I self-identify as low vision because I particularly value, enjoy, and make use of my remaining vision.

Clinical criteria for low vision: Acuity and visual field

Visual acuity refers to the ability to see fine details. Chapter 2 is devoted to a discussion of acuity. Letter acuity on the eye chart is the traditional clinical measure of vision, dating from the first such chart introduced by the Dutch ophthalmologist Herman Snellen in 1862. Values of letter acuity are often used to establish a boundary between normal vision and low vision and between low vision and blindness. Values of visual acuity are often given as a fraction such as 20/20 or 20/200 in the United States, called a Snellen fraction or Snellen ratio. In metric notation, the corresponding Snellen ratios are 6/6 and 6/60. In this book, I'll often include corresponding metric notation for acuity in parentheses. I'll describe the meaning of Snellen ratios in detail in the next chapter. Here, I'll discuss some reference points on the Snellen scale for classifying vision status.

A Snellen acuity of 20/20 (6/6) is the conventional standard for normal vision. In reality, many people can recognize letters smaller than those on the 20/20 line of the eye chart. The population average in the United States is closer to 20/16 (6/4.8) and more than half the population have acuity better than 20/20. Some people with eagle-eyed vision have acuity better than 20/10 (6/3), meaning that they can read letters on the acuity chart that are less than half the size of the letters on the 20/20 line.

On one memorable occasion, my wife Wendy came home from an eye check-up and reported to me that she had excellent vision: "I have 20/20 vision in both eyes!" I smugly replied, "That's not so great. Many people have better than 20/20 vision." Not to be outdone, she countered in jest, referring to my low vision, "Who are you to talk?"

According to the WHO (2019), the acuity boundary for low vision (they use the term "visual impairment") is an acuity less than 20/40 (6/12) (i.e., acuity letters more than two times larger than the standard for normal vision). If your acuity is 20/40 or worse, you are likely to run into trouble reading small print in newspapers or on electronic devices. In many U.S. states, acuity better than 20/40 is required for driving, so if your acuity is less, you are at risk of losing your driver's license. We'll return to the issue of driving and visual acuity in Chapter 8.

The WHO's definition of blindness is an acuity worse than 20/400 (6/120). It is certainly the case that people with an acuity less than this level experience major visual impairment and typically benefit from nonvisual strategies for dealing with daily activities. But, many people with acuity less than 20/400 continue to read visually for some purposes, given adequate magnification, and to rely on vision for mobility and other activities. While defining blindness as vision poorer than 20/400 is convenient for studies in epidemiology, I prefer to classify those of us with acuity less than 20/400, but with remaining useful vision, as having low vision. Indeed, people with acuities as low as 20/2,000 (who require acuity letters 100 times larger than the 20/20 letters) are sometimes able to read highly magnified print on a large-screen display.

In the United States, the acuity criterion for legal blindness is 20/200 or less (acuity letters at least 10 times larger than the 20/20 letters). The designation of legal blindness is used for statutory purposes, such as eligibility for social security benefits or tax deductions. Many people who are "legally blind" and have functionally useful vision are classified as having low vision in this book. The categorization of people as "seeing" or "legally blind" has tended to obscure the many gradations of low vision and the functional value of residual vision. Some people with low vision dislike being labeled "legally blind" because they feel there is a stigma or because they feel the designation may disqualify them from access to jobs or other activities. Others find it desirable to be designated "legally blind" to qualify for certain benefits.

Under some conditions, people who are legally blind can meet the visual requirements for restricted-use driver's licenses.

When acuity is too low to be easily measured on an acuity chart, eye doctors will often use qualitative descriptions of remaining vision such as "finger counting," "hand motion," or "light perception." These descriptors tend to be imprecise and may often devalue the functional benefits of very low vision. To address this deficiency, the term *ultra-low vision* was coined in 2010 by Gislin Dagnelie and Duane Geruschat at Johns Hopkins University in Baltimore. They were interested in characterizing and finding methods to measure vision that is too impaired to be measurable with standard letter acuity charts, typically acuities worse than 20/1600. Some of the new technologies being explored for vision restoration, such as retinal implants, improve vision from total blindness or light perception to ultra-low vision. There is ongoing research on appropriate methods for measuring ultra-low vision. We'll return to a discussion of vision restoration in Chapter 10.

A definition of low vision based on acuity excludes some people with good central vision who have serious peripheral visual-field loss. For this reason, definitions of low vision often include field restriction as well. For example, the International Classification of Diseases (ICD-10) defines a visual field restricted to 60° as "mild" visual impairment and a visual field of less than 10° as blindness. In the United States, a visual field of less than 20° qualifies as legal blindness even if visual acuity is in the normal range. We will discuss peripheral field loss in detail in Chapter 4.

Prevalence

In the field of public health, *prevalence* refers to the number of cases of a condition present in a particular population at a given time, while *incidence* refers to the number of new cases of the condition per year. Epidemiology researchers have estimated the prevalence and incidence of impaired vision worldwide and in specific countries. These studies are difficult, typically relying on counts of cases in limited samples of people with extrapolation to the population at large. Adding to the challenge are the different definitions of visual impairment and the methods for determining the vision status of the sampled individuals. Population-based studies endeavor to sample as many individuals as possible from a specified demographic group. For example, in the Salisbury Eye Evaluation (SEE) study, conducted in Salisbury, Maryland, from 1993 to 1995, 2,520 residents in the age range from 65 to 84 years agreed to undergo an eye exam including acuity testing. Overall, 4.5% of the participants had acuity worse than 20/40, with 4% in the age range from 65 to 74 years and 16% in the range from 80 to 84 years. These numbers demonstrate the high prevalence of vision impairment among seniors and its increase with age.

In 2021, Rupert Bourne and members of the Vision Loss Expert Group published updated estimates of the worldwide prevalence of vision impairment. Their estimates were based on statistical modeling using data from population-based studies from several countries in the period 1980–2019. Table 1.2 shows prevalence estimates for the year 2020, using their acuity-based categories of visual impairment and blindness.

Bourne et al. (2021) estimated that in 2020, 596.3 million people worldwide were visually impaired, representing 7.55% of the world population of 7.89 billion. The Vision Atlas,[2] maintained by the International Agency for the Prevention of Blindness (IAPB), reports updated estimates for the prevalence of vision impairment worldwide.

A large majority of this group, 553 million, have acuities in the range from 20/40 to 20/400. About 43.3 million are classified "blind" with acuities worse than 20/400. From these numbers, it is clear that the vast majority of people with visual impairment retain some level of vision and could be characterized as having low vision. Bourne and colleagues further estimated that about 55% of the visually impaired population are female. The gender imbalance is primarily due to the greater longevity of women and the rising prevalence of visual impairment with age.

Tiffany Chan (2018) and colleagues at Johns Hopkins University estimated the prevalence of visual impairment in the United States in 2017

Table 1.2 Global estimates of visual impairment (2020)

Category	# in Millions	% of World Population	# per Thousand
Mild: 20/40–20/60	258	3.3	32.7
Moderate to severe: 20/60–20/400	295	3.7	37.3
Blind: Worse than 20/400	43.3	0.55	5.5
Total	596.3	7.55	75.5

[2] https://www.iapb.org/learn/vision-atlas/#main.

Table 1.3 Estimates of visual impairment in the United States—2017 and 2050

Category of visual impairment	Prevalence in millions/% of population (2017)	Prevalence in millions/% of population(2050)
Worse than 20/40	5.7/1.75%	9.6/2.19%
20/200 Or Worse (legal blindness)	1.3/0.4%	2.3/0.53%

and projected prevalence for 2050. They based their analysis on best-corrected acuities obtained in the 2007–2008 National Health and Nutrition Examination Survey conducted by the National Center for Health Statistics. They used statistical modeling and census projections to make their estimates. Table 1.3 summarizes their prevalence estimates for the years 2017 and 2050. For 2017, they estimated that 5.7 million Americans had visual impairment (acuity worse than 20/40), of which 1.3 million were legally blind (acuity of 20/200 or worse). Although not included in their analysis, previous estimates indicate that about 20% of the legally blind population are totally blind, that is, have no useful pattern vision, which would be about 260,000 in 2017. A 2021 published study, led by Abraham Flaxman at the Institute for Health Metrics and Evaluation at the University of Washington, also made prevalence estimates for the year 2017 in the United States. The authors performed a meta-analysis of data from several surveys and population-based studies. Their estimate of the total number of people with visual impairment was 7.08 million, higher than the 5.7 million estimated by Chan et al. Their estimate of 1.08 million people who are legally blind was a little lower than the 1.3 million estimated by Chan et al. Differences such as these are not surprising, given the challenges in collecting and analyzing prevalence data for impaired vision.

The prevalence estimates in Tables 1.2 and 1.3 are surprising to most people. They reveal the vast scope of visual impairment worldwide and in the United States. Prevalence studies are important because they inform policymakers about the need for vision screening, rehabilitation services, and social programs. They also let those of us with low vision know that we are not alone. Because vision impairment is sometimes a hidden and often neglected condition, many people with normal vision are unaware of the low-vision status of their neighbors and friends.

A global initiative to eliminate avoidable blindness

Comparison of Tables 1.2 and 1.3 reveals a big difference in the prevalence of impaired vision worldwide and in the U.S. Allowing for some differences due to methods and definitions, it seems clear that the global prevalence (about 7.5%) is much higher than the U.S. prevalence (about 2%). Why might this be the case?

A substantial proportion of vision impairment worldwide is preventable or treatable. Access to eye care is more widely available in wealthy nations than in poorer countries. In 1999, the WHO and the IAPB launched an initiative called VISION 2020: The Right to Sight: A Global Initiative to Eliminate Avoidable Blindness. The goal was to provide treatment for the leading causes of preventable blindness in parts of the world where such treatment has not been readily available. The major treatable disorders included uncorrected refractive error (lack of eyeglasses), cataract, trachoma, and river blindness (onchocerciasis).

The global prevalence estimates from Bourne and colleagues in Table 1.2 include people who have impaired vision for lack of eyeglasses. These estimates are based on measures of *presenting* acuity rather than *best-corrected* visual acuity. "Presenting" visual acuity refers to measures taken with whatever glasses (or lack thereof) the individual brings at the time of testing. "Best-corrected" acuity refers to results after the individual has been fitted with appropriate glasses or contacts. In many countries worldwide, the prescription and provision of glasses is not routine. Many individuals live their daily lives with impaired vision due to lack of an appropriate optical prescription. In the United States and other countries with access to good health care, the prevalence of impaired vision is based upon best-corrected visual acuity. U.S. prevalence estimates of impaired vision, such as those in Table 1.3, usually do not include deficits in acuity that can be remedied by glasses or contacts. It is assumed that most people in wealthy countries have access to appropriate lens prescriptions. It is notable, however, that the SEE study, mentioned earlier, found that about one third of the visually impaired individuals in their sample could be optically corrected to an acuity better than 20/40. This finding indicates that mild vision impairment due to inadequate optical prescriptions exists in the United States. It is also noteworthy that people with low vision can often benefit from improved prescription of glasses. In a study conducted in low vision clinics at the Wilmer Eye Institute of Johns Hopkins University, nearly 28% of entering low-vision patients improved by at least two lines on the acuity chart with best prescriptions (Guo et al., 2020).

Bourne and colleagues estimated that in addition to the nearly 600 million people worldwide with vision impairment, 510 million more are unable to focus clearly on nearby objects, such as text in a book, due to uncorrected presbyopia. Presbyopia is the normal age-related decline in the ability to focus on near objects, easily corrected with bifocals or reading glasses. A 2018 article in *The New York Times* by Andrew Jacobs described "a simple way to improve a billion lives: eyeglasses." The article gave examples of typical disabilities due to the lack of eyeglasses—children in India whose education is hampered because they can't see the blackboard, Nigerian truck drivers involved in preventable road accidents, and Bolivian coffee farmers who have trouble finding the ripe beans. Farzana Sehrin (2024) and colleagues from Bangladesh Rural Advancement Committee demonstrated the economic benefits of providing inexpensive reading glasses to workers. They recruited workers from several villages in Bangladesh who did not wear glasses, who had below normal acuity for targets at a near viewing distance (40 cm), and who were engaged in jobs requiring near vision, such as tailors, carpenters, and shopkeepers. An intervention group was provided with inexpensive reading glasses. A control group received reading glasses only after the eight months of the intervention. The critical measure was a comparison of self-reported monthly incomes after eight months between the groups who received reading glasses and the controls who did not. The researchers found that the intervention group with reading glasses had 35.3% more income than the control group. The researchers concluded that provision of inexpensive reading glasses (less than $2 per pair) had major economic benefits for those with the glasses. A follow-up article in *The New York Times* by Andrew Jacobs (2024) described an interview with a tailor who participated in the intervention. As the tailor grew older, increasing presbyopia made it more and more difficult for him to thread needles and stitch clothing; his work slowed down, and his income declined. He reported that in the short time after receiving the glasses from the research team, his income had doubled.

While cataract surgery is commonly available to most people in developed countries, it remains a major cause of impaired vision worldwide. There is an international effort to provide affordable access to cataract surgery in low-income countries. In a 2015 article in *The New York Times* entitled "In Five Minutes, He Lets the Blind See," Nicholas Kristof reported on the work of Sanduk Ruit, an ophthalmologist in Nepal. Dr. Ruit has developed a simple form of cataract surgery that costs only $25 per eye and can be accomplished with modest equipment. The surgery has 98% success at six-month follow-up. Kristof reported on the case of Thuli Maya Thing, a 50-year-old woman whose daily activities were seriously disrupted by sight-impairing cataract. Because of her inability to fetch water, gather firewood, and cook over an open fire, her family often went hungry. Her vision was restored to 20/20 acuity the day after Dr. Ruit's surgery. It is realistic to hope that the prevalence of sight-impairing cataracts worldwide will be reduced in the near future.

Two infectious eye diseases—trachoma and onchocerciasis (river blindness)—are virtually unknown in developed countries but continue to account for severe vision impairment in parts of the world. Trachoma is the leading infectious cause of vision impairment. The infection results in scarring of the inside of the eyelids. The lids turn inward so that the lashes scratch the cornea, eventually leading to permanent corneal damage and loss of vision. Trachoma is spread by bacteria from contact with facial secretions (especially among children) or on clothing or by flies. It can be prevented by improved sanitation. It can be treated by antibiotics (especially Zithromax, donated in large quantities by the manufacturer Pfizer) or by eyelid surgery. Trachoma is essentially nonexistent in the United States where it was prevalent in the early 20th century. Immigrants arriving at Ellis Island were routinely screened for trachoma. Helen Keller's famous teacher and companion Anne Sullivan Macy had low vision resulting from trachoma.

River blindness is the second leading infectious cause of vision impairment. It is caused by parasitic worms (*onchocerca volvulus*). The larvae of these worms are spread by a type of black fly that breeds near rivers, accounting for the name river blindness. The flies ingest larvae when they bite an infected person and then transmit the larvae when they bite someone else. The larvae penetrate the skin and eventually reproduce as worms in the human host. The infected person exhibits an inflammatory response in the skin and eyes. Longstanding and intense cases can result in blindness. The condition can be treated with the anti-parasitic drug ivermectin and may require periodic doses over several years. The vast majority of river blindness occurs in rural areas of sub-Saharan Africa. Progress in reducing prevalence has been accomplished through spraying insecticides and through community administration of ivermectin with major donations of the drug by the manufacturer Merck.

While the aspirational goal of Vision 2020, to entirely eliminate avoidable blindness, was not achieved, there has been major progress. For example, several countries have eliminated trachoma and river blindness as public health problems.

Impact of aging

A remarkable finding from the prevalence estimates in Table 1.3 is that the number of people with visual impairment in the United States is expected to nearly double by the year 2050. Wouldn't we expect the prevalence of vision impairment to decline with advances in medical treatments for eye diseases? There are two major reasons for the projected growth in prevalence: the U.S. population is rising (from 325 million in 2017 to a projected 438 million in 2050), and the U.S. population is aging. The leading causes of visual impairment in the United States are age-related diseases—macular degeneration, glaucoma, diabetic retinopathy, and cataract.

The prevalence of impaired vision rises steeply with age. According to the Flaxman study cited earlier, 77% of those with vision impairment are over the age of 40, and 87% of those who are legally blind are older than 40 years. For those over 85 years, 20.7% have vision impairment and 5.5% are legally blind (acuity of 20/200 or worse).

When I present statistics on the prevalence of impaired vision and aging to my undergraduate students, I point out that by 2050, many of them will be approaching senior status and that a significant proportion of them are likely to experience visual impairment firsthand. I'm not trying to scare them, but I am trying to raise awareness about the societal significance of impaired vision.

Aging is also associated with increased prevalence of many health disorders in addition to impaired vision. In the SEE study of people aged 65 to 84 years, each individual reported an average of two health issues (comorbidities) from a standard list of 13 conditions, including arthritis, heart disease, and cancer, in addition to sensory impairment. From this finding, it is evident that many older people with low vision have multiple disabilities.

By a recent estimate, the prevalence of hearing impairment in the United States is twice that of vision impairment, and there are many older people with concurrent impairments in vision and hearing. According to a review by Minhas et al. (2022), between 10% and 20% of people 80 years and older in the United States have dual-sensory loss. Just as vision impairment may go unacknowledged, concurrent hearing difficulty may also be ignored. Even when dual sensory loss is recognized, strategies that are helpful for people with hearing impairment may not be effective for people who also have low vision. For example, TV subtitles that help with hearing impairment may not be legible for people with low vision.

While age-related hearing impairment and vision impairment usually result from different causes, Usher syndrome is an inherited disorder that affects both hearing and vision. Usher manifests early in life. In its most severe form (Usher 1), it is the leading cause of deafblindness. In the milder forms (Usher II and III), hearing impairment is accompanied by a form of retinitis pigmentosa that results in progressive vision loss.

Balance disorders pose another challenge for people with low vision. When combined with vision impairment, difficulties with balance increase the risk of falling. A study by Stephen Lord and Julia Dayhew (2001) at the Prince of Wales Medical Research Institute in Sydney, Australia, showed that visual impairment is an important and independent risk factor for falls. Injuries from falling can be life-threatening, especially in old age. Ursula White and colleagues (2015) at the Queensland University of Technology in Brisbane, Australia, reviewed findings showing that fear of falling itself tends to restrict daily activities, sometimes resulting in reduced social interaction and depression.

Causes

There are many different eye diseases and disorders and a bewildering number of names for them. To complicate matters, some eye diseases have multiple names, representing stages or variants of the pathology. For example, the wet form of age-related macular degeneration (AMD or ARMD) is also known as exudative macular degeneration, as choroidal neovascularization (CNV) (its prominent symptom), or as wet AMD or wet ARMD. The dry form of age-related macular degeneration is termed dry AMD or dry ARMD, and an advanced form is called geographic atrophy (GA).

Many informative resources are available for describing the symptoms, anatomical characteristics, and treatments of the major forms of eye disease. For example, the National Eye Institute (a component of the United States National Institutes of Health) provides information about many eye conditions and diseases.[3]

A few major eye diseases account for the vast majority of vision impairment. Table 1.4 compares the percentage prevalence of vision impairment worldwide and in the United States due to four major eye diseases.

In later chapters, I will describe some details of these diseases that are pertinent to understanding their distinct visual consequences. Here, I will mention several major differences between the United States and the world as a whole in the percentages of vision loss due to major eye diseases.

Table 1.4 indicates that cataract continues to be a major cause of visual impairment. Worldwide, cataract accounts for about 35% of blindness as defined by WHO, while in the U.S., only 12.6% of legal blindness is due to cataract. Surgery for removal of cataracts is widely available in developed countries, but not so in less-developed countries. As discussed earlier, cataracts are considered to be a treatable form of vision impairment, and now,

[3] https://www.nei.nih.gov/learn-about-eye-health/eye-conditions-and-diseases.

Table 1.4 Percentage prevalence of causes of visual impairment worldwide and in the United States

A. Worldwide (Flaxman et al., 2017)		
Eye conditions	**Acuity below 20/400 (WHO definition of "blind")**	**Acuity 20/60–20/400**
AMD	5.9	4.4
Cataract	35.1	25.2
Diabetic retinopathy	1.1	1.3
Glaucoma	8.5	2.1
Other	29.1	14.6
Refractive error	20.3	52.4
B. United States (Eye Diseases Prevalence Research Group, 2004)		
Eye conditions	**Acuity below 20/200 (legally blind)**	**Acuity 20/40–20/200**
AMD	47.2	21
Cataract	12.6	57.8
Diabetic retinopathy	5.9	6.1
Glaucoma	9.4	4.3
Other	25.2	10.8
Refractive error	NA	NA

there are international efforts to provide affordable access to cataract surgery in low-income countries.

There is a huge disparity in the worldwide and U.S. proportion of vision impairment due to AMD. Nearly 50% of legal blindness in the U.S. is due to AMD, compared to only about 6% worldwide. The risk for AMD rises rapidly with age. In the early 20th century, when life expectancy in the United States was only about 40 years, AMD was rare. But, with increased longevity and the baby boomer bulge in the population of seniors in the United States, the prevalence of AMD has increased rapidly. I'll have more to say about macular degeneration and its implications for activities of daily living in Chapter 5.

There are also racial differences in the causes of impaired vision. In the United States, AMD is the leading cause among whites and cataract and glaucoma among blacks. The prevalence of AMD is higher among whites than blacks in the U.S., but roughly comparable between whites and Americans of Chinese ethnicity. Curiously, data from the Beijing Eye Study imply that the prevalence of AMD is substantially lower in China than among Chinese

Americans. It would be valuable to understand the risk factors that underlie this difference.

Diabetic retinopathy has substantially higher prevalence as a cause of visual impairment in the U.S. than worldwide. This difference is related to the high proportion of people with obesity and the corresponding high risk for diabetes in the United States. According to the Centers for Disease Control, the prevalence of adult obesity in the United States in 2015 was 39.8%. People with diabetes have an increased risk of vision impairment.

Attitudes

In her book "*For the Benefit of Those Who See: Dispatches from the World of the Blind*," Rosemary Mahoney (2014) described how historical attitudes toward blindness have been dominated by fear, prejudice, and ignorance. She described her own "morbid fear" of blindness and the unease of many sighted people when encountering someone who is blind. She identified three ways in which the blind are portrayed in the Bible and in Greek and Roman mythology—as mystical soothsayers, subjects of pity, or objects of derision. At the root of many of these caricatures is the belief that blindness is a punishment for moral failing on the part of the afflicted person or their family.

Fear of blindness remains prevalent in modern American society. A 2014 opinion poll conducted by Zogby Analytics queried public attitudes toward vision loss. Losing eyesight was judged to have greater impact on daily life than loss of memory, hearing, or speech. The poll found that blindness ranked among the top four "worst things that could happen to you" along with cancer, Alzheimer's disease, and HIV/AIDS.

Most people have casually thought about the question: would you rather become blind or deaf? In a survey of 250 adults in the United Kingdom, conducted in 2016 by Jamie Enoch (2019) and colleagues at the City University of London, participants were asked to rank the value of the five traditional senses (sight, hearing, touch, taste, and smell) plus three additional senses associated with balance, pain, and temperature sensation. Out of the 250 participants, 220 ranked sight first, followed by hearing and then balance.

Advocates for funding of eye and vision research sometimes capitalize on the public's fear of blindness. I have received fundraising appeals from worthy organizations that described vision loss in the most fearful and dreadful terms. As a person with very low vision myself, I find fundraising appeals capitalizing on fear of blindness to be demeaning. While I fully support research to maximize vision and its rehabilitation, I recognize from my personal experience and interactions with many others that it is possible to live a full and productive life with impaired vision. Life with vision loss, while sometimes challenging, need not be viewed as an unmitigated catastrophe.

Public attitudes toward low vision are fraught with ignorance and misinformation. Sometimes people simply accept impaired vision as an unavoidable consequence of aging; they fail to take measures to forestall it and fail to take advantage of strategies to overcome it. Sighted people typically think that low vision is just like the blur when they take off their glasses. Isn't low vision usually correctable by lenses? Most of us with low vision have had the experience of being yelled at by a stranger on the street "you'd better get new glasses" when we trip or bump into something.

Mocking portrayals of low vision have appeared in the media. Mr. Magoo was a Hollywood cartoon character—an old guy with very thick glasses. He first appeared in 1949 voiced by Jim Backus. Mr. Magoo re-emerged in 1997 in a live-action film starring the comedian Leslie Nielsen. Mr. Magoo's thick glasses apparently did not correct his severe shortsightedness. He exhibited bumbling incompetence due to his poor vision, making mistakes such as confusing toothpaste for sun lotion and trying to withdraw cash from a soda machine. I'm afraid that I've made mistakes that rival Mr. Magoo, like dumping the kitty with the kitty litter into the trash (fortunately, the kitty jumped clear). On one memorable occasion, I ventured into an empty washroom. I found and entered the stall, closed the door, and sat down. A moment or two later, I heard someone else enter the washroom and the unmistakable click-clack of high heels. I waited in silence, embarrassed and fearful of being discovered and deemed a pervert, a man in the women's washroom. She did her thing and then left. As soon as she was safely gone, I left the stall, washed my hands at record speed, and slipped out of the washroom, hoping not to be noticed. Such incidents are embarrassing at the time. They can be humorous in the retelling but not when used as ridicule by someone else. The 1997 Magoo film was protested by the National Federation of the Blind and others for exploiting and stigmatizing vision impairment for entertainment value.

Occasionally, there have been unrealistic depictions of blind people in films or on TV such as the Ferrari driving exploits of Colonel Frank Slade (played by Al Pacino) in the 1992 movie *Scent of a Woman*. But, there have rarely been positive or realistic depictions of people with low vision in the movies or on TV. Unlike other forms of disability which have received some realistic portrayals in modern media, low vision remains largely unrecognized in contemporary movies or television.

Many people with low vision succeed in public and private life, often without public recognition of their impairment. There are some examples of people with low vision whose visual impairment is more widely known.

Marla Runyan, a track and field star who represented the United States in the 2000 Olympics in the 1,500-meter race, has Stargardt disease. This is an early onset form of macular degeneration that results in a loss of central vision. In a YouTube video,[4] Marla described her winning run at the Twin Cities Marathon in 2006. The major problem posed by her low vision was her inability to read time splits on the large clocks posted on the race course.

Earlier, I referred to Anne Sullivan Macy, Helen Keller's teacher, who had low vision resulting from trachoma. As depicted dramatically in the movie *The Miracle Worker*, Anne played a key role in Helen's education. Anne was a lifelong companion of Helen and played a major role supporting Helen's national and international success. A few years ago, I visited Helen Keller's birthplace in Tuscumbia, Alabama. Keller Johnson-Thompson, Helen's great grandniece, kindly showed me, Wendy, and my former PhD student and colleague MiYoung Kwon around Helen's childhood home named Ivy Green. The home is now maintained by The Helen Keller Foundation. The photo in Figure 1.1 shows me with Keller Johnson-Thompson standing by the famous water pump where Helen first learned the word "water."

The growing awareness of low vision has resulted in the creation of self-help groups in many communities, some organized by national organizations such as the Foundation Fighting Blindness and others organized by local rehabilitation services. These groups allow people with low vision to share their experiences, particularly their strategies for coping with activities of daily living.

Everyone understands that people with visual impairment face challenges in their daily lives. Data from population-based studies, such as the SEE and the Beaver Dam Eye studies in the United States and the Blue Mountains Eye study in Australia, provide detailed evidence of these challenges. For people with acuity less than 20/40, there is evidence of measurable difficulty in activities of daily living, social functioning, and religious participation. Loss of each line on the acuity chart is associated with greater use of community services and an increase in falls and hip fracture.

People with visual impairment face problems in employment, sometimes because jobs are highly dependent on good vision and sometimes because of discrimination. A widely reported unemployment rate of 70% for people with vision impairment implies bleak prospects for finding work. But, a 2019 report by Michele McDonnall and Zhen Sui debunked the 70% unemployment rate. The misunderstanding comes from two confusing concepts—the rate of employment and the rate of unemployment. The *rate of employment*

[4] https://www.youtube.com/watch?v=zlBuyRoyDMg.

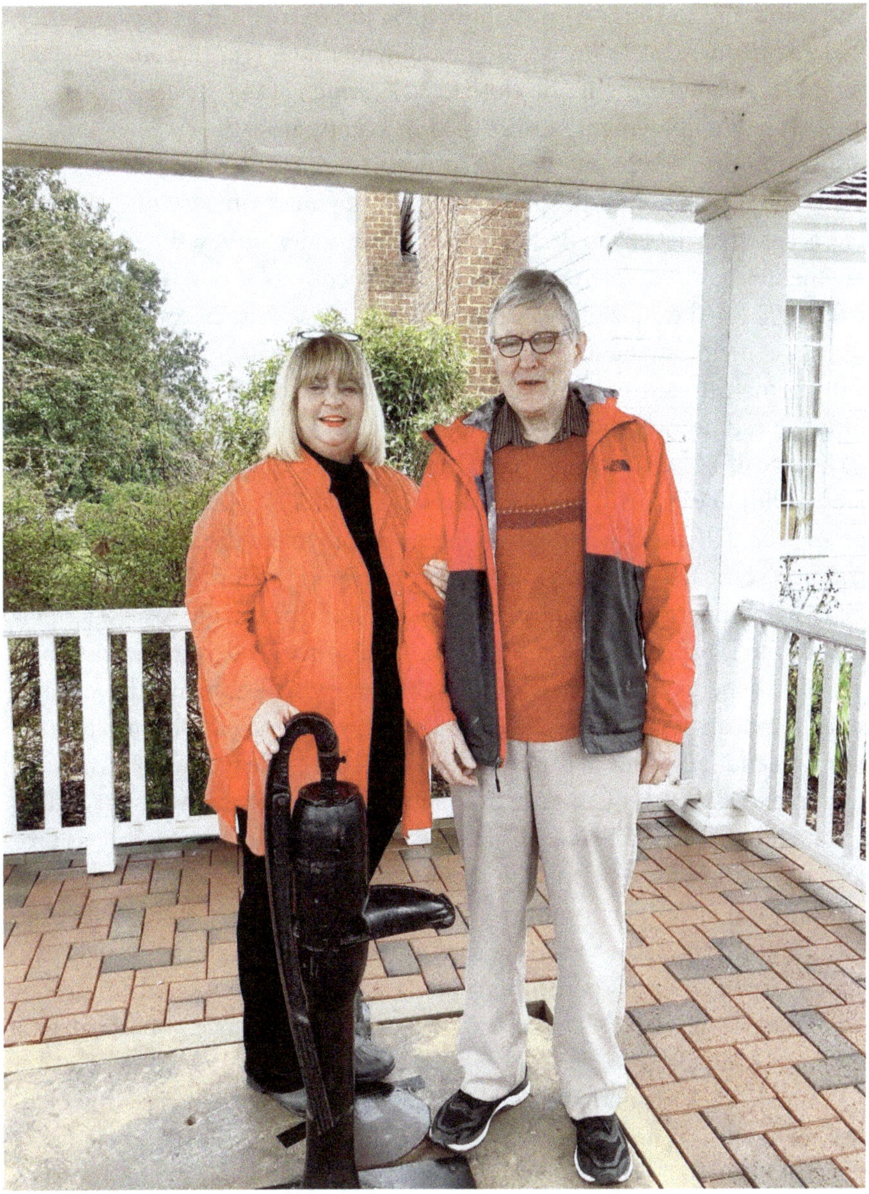

Figure 1.1 The author, Gordon Legge, and Keller Johnson-Thompson standing by the water pump at Helen Keller's birthplace, Ivy Green, in Tuscumbia, Alabama.

refers to the proportion of the population in the labor market, either working or looking for a job. McDonnall and Sui analyzed several data sources. Based on the American Community Survey which uses data from the U.S. census, the employment rate for people with visual impairment (including both blind and low vision) was about 44% in 2017. Of the remaining 56%, the large majority were not seeking employment. (A report from the 1980s estimated an employment rate close to 30%, which led to the erroneous estimate of an unemployment rate of 70%.) By comparison, the *employment rate* for the non-disabled population was about 77% in 2017. *The unemployment rate* is the proportion of people seeking employment who are unemployed. Again, based on data from the American Community Survey, the 2017 unemployment rate for people with vision impairment was about 10% compared with 4.8% for the non-disabled population. These figures reveal a disparity between employment opportunities for people with vision impairment and the mainstream public, but the disparity is much less severe than the mistaken estimate of a 70% unemployment rate.

Historically, many jobs had visual prerequisites that unfairly disqualified people with low vision. The *Americans with Disabilities Act* (ADA) now protects visually disabled people from unfair employment discrimination. But, common sense tells us that some jobs require "good vision." What should be the visual standards for airline pilots, truck drivers, prison guards, police officers, or food inspectors? Vision criteria are also set for driver's licenses and disability benefits. The methods for establishing visual standards have major social implications for those affected. Typically, criteria have been set by the intuition and judgment of experts without a solid evidence base. It would be desirable to establish more scientifically valid and equitable ways for setting vision requirements. Chris Johnson (2008) at the University of Iowa has proposed a method for determining the visual requirements for vision-critical jobs and for including appropriate accommodations. His method assesses how several aspects of vision (including acuity, extent of the visual field, color vision, and depth perception) interact with environmental conditions (such as lighting, fog, or smoke) and level of job experience in performance of essential job tasks.

Why does low vision have such a low profile? Low vision certainly qualifies for inclusion under the ADA. The definition of disability includes "a physical or mental impairment that substantially limits one or more major life activities." The ADA has raised the profile of disability in general, but low vision continues to be poorly understood. Considered collectively, the population of people with disabilities is large but is fragmented into groups with different needs. Dating back to the 19th century, the needs of people with disabilities were first addressed by the medical community using what is known as the "medical model" of disability. The medical approach is to cure or "fix" the problem, such as impaired vision, by addressing the disorder. But, cures are frequently not possible. Many people remain with lifelong disabilities. A second approach, the rehabilitation model, is to provide the disabled person with tools to cope with their disability. Tools might include job training, provision of assistive technology, using nonvisual strategies for accomplishing daily tasks, and laws providing financial benefits. The rehabilitation approach gained momentum after World War II to address the needs of injured veterans, including those who were blind. A third and more recent approach is the demand for social justice and civil rights. According to this view, society has an obligation to enhance accessibility for people with disabilities, including all forms of vision impairment. Accessibility means removing barriers to effective functioning in public and private places, transportation, education, employment, communications such as the internet, and generally all spheres of modern culture. It is not sufficient to provide only medical treatment and rehabilitation (although these remain crucial and desirable); modifications should be made to enable people with disabilities to enjoy full participation in mainstream society.

The disability rights movement began in the 1960s and 1970s, motivated primarily by activists in wheelchairs. Students at the University of California at Berkeley initiated the Independent Living Movement in the 1960s. They advocated for removal of architectural barriers on campus and in the community. Disability rights gained momentum in the 1970s and 1980s. Gallaudet University in Washington, DC, is dedicated to the education of students who are deaf or hard of hearing. In 1988, students at the university closed the campus for six days protesting the selection of a hearing president rather than two deaf candidates. The protests culminated in the appointment of the university's first deaf president. In 1990, during the Wheels of Justice March in Washington, protesters left their wheelchairs and crawled up the steps of the Capitol. They were protesting segregation and discrimination against wheelchair users and advocating for the ADA (which was signed into law only a few months later). Switzer (2003) describes the history of the disability rights movement in the United States. A revealing depiction of the disability rights movement is given in the movie *Crip Camp: A Disability Revolution*.

Advocacy groups for the blind have also played a role in seeking social justice. They include the National Federation of the Blind (NFB) and the American Council of the Blind (ACB). These groups have sometimes differed in their approach to advocacy. I encountered their disagreement regarding the accessibility of United States currency bills. In 1994, I served on a national advisory committee to the U.S. Treasury Department addressing accessibility of currency bills by people with vision impairment. U.S. currency bills of different denominations are the most uniform of any country. They all look very much alike and are difficult for people with low vision to distinguish. They can't be distinguished by size or any other tactile feature, posing problems for people who are blind. One of our committee recommendations was to enhance the legibility of numerals on the bills to facilitate recognition by people with low vision. This recommendation was implemented as the large, bold numerals on more recent U.S. currency bills except the $1 bill. Our committee also recommended the inclusion of tactile features so that blind users could distinguish the bills by touch. The U.S. Treasury Department resisted this recommendation on the grounds of the cost of production and possible trouble for the vending industry. Subsequently, the ACB brought suit in district court against the Treasury Department, arguing that the government was in violation of Section 504 of the Rehabilitation Act in its continuing failure to distribute currency bills that are accessible by blind people. Representatives of NFB objected to the inclusion of sizing or other tactile features on the grounds that blind people are already capable of handling money and that special tactile features would tend to stigmatize blind citizens. In a series of rulings in 2006, 2007, and 2008, the court decided in favor of the ACB and plans were implemented to include tactile features for currency identification in a future design. It was expected that the bills will contain tactile rectangles with the number and spacing of the rectangles indicating denomination.

Although NFB and ACB advocate on behalf of all people with vision impairment, their focus is primarily on people who are blind. There has been very little advocacy specifically by people with low vision. One reason is that activists tend to be students or working-age adults. People with low vision in these groups are widely dispersed and rarely organized. The majority of people with low vision are older. Many are retired, and many have acquired their low vision later in life. While enhanced environmental accessibility is important in determining the quality of life (QOL) for older people, access to educational and employment opportunities is less crucial. Moreover, across all age groups, people with low vision often do not identify as part of a disability rights group. In short, the demographics of low vision tend to contribute to its low profile in society.

Quality of life (QOL) with low vision

What are the attitudes of visually impaired people themselves concerning their life situation? How do they value their quality of life? We can ask them. I teach a class on visual impairment to advanced undergraduate students. Some of them take my class because they are interested in health careers such as optometry, medicine, nursing, mental health, and occupational therapy. Most of them have normal vision, and some have had little or no contact with visually impaired people. At least once during the course, a panel of people with low vision visits the class and discusses their life experiences, including trials, tribulations, and joys. A retired nun described her disappointment when she learned that her vision loss from macular degeneration could not be treated or cured and later the joy she experienced as a peer counselor for other sisters with low vision. A college student with low vision described how he tried to hide his vision impairment in high school to fit in, and how his efforts led to embarrassment and isolation. But, later, in college, he “came out” about his impairment, a change in attitude which was liberating for him. My students love the interaction with the panelists and consider the sessions a highlight of the course. Hearing directly from people with low vision is crucial to understanding the impact of vision impairment.

My students often ask when or if they should offer help to a stranger with vision impairment. Does the person want help? Will the person be insulted? My answer is that offers of assistance are usually appreciated, but not always needed. People with vision impairment vary in their desire for independence. It is generous and appropriate to offer assistance to someone who seems uncertain about crossing a street or who is searching for a room in a large building. The person can always decline the offer. Turning the tables, people with low vision sometimes need to seek assistance. We know the stereotype that men don’t like to ask for directions. But, those of us with low vision learn to overcome our reticence. As a graduate student, I was lost on campus in search of an obscure classroom. I asked a pretty girl if she knew where it was. Luckily, she was searching for the same classroom. Eventually, we found it together. Later, I asked her for a date. And, lo and behold, one thing led to another, and she became my wife.

There are many autobiographical accounts of life with blindness or low vision. Books I find particularly insightful are *The Story of My Life* (Helen Keller, 1905), *And There Was Light* (Jacques Lusseyran, 1998), *Touching the Rock* (John Hull, 1990), *The Beauty of Dusk* (Frank Bruni, 2022), and *The Country of the Blind* (Andrew Leland, 2023). In *Crashing Through* (2007), Robert Kurson tells the compelling story of Mike May, a man who experiences restored vision after 40 years of near total blindness. I’ll have more to say about Mike May in Chapter 10.

Personal testimonials are valuable, but researchers would also like a numerical measure of the self-perception of the impact of vision impairment. A numerical index of QOL can be useful for assessing improvements due to treatments, rehabilitation programs, or assistive technology. A numerical measure could also be used to compare the impact on QOL of vision impairment and other health conditions.

Several methods are in use for measuring QOL in the presence of adverse health conditions. These include questionnaires, rating scales, and an interesting method called the time-tradeoff (TTO) method. In the TTO, a participant is asked to compare living their remaining lifespan with a given condition to living a shorter lifespan with full health. For example, suppose you are 60 years old with a life expectancy of 30 more years. How would you respond to a question like this: "You are given a choice of living 30 more years with a debilitating illness that keeps you bedridden or fewer than 30 years in good health. How many years would you be willing to trade away for sustained good health?" Suppose you say you would trade 10 years, leaving you only 20 more years of life in good health, instead of 30 years bedridden. (This is not to suggest that anyone would or should elect this tradeoff, but it is used only as an example.) According to the TTO method, your perception of QOL as a bedridden patient is 2/3 (20 years of good health divided by 30 years bedridden). The numerical value of QOL obtained in this way, termed "health utility," is typically placed on a scale from 0 (death) to 1.0 (full health). Several studies have asked participants with specific forms of low vision how many years of remaining life they would trade for restoration of normal vision. The results are used to estimate the reduction in QOL associated with the eye condition. Box 1.1 describes the results of one such study of people with age-related macular degeneration. Estimates of QOL for people with the same eye condition may vary widely. People who are well-adapted to their low vision with good coping skills and family support will likely judge their QOL to be better than a peer with the same eye condition who may be depressed or who faces more challenges in coping with daily life. Research studies try to deal with individual variability by assessing QOL in a large group from which an average value can be obtained.

Box 1.1 Using the time-tradeoff method to estimate quality of life with macular degeneration

J.D. Stein from the Wills Eye Hospital in Philadelphia and colleagues published a report in 2003 in which they used the TTO method to estimate QOL with AMD. Their participants included individuals with mild, moderate, and severe forms of AMD, defined by levels of visual acuity (see Table 1.5). The 115 AMD patients were drawn from the medical practices of two of the authors. The AMD participants were first asked to estimate

Table 1.5 Average utility scores for participants with AMD, medical professionals, and community members (adapted from Stein et al. (2003). Quality of life with macular degeneration: Perceptions of patients, clinicians, and community members. *British Journal of Ophthalmology*, *87*(1), 8–12).

Disease status (acuity)	AMD patients	Medical professionals	Community members
Mild(20/30)	0.83	0.93	0.96
Moderate(20/40–20/100)	0.73	0.88	0.92
Severe(20/200 or worse)	0.56	0.82	0.86

the number of years they expected to live. For instance, a 60-year-old might have estimated 30 years. They were then asked to assume there was a permanent cure for their AMD that would restore them to healthy, normal eyesight, but the cure would shorten their lifespan. What would be the maximum number of years of their remaining life they would be willing to give up to obtain this cure? For example, if the 60-year-old was willing to give up five years so that her remaining lifespan would be 25 years with full eyesight; the associated health utility of her AMD condition would have a numerical value of 25/30 = 0.83.

The authors also asked two groups with normal sight to first estimate the number of years they expected to live and then to imagine they had mild, moderate, and severe forms of AMD: How many of your expected years would you be willing to trade away for a permanent cure of your imagined AMD condition? The two normally sighted groups included 62 medical professionals (but not ophthalmologists) and 142 community members recruited from the general public. The purpose of testing the normally sighted groups was to assess their perception of the reduction in QOL associated with AMD.

Average estimates of health utility from the three AMD groups and two normally sighted groups are given in Table 1.5. Values closer to 1.0 correspond to better QOL. From the table, we see that the normally sighted medical professionals and community members agree in estimating higher utility values than the AMD groups. This means that they judge the QOL with AMD to be higher than the self-perceptions of the AMD patients themselves. This difference may represent misunderstanding by the sighted subjects of the practical and mental-health challenges faced by people with macular degeneration. The patients with severe macular degeneration (acuity 20/200 or worse) had an average utility score of 0.56. In the context of the TTO procedure, this means that, on average, they would be willing to exchange almost half of their remaining years of life for restored normal vision.

The Stein et al. study had some limitations. The two normally sighted groups were much younger than the AMD groups, and we are not told what information they had about mild, moderate, or severe AMD. We also understand that individual judgments in the TTO procedure are dependent on individual circumstances that could vary on a day-to-day basis. Despite these limitations, the study reveals that the impact of AMD on self-perceptions of QOL depends substantially on the severity of vision impairment. It also suggests that fully sighted people may underestimate the life challenges of living with macular degeneration.

QOL measures can also be used to evaluate the impact of vision treatments or rehabilitation. While gains in acuity and other clinical measures are commonly used to evaluate the effectiveness of vision therapies, changes in QOL speak more directly to the patient's experience. Imagine, for example, administering the TTO procedure to a group of participants undergoing a new treatment for macular degeneration. If the treatment results in an improvement in QOL indicated by a higher TTO score, the change in QOL score can be used as a numerical indicator of the improvement. It remains an interesting question how well improvements in QOL are mirrored by (correlated with) changes in acuity or other clinical tests of vision. Rehabilitation programs or adoption of assistive technology will often have little or no effect on acuity but may result in measurable improvements in QOL.

QOL estimates have also been used by health economists to compute cost efficiency of treatment options. Suppose a group with a particular form of macular degeneration shows an average improvement from 0.6 to 0.8 on the TTO test following a new treatment. Suppose also that the gain is expected to last for an average of 30 years, such as from age 60 to the end of life at age 90. The improved QOL of 0.2 can be multiplied across the 30 years life expectancy to yield a cumulative gain of 0.2 times 30 = 6.0, a quantity term "quality adjusted life years" or QALY for short. Using the TTO terminology, the cumulative effect of the treatment is equivalent to six years of normal, healthy vision. If the average cost of the treatment is known, say $60,000, we can say that the cost effectiveness of the treatment is $10,000 per QALY. The lower the cost per QALY, the more cost-effective is the treatment.

Mental health affects a person's quality of life. Social isolation, depression, or even cognitive decline may accompany low vision. Many studies have shown higher prevalence of depression among people with vision impairment than among controls with normal vision. Nevertheless, it has proven difficult to establish associations between severity of depression and visual acuity or other clinical measures of vision impairment. To examine this issue, Zhang and colleagues (2013) analyzed data from a nationally representative sample of 10,480 people in the U.S., aged 20 years and above. The data, taken from the National Health and Nutrition Examination Survey (NHANES), included measures of depression (on the PHQ-9 scale), measures of visual acuity, and also ratings of difficulty in daily visual functioning. Questions about visual functioning were adapted from the National Eye Institute Visual Function Questionnaire (NEI-VFQ) and assessed difficulty with six daily activities: reading, driving, hobbies requiring close work, negotiating steps in dim light, noticing objects to the side while walking, and finding objects on a crowded shelf. The study found no statistically significant association between depression scores and visual acuity. Instead, there was a significant association between depression scores and difficulty ratings with the six daily activities. In other words, the extent of depression was related to difficulties in accomplishing everyday tasks and not with vision status per se. Some people with very low acuity may have found strategies to deal effectively with visually challenging activities and would not be at risk for depression. Others with better acuity might not have developed effective coping strategies for daily activities and be more vulnerable to depression.

What's next?

We've now defined *low vision* as a category, distinct from normal vision and total blindness. We've emphasized a wide range of conditions comprising low vision and its surprisingly high prevalence. We've discussed the reasons why low vision has a low profile and why it is often misunderstood.

Because low vision lies in the middle ground between normal vision and no vision, it has the status of the proverbial glass half full or half empty. Yes, low vision poses problems for reading, mobility, and social interaction. But, the retention of vision, even when it is very low, is a gift to be cherished. There is pleasure and functional benefit associated with vision at any level. This is why a focus on rehabilitation and research on low vision is so important, and why personal insights into one's own low vision can be valuable.

In the next four chapters, I'll examine four aspects of vision that are typically used to describe low vision—acuity, contrast sensitivity, and the status of central and peripheral visual fields. The diversity of low vision arises because different eye disorders impact these aspects in different ways.

2

Acuity

Size Matters

Low vision is often described in terms of reduced acuity, reduced contrast sensitivity, and visual-field loss. Traditionally, visual acuity has been the primary measure of vision status. In this chapter, I'll discuss visual acuity—how it is measured and the impact of reduced acuity on what can be seen. The following chapters will deal with reduced contrast sensitivity and visual-field loss in low vision. Although I'll discuss the three aspects of vision impairment in separate chapters, most people with reduced acuity have reduced contrast sensitivity as well. And many people with visual-field loss also have reduced acuity and reduced contrast sensitivity.

• • • • •

Acuity refers to the ability to recognize small details in visual patterns such as distinguishing an O from a C on an eye chart. A person's letter acuity is found by measuring the smallest letter size for which they can make such distinctions. The better your acuity, the finer the details you can see, and the sharper is your vision.

Measures and charts

Figure 2.1 illustrates that the ability to see pattern details depends on both the size of the pattern and the viewer's distance from the pattern. Letters and numbers on the license plates of cars in North America are about 3 inches (76 mm) in height and can be easily recognized by people with good acuity from a distance of 60 feet (18 m). But to see 12-point Times Roman text in a book, people with good vision typically adopt a comfortable reading distance of about 16 inches (40 cm). In short, visual limitations due to acuity are determined by the ratio of object size to viewing distance. This ratio is termed the *visual angle* subtended by the object. Box 2.1 provides numerical examples for those who are interested.

Low Vision. Gordon E. Legge, Oxford University Press. © Oxford University Press (2026).
DOI: 10.1093/9780198946960.003.0003

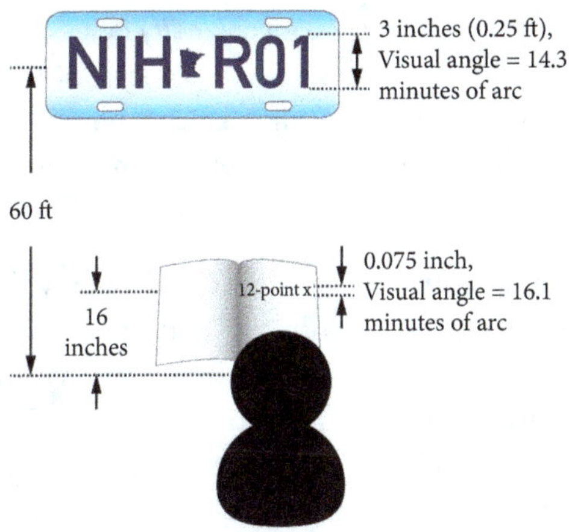

Figure 2.1 Drawing of a person looking at a license plate from a distance of 60 feet (18 meters) or a page of text in a book 16 inches (40 centimeters) away. The drawing illustrates that from the person's perspective, the characters on the license plate and the characters in the book have nearly the same visual angle.

Box 2.1 Computing visual angles

Characters on license plates in North America are typically 3 inches (0.25 feet) high. Viewed from a distance of 60 feet, the ratio of size to distance (both measured in feet), approximating the visual angle, is 0.25/60 = 0.0042 radians. (In geometry, angles are often measured in radians. One radian is approximately 57.3 degrees.) We can convert radians to degrees of visual angle by multiplying by 57.3 to get 0.24 degrees. Multiplying by another factor of 60, we get the corresponding value in minutes of arc as 14.3. This value is almost three times larger than the letters on the 20/20 line of the acuity chart, which subtend 5 minutes of arc, so the license plate characters viewed from 60 feet should be legible for someone with 20/20 acuity.

Suppose the same person reads 12-point Times Roman print in a book. A lowercase x in 12-point Times Roman is actually 5.4 points in height, equivalent to 0.075 inch (1.9 mm). This time, the size/distance ratio, approximating the visual angle of the x, is 0.075/16 = 0.0047 radians, equivalent to 16.1 minutes of arc. These letters will also be legible to the reader with 20/20 acuity. Notice that the visual angle for the x on the page, viewed from 16 inches, is not very different from the visual angle for the 3-inch characters on the license plate viewed from 60 feet. From a vision science perspective, the visual acuity requirements are similar for the two cases.

Exact measures of visual angles require trigonometry ratios, but the simple ratio of size to distance is good for most calculations relevant to acuity. If we use trigonometry to compute the visual angle, rather than the simple ratio of size to distance, the difference in the resulting value is less than 1% for the small angles in the examples given here.

My son Alex, at the age of five years, understood that my ability to see things with my low vision depended on both size and distance. When asked how well I can see, he said, “Dad can see some things. He can see little things close up, or big things far away, but not little things far away.” When he wanted me to look at something, he would put the item up against my glasses; he wanted to be sure it was close enough for me to see it.

The roles of size and distance in determining acuity are reflected in the familiar Snellen notation used on the letter-acuity chart, such as 20/20 or 20/200. Traditionally, the numerator (top number in the ratio) represented a standard testing distance for acuity, typically 20 feet. The European standard testing distance was 6 meters, with corresponding Snellen ratios such as 6/6 or 6/60. These test distances were chosen somewhat arbitrarily as representative of distance vision. If your glasses are prescribed for good focus at 20 feet (or 6 meters), you can focus all greater distances.

The denominator (the lower number) in the Snellen ratio indicates the letter size as a visual angle. By convention, letters on the 20/20 line subtend 5 minutes of arc (1/12 degrees). The critical features distinguishing letters on the 20/20 line, such as the gap in the C that distinguishes it from an O, subtend 1 minute of arc. The value of the denominator in the Snellen ratio indicates how much larger (or smaller) the letters are on other lines on the eye chart. For example, letters on the 20/60 line are three times larger than the letters on the 20/20 line and therefore subtend a visual angle that is three times larger; they subtend 15 minutes of arc. An alternative, and equivalent, interpretation of the denominator of the Snellen ratio is the distance at which a person with 20/20 visual acuity can read the letters on that line. For instance, a person with 20/20 acuity will be able to read the letters on the 20/200 line from a distance of 200 feet.

In practice, many visual-acuity charts have been designed for testing at viewing distances other than 20 feet. The important design principle is to ensure that letters on the line marked 20/20 (or 6/6) are scaled in size so that the size/distance ratio at the recommended testing distance yields a visual angle of 5 minutes of arc, with letter sizes on the other lines scaled in size appropriately.

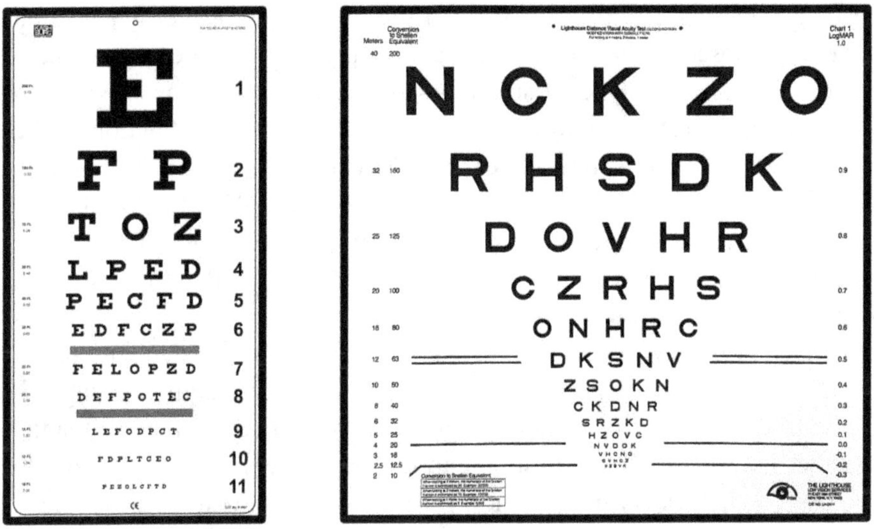

Figure 2.2 Comparison of the traditional Snellen chart (left) and the Early Treatment of Diabetic Retinopathy Study (ETDRS) chart (right).

The traditional Snellen acuity chart, shown on the left in Figure 2.2, is adequate for screening patients with near-normal acuity but has drawbacks for testing low vision. Its largest symbol, usually a big E, is a 20/200 letter, so it can't be used to measure the acuity of people with poorer vision. The progression of print sizes is irregular, making it difficult to calibrate for nonstandard viewing distances; nearer distances often become necessary for people with low acuity. A third problem is that the chart has fewer letters on rows at the large-print end of the scale, typically only one letter on the 20/200 line, which makes the task easier and reduces precision. I took advantage of this latter characteristic of the Snellen chart many years ago. I was undergoing a medical exam as part of my application for a U.S. green card. (I was born in Canada and working in England at the time.) The exam included an acuity test. The London doctor nodded vaguely toward the eye chart and asked me to read from the top. Given my very low vision, I couldn't see the eye chart, let alone read the letters. But I did know that most such charts had a big E at the top. So I just said "E." He said "Good," and checked the box indicating that I passed the vision screening.

In 1976, Ian Bailey and Jan Lovie, then at the National Vision Research Institute of Australia, proposed new design principles for acuity testing. Their design principles standardized the visual task so that letter size became the only significant variable from one line to the next. They recommended that acuity charts should have 1) an equal number of test letters at each size, and spacing proportionate to letter size; 2) the font and subset of letters used should be chosen so that the characters are equally legible when viewed near the acuity limit; and 3) letter size should decrease in a regular progression such that each step down in print size would be a constant fraction of the size of the letters on the next larger line. They recommended a reduction to 4/5 of the preceding larger line (more precisely, to 79.4% of the preceding line, equivalent to a reduction by 0.1 log units). Three steps down in print size using this fraction results in letters half the size of the reference line. For example, use of this principle would mean that three lines down from the 20/40 line is the 20/20 line. A major advantage of the standardization of the task and this geometric progression of print sizes is that testing can be done at nonstandard distances, with easy numerical correction for the distance chosen. It is often desirable to test people with low vision close to the chart so that they can read a few lines near the top. Using a closer viewing distance increases the angular size of the letters, bringing some of them within the acuity limit of the person with low vision. Employing the proper compensation for the shorter distance, a valid measure of acuity can be obtained.

In 1982, Frederick Ferris at the U.S. National Institutes of Health and colleagues incorporated these design principles into a new visual-acuity chart known as the Early Treatment of Diabetic Retinopathy Study (ETDRS) chart, shown on the right in Figure 2.2, named after the clinical trial for which it was designed. This chart has become the de facto standard for clinical trials and most vision research. It uses 10 capital letters (N C K Z O R H S D V) from a font designed for vision testing by Louise Sloan in 1959. The Sloan letters were recommended as a U.S. standard for vision testing by the National Research Council Committee on Vision in 1980. The ETDRS chart has five letters per line. The standard test distance is 4 meters (13 feet). The chart lists print size in three types of notation—logMAR units, the corresponding denominator of the Snellen ratio in the 20/xx format, and the viewing distance in meters at which the letters subtend 5 minutes of arc. For example, the big letters on the top line of the ETDRS chart have an angular letter size equivalent to 20/200 letters, a corresponding logMAR size of 1.0, and would subtend 5 minutes of arc at a viewing distance of 40 meters. The print sizes on the chart range from 20/200 to 20/10 (with corresponding logMAR values from 1.0 to −0.3). Print sizes on successively smaller lines are four-fifths the size (0.1 log unit) of the line above it.

People with low vision often need to be tested at distances less than the standard 4 meters in order to extend the range of angular print sizes. A common testing distance for low vision is 1 meter. At this testing distance, the letters on the top line of the chart have an angular print size of 200 minutes of arc, equivalent to a Snellen ratio of 20/800.

Several computerized and chart-based tests have been developed to extend the range of measurable acuity into the ultra-low vision range. For example, the Berkeley Rudimentary Vision test, developed by Ian Bailey (2012) and colleagues at the University of California at Berkeley, extends the range to at least 20/8000. The test requires identification of the orientation of an uppercase E (termed a Tumbling E) printed on cards: Is the E oriented with the legs pointed up, down, left, or right? The largest E is 5.7 inches in height (145 mm). At the near testing distance of 10 inches (25 cm), it has a Snellen ratio of 20/8000.

Measures of visual acuity can be confusing because there are several alternative scales and several different recommended viewing distances. Let's review the scales you are likely to encounter.

The Snellen notation 20/20, 20/200, and so forth, has its metric equivalent based on a 6-meter testing distance. 20/20 corresponds to 6/6 metric, 20/40 corresponds to 6/12 metric, and so forth. Decimal acuity is simply the Snellen fraction converted to a decimal. For example, 20/20 corresponds to a decimal acuity of 1.0 and 20/200 corresponds to a decimal acuity of 0.1.

The ETDRS and many other modern acuity tests convert angular letter size to a logarithmic unit, called logMAR for logarithm of the Minimum Angle of Resolution. Letters on the 20/20 line subtend 5 minutes of arc, and their critical features (such as the gap in the C) subtend 1 minute of arc. These letters are regarded as having a baseline or unit size. The logarithm of one is 0.0, so the logMAR value associated with 20/20 letters is 0.0. Letters on the 20/200 line are 10 times larger than letters on the 20/20 line. The logarithm of 10 is 1.0, so the logMAR notation for the 20/200 letter size is 1.0. When a geometric progression of print sizes is used so that each letter size is 79.4% (~4/5) the size of the line above, the change corresponds to 0.1 log units. Print sizes on the ETDRS chart therefore proceed in steps of 0.1 logMAR. Table 2.1 lists some angular print sizes using these different scales. The table illustrates that poorer acuity corresponds to smaller values of decimal acuity and larger values of logMAR acuity.

Clinical trials of new eye therapies often use changes in acuity as an outcome measure. Improvements in acuity may be stated in terms of the change in Snellen ratio (e.g., an improvement from 20/200 to 20/100), or as the equivalent in logMAR acuity, from logMAR 1.0 to 0.7. Sometimes, the improvement is stated in terms of the number of lines on the ETDRS chart. For example, an improvement in acuity from 20/200 to 20/100 would correspond to an improvement of three lines or 0.3 logMAR.

Table 2.1 Acuity values in different scales

Snellen (U.S.)	Snellen (metric)	Decimal	logMAR	Description
20/10	6/3	2.0	−0.3	Excellent acuity
20/20	6/6	1.0	0	Conventional standard for normal acuity
20/40	6/12	0.5	0.3	Boundary for low vision
20/63	6/19	0.32	0.5	Older boundary for low vision
20/100	6/30	0.2	0.7	Moderate low vision
20/200	6/60	0.1	1.0	U.S. boundary for legal blindness
20/400	6/120	0.05	1.3	WHO* boundary for blindness
20/2000	6/600	0.01	2.0	Ultra-low vision

* World Health Organization

What do acuity values tell us about what people can actually see?

The size of an object and its distance from the viewer jointly determine whether a person with a given level of acuity can see the distinguishing features of the object. In particular, as we saw earlier, the ratio of object size to viewing distance must exceed some critical value for a person to recognize letters, numerals, or similar symbols. The critical value is determined by the person's acuity. If you are looking at text on a computer screen from a distance at which you can just barely make out the letters, it is likely that the ratio of the size of letters on the screen to your viewing distance is at your acuity limit. You can enhance the visibility of the text by enlarging the size of the letters on the screen (zoom) or by getting closer to the screen. Both operations enhance the visibility of the text for you by increasing the ratio of the letter size to viewing distance; both magnify the angular size of the text letters. In a study conducted in my laboratory at the University of Minnesota, led by Christina Granquist (2018), we found that most people with low vision use both zoom and shorter viewing distance to magnify text on computer screens, but usually rely more on zoom.

Acuity testing with letter charts relies on keeping the viewing distance constant while the subject reads smaller and smaller letters until the critical size/distance ratio is reached. But acuity also determines the greatest distance at which objects of a given size—faces, playing cards, or alphabet letters—can be recognized. For instance, if we know a person's acuity, we should be able to use the corresponding size/distance ratio to estimate the maximum distance at which they could recognize letters of a given size. Box 2.2 gives a formula you can use to test this for yourself.

Box 2.2 Predicting acuity distance

Try this simple test and apply the formula to predict the maximum distance at which you can recognize a sample of text. You will need a tape measure or other device for measuring distances.

Suppose you know your acuity as a Snellen ratio such as 20/20 or 20/200. Express this ratio as a decimal (termed "decimal acuity") and represent it by A. The value of A for 20/20 is 1.0, and for 20/200 is 0.1.

Measure the height of letters on a sign, on the computer screen, in newspaper headlines, or any other source you like. Refer to this height as Y in inches. Then, your acuity limits the maximum viewing distance D at which you should be able to recognize the letters. Use the following formula to estimate D in inches:

$$D = 688 \times Y \times A$$

For example, if letters are 5 inches high and your acuity is 20/200, then Y = 5 and A = 0.1. Then:

$$D = 688 \times 5 \times 0.1 = 344 \text{ inches} = 28.4 \text{ feet}$$

This means that if you have 20/200 acuity, you would not be able to recognize the 5-inch letters beyond about 28 feet. Depending on viewing conditions and the font and context of the letters, your maximum distance for recognizing the letters might be somewhat less. Try using the formula on a sample of text. Measure the height of the text letters and back away, to find your maximum reading distance, being sure to keep the text upright and in your line of sight.

Although this example is given in inches, the same formula works if the letter size Y and viewing distance D are given in the same units, whether centimeters, meters, or other units. The formula works for acuities expressed as Snellen ratios in the form 20/X or in metric notation 6/X.

The multiplier 688 in the above formula arises from the conversion of angular letter sizes in Snellen ratios to distances in linear units and has been slightly rounded to simplify computation.

As another application of this formula, for anyone with normal acuity of 20/20, the value of A is 1.0, so there is a very simple relationship between acuity distance D and letter size Y: D = 688 × Y. As an extreme example, the uppercase letters on the famous Hollywood sign on the hill overlooking Hollywood, California, are 45-feet high. At what distance would these letters be at the acuity limit for someone with 20/20 vision? Applying the foregoing formula, D = 688 × 45 = 30,960 feet, which converts to about 5.9 miles.

Using this principle, 6-inch-high letters could be recognized at a distance of 100 yards (the length of a U.S. football field) by a person with 20/20 vision, at 10 yards by a person with 20/200 vision, and at 1 yard by a person with 20/2000 vision. In practice, the ideal lighting and other testing conditions associated with typical acuity measures in the eye clinic rarely occur in most everyday environments. On the football field, for example, the lighting may be uneven, the observer may be in motion, or the 6-inch letters 100 yards away may be crowded by other letters or in an unusual font. So, although clinical acuity measures do provide predictions for maximum distances for recognizing letters, in everyday life, these predictions yield an upper bound. Actual distances for high-confidence recognition will often be less, perhaps only half the maximum predicted distance. Nevertheless, a person's measured acuity is an important indicator of their range of vision.

Reading highway signs is a situation in which the size/distance ratio of characters is particularly important. What letter size on highway signs is necessary to be legible from desirable distances? The U.S. Federal Highway Administration's *Manual of Uniform Traffic Controls and Devices* (MUTCD, 2009) indicates that letter size on highway signs should be 1 inch larger for each 30 feet of maximum desired viewing distance. (The ratio of 30 feet per inch of letter height is termed the *Legibility Index*.) For example, if letters need to be legible for drivers at a distance of 900 feet, the letters should be at least 30 inches in height. Converting this letter size and distance into a visual angle, the letters would subtend approximately 9.6 minutes of arc, close to the limit for someone with acuity of 20/40. This means that in very good viewing conditions, the 30-inch letters should be legible from a distance of 900 feet for drivers with acuity better than 20/40. A driver with acuity worse than 20/40 would not be able to read the sign until their vehicle is substantially closer than 900 feet. We'll return to low vision and driving in Chapter 8.

Letters and numerals on sports scoreboards provide another example of large characters viewed at a great distance. The manual baseball scoreboard in Chicago's Wrigley Field is located above center field. It is about 400 feet from home plate and 460 feet from the stands behind home plate. The scoreboard numerals are painted on steel plates and are about 16 inches in height. If we apply the Legibility Index from highway signage, letters 16 inches in height should be legible from 30 × 16 = 480 feet. The Wrigley Field scoreboard numerals meet this criterion for the fans behind home plate. The visual angle subtended by 16-inch letters viewed from 460 feet is about 10 minutes of arc. Letters of this size on an eye chart would be at the limit for someone with acuity of 20/40. People with acuity worse than 20/40, seated behind home plate at Wrigley, would not be able to read the scoreboard numerals. Wrigley Field was built in 1937, and the scoreboard has been in use since then. I attended a game there with my father when I was a child. I couldn't read the scoreboard. I do remember the visiting team hitting four home runs in one inning.

Acuity values tell us that someone with 20/40 acuity has better vision than someone with 20/100 acuity, or that someone with 20/200 acuity has better vision than someone with 20/400 acuity. But, in everyday life, what do these numbers tell us about what can or cannot be seen?

Figure 2.3 provides a demonstration of the impact of reduced acuity when viewing another person at a distance of 4 meters (13 feet). The figure shows several versions of a photo of my lab manager, Rachel, standing next to an ETDRS acuity chart. She's a key member of my lab and does much of the acuity testing. The original image shows that she is wearing a striped sweater and a necklace with a pendant. She has a ring on her finger and she is wearing a watch. Suppose an observer is standing at the typical 4-meter (13 feet) testing distance from the chart. What features of Rachel would be visible to observers with different levels of acuity? To answer this question, we blurred the images by several amounts to simulate reduced acuity. Having the chart in the image allows us to associate different levels of acuities with gradations of blur. Let's consider the loss of visual information about Rachel from 20/40 to 20/640. The images have been scaled for viewing at a typical reading distance, but represent what details an observer would see from a 4-meter viewing distance.

When acuity is reduced to 20/40, Rachel is still easily recognizable, but her freckles have disappeared and the ring on her finger is no longer visible. We can still see her watch. We can work out that she has a necklace from the more visible pendant. This is the acuity at the boundary for low vision.

At 20/80, Rachel's facial features are less distinct and it is hard to recognize her. The fingers on her hand are no longer distinct and the stripes on her sweater are blurry. This acuity might be termed mild to moderate low vision.

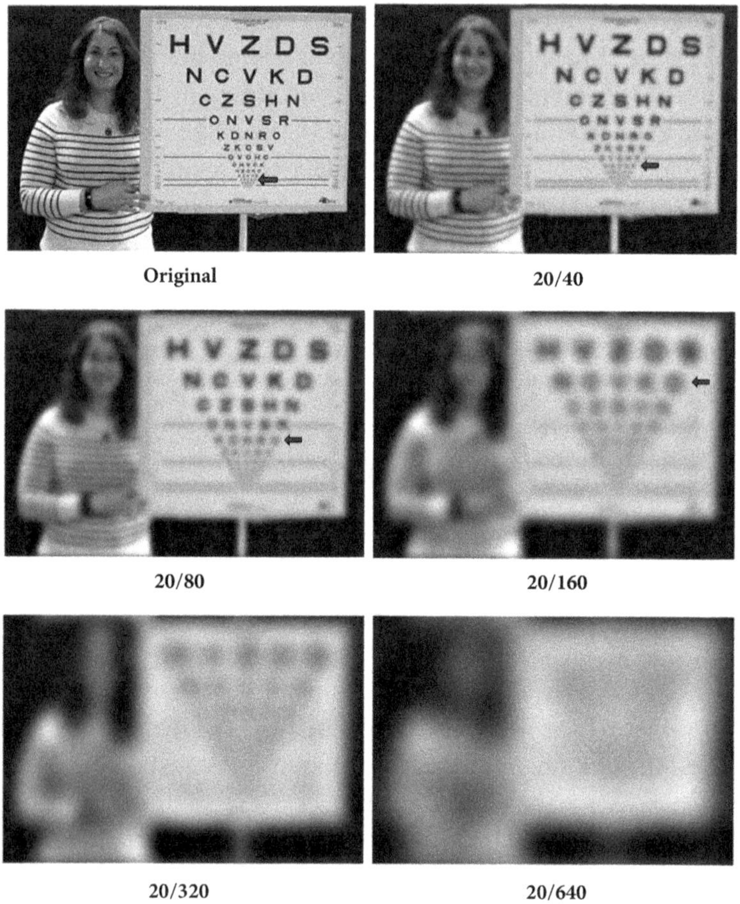

Figure 2.3 Examples of visibility with several levels of artificial acuity reduction. An original image shows a woman standing next to an ETDRS acuity chart. Five additional panels blur the image to show what features would be visible for observers with acuities of 20/40, 20/80, 20/160, 20/320, and 20/640. The images show details that could be seen by the observers standing 4 meters (13 feet) from the woman and the chart. The images have been rescaled for viewing at a typical reading distance. Arrows indicate the lines on the ETDRS chart corresponding to acuities of 20/20 (original image), 20/40, 20/80, and 20/160. Since the top line on the chart is 20/200, there are no lines matching the size of acuity letters for acuities of 20/320 or 20/640. The examples are shown in grayscale to avoid artifacts produced by blurring of color images.

At 20/160, we can no longer see the expression on Rachel's face. The stripes on her sweater are gone. There is something on her arm, but we can't tell that it's a watch. We can't tell much about her hair. Only the top line on the ETDRS chart (the 20/200 line) is legible. The 20/160 line is hard to read, so this degree of blur might actually correspond to an acuity of about 20/180, close to the boundary of 20/200 for legal blindness in the United States.

At 20/320, no lines on the ETDRS chart are visible at the 4-meter viewing distance. We can no longer see Rachel's facial features. We know it's a person, but determining gender is difficult. We can't tell much about her clothing. This is moderate to severe low vision.

At 20/640, we can see the outline of the chart. It's hard to tell that there is a person next to it. This is severe low vision. Despite not being able to discern a person 4 meters away, this level of vision is still valuable in many situations.

The examples in Figure 2.3 indicate that someone with acuity of about 20/80 might need to be less than 4 meters away from a person to recognize them. Someone with lower acuity would need to be even closer. Someone with better acuity might be able to recognize a person from a greater distance. In general, we would expect at least a rough correspondence between a viewer's acuity and the maximum distance at which they can recognize another person.

Face recognition is the primary visual method for identifying people. There has been an enormous amount of research on face recognition by psychologists, neuroscientists, and computer scientists. There is a region in the temporal lobe of the brain's right hemisphere, known as the fusiform face area, which is thought to be specialized for recognizing faces (Kanwisher, 2010). It is known that there is a wide range of abilities for recognizing faces among people with normal acuity, ranging from super recognizers with phenomenal memory for faces to people who are face blind (they have prosopagnosia). For more about face blindness and a test of face recognition ability, visit the Prosopagnosia Research Center—Faceblind.[1]

There have been several studies of the impact of low vision on face recognition. I'll mention one of them now, and others in later chapters. In 1991, Mark Bullimore and colleagues at the University of California at Berkeley investigated how the maximum distance for recognizing people's faces depends on acuity. They tested four normally sighted subjects. They also tested 15 subjects with age-related macular degeneration (AMD) with acuities ranging from 20/37 to 20/300. The subjects first learned the names of eight individuals (four male and four female) from studying black-and-white photos close enough to be easily recognized. The subjects were then tested with additional photos of the eight individuals, projected on a display screen, at several viewing distances. By varying the viewing distance and the size of the images on the display screen, the researchers simulated viewing of real

[1] https://www.faceblind.org/.

human faces at increasing distances. The subjects were asked to name the individuals in the test photos. The data were analyzed to estimate the maximum distance at which a subject would be able to identify half of the images correctly (50% correct recognition). For the four normally sighted subjects, the average maximum distance was 60 feet (18 m). Two of the subjects with macular degeneration could not achieve 50% correct recognition at any test distance. For the other 13, the maximum distance for recognition ranged widely but averaged about 5 feet (1.5 m). As expected, people with better acuity were able to recognize faces at greater viewing distances. For the AMD subjects, the maximum distance for recognition correlated more closely with word acuity than letter acuity. Word acuity refers to the smallest print size for reading words rather than naming letters on the eye chart. Bullimore and colleagues considered word acuity to require more complex visual processing than letter acuity, accounting for the closer association with face recognition. This study demonstrated a relationship between clinical measures of acuity and face recognition in low vision. It also demonstrated that some people with low vision are unable to recognize faces and that face recognition is a more complex task than letter recognition.

Difficulty in recognizing friends and acquaintances is a major challenge for people with low vision and a source of social anxiety. With my very low vision, I'm unable to recognize faces at any distance. I rely on voices rather than faces for recognizing people. When I pass someone in the corridor in my building at work, if they don't speak to me, I don't know if they are a fellow faculty member, staff member, student, or a stranger. I can usually tell their gender. Sometimes other cues such as body size, clothing, or the context are enough for me to have a good guess. But I have certainly been embarrassed by mistakenly greeting someone by the wrong name. Happily, many of my students and colleagues identify themselves to me by voice when we meet in the corridor or elsewhere on campus.

Acuity limitations affect many other activities of daily living. In a survey study in my lab led by Yueh-Hsun (Walter) (Wu et al., 2024), we investigated the relationship between measured values of acuity and everyday function. Participants with a wide range of acuities were asked yes–no questions about their everyday visual experience. The 100 questions posed scenarios that refer to objects of stereotypical size viewed from typical distances. For example, "When stopped at a crosswalk in a residential area, are you able to read the street sign of the road you are about to cross?" The scenarios ranged from those requiring very good acuity to others requiring very low acuity. By analyzing data from 385 participants, we found that specific visual scenarios were associated with particular acuities. To illustrate, our data indicated that people with acuity near 20/200 are about equally likely to say "yes" or "no" for these three scenarios:

- Q. When standing an arm's-length away from a red brick building, are you able to make out the individual bricks?
- Q. When looking at a bunch of bananas on a table in front of you, are you able to count the individual bananas?
- Q. When you are standing, can you tell whether the trousers you are wearing are solid in color or have pin stripes?

People with acuities better than 20/200 are more likely to say "yes" to these questions and those with acuities poorer than 20/200 are more likely to say "no." This means that these scenarios are near the limit of vision for people with 20/200 acuity.

Measuring print size in points

I have emphasized the importance of taking viewing distance into account in acuity testing; the ratio of letter size to viewing distance determines whether a letter is at or above the acuity limit and determines the size of the letter's image on the retina. But typographers and software designers don't have precise knowledge of the reading distances of their users. They specify the size of letters in terms of physical measures such as inches, millimeters, or points.

In modern practice, there are 72 points in 1 inch. The traditional unit for measuring print size in books and computer software is termed *body size.* Body size for a given font is the vertical distance between the top of ascenders in letters such as "b" and the bottom of descenders in letters such as "q" plus a small gap to ensure space between the descenders of one line and the ascenders on the line below it. When large-print books are listed as having 16-point or 18-point print, or a Word processor has a menu of font sizes for documents, it is the body size being referred to. Most letters in a font are actually smaller than the body size. The height of a lowercase x is sometimes used as a measure of character size and is more representative of letters in narrative text than body size. For example, 12-point Times Roman has a body size of 12 points (equal to 12/72 = 0.167 inch [4.2 mm]). The x-height in Times Roman is only 45% of the body size or just 5.4 points (equals 0.075 inch or 1.9 mm).

Specifying print size in points (either body size or x-height) does not take viewing distance into account. Knowing the viewing distance is necessary to determine if a given print size in points is within a reader's acuity limit. As described in Box 2.1, if someone views 12-point Times Roman text from a distance of 16 inches, the x-height, expressed as a visual angle, is about 16 minutes of arc, just a little larger than the size of 20/50 letters on an acuity chart. A person with acuity worse than 20/50 would have difficulty reading 12-point Times Roman text from a distance of 16 inches or more.

Comparing acuity in adult humans to animals and infants

How does the acuity of humans compare with the acuity of other species? Animal vision has evolved to be functional in the creature's ecological niche and can differ from human vision in many ways—in acuity, color vision, and depth perception, and the ability to function in daylight or at night. Human evolution has favored the development of high visual acuity in daylight. Human visual acuity is superior to most creatures, but not all.

How do we measure acuity in animals? We can't ask them to read the letters on the Snellen or ETDRS charts. Animals can be trained to respond selectively to visual patterns. Even cats can be trained with food rewards to press a key with their nose to indicate the presence of a visible pattern on one of two displays. A typical pattern for measuring acuity in animals (and also preverbal human infants) is called a grating pattern. It consists of a series of black-and-white stripes, like the stripes on a zebra or the stripe pattern on a shirt. To test acuity, the stripes of the grating pattern can be made narrower and narrower until the animal can no longer distinguish the individual black-and-white stripes from a uniform gray at the testing distance. The narrowest stripes that can be detected from a specified viewing distance determine the *grating acuity* for the animal or human in question.

It is possible to establish the correspondence between acuity measured with grating patterns and acuity measured with letters on an eye chart. As a technical aside, here is how we establish this correspondence. Grating acuities are usually expressed as the highest spatial frequency, in cycles per degree, of a grating visible to an observer (known as the high spatial frequency cutoff). It is often assumed that a human letter acuity of 20/20 corresponds to a grating acuity of 30 cycles per degree and that letter acuities scale in proportion to grating acuity. If so, we can convert grating acuities to letter acuities. For example, a grating acuity of three cycles per degree would correspond to a

Table 2.2 Comparing human and animal acuities*

Creature	Acuity	Description
Eagle	20/4	Ultra-high vision
Human adult	20/10	High normal acuity
Human adult	20/20	Standard for normal acuity
Human infant(12 months)	20/90	Mild low vision
Cats and dogs	20/70	Mild low vision
Human infant(4 months)	20/200	Legal blindness
Frog	20/200	Legal blindness
Human infant(at birth)	20/600	Severe low vision
Rat	20/600	Severe low vision
Honeybee	20/1800	Ultra-low vision

*For data on the development of acuity in human infants, see Mayer et al. (1995). For interesting papers on animal vision, see the review by Caves et al. (2018), and for specific animals, see Blake (1988) for cats, Miller and Murphy (1995) for dogs, Reymond and Wolfe (1981) for eagles, Lettvin et al. (1959) for frogs, and Srinivasan (2011) for honeybees.

letter acuity of 20/200, and a grating acuity of 10 cycles per degree would correspond to a letter acuity of 20/60.

The letter acuities shown in Table 2.2 for animals and infants were derived in this way, sometimes rounded to simple Snellen ratios. Of course, just as human visual acuity varies to some degree across the population, the acuity for animals will vary across individuals and breeds. The values in the table should therefore be considered as rough approximations.

We often hear about the superior acuity of raptors, such as hawks or eagles. Behavioral measurements of eagle acuity do indeed show that they have superior acuity to humans. The acuity of 20/4 for eagles, listed in the table, implies that eagles would be able to resolve an acuity target at five times the distance of a human with 20/20 acuity or 2.5 times the distance of an "eagle-eyed" human with acuity of 20/10.

Behavioral measurements of dogs and cats indicate that their acuity is about 20/70, substantially lower than human adult acuity and would be considered mild low vision for humans. Dog guides that assist visually impaired humans function very effectively despite their "low vision."

It's astonishing to realize that honeybees have visual acuity so low that it would be considered ultra-low vision for humans. It is known that honeybees and frogs have some specialized visual capacities for the detection of movement, color, and the polarization of light, which help compensate for their low acuity.

The low acuities of rats (20/600) and honeybees (20/1800) give me comfort. My visual acuity is very low, lying somewhere in the rat–honeybee range. These animals function effectively in their ecological niches. They give me reason to appreciate the value of my very low vision.

Behavioral methods, similar to those used to assess animal acuity, can be used to assess the acuity of preverbal human infants. Davida Teller developed a method called forced-choice preferential looking, described in her 1997 review article. Given a choice between a blank display and a display with stripe patterns (grating patterns), babies prefer to look at the stripes. In Teller's method, a card is shown to the infant, with a grating pattern displayed on the left or right side and the other side blank. By monitoring the gaze direction of the infant, an examiner can determine if the grating pattern is visible to the infant. Just as letters are made smaller on the eye chart to test acuity in human adults, a series of cards can be shown with the stripes in the grating patterns made narrower and narrower until an infant no longer looks reliably at the side of the card with the stripes. In this way, the infant's grating acuity can be measured. As indicated in Table 2.2, newborn infants have very low acuity of about 20/600. Human vision develops rapidly in the first year of life, increasing from about 20/200 at four months of age to 20/90 (mild low vision) at twelve months. Happily, for most infants, the most important visual patterns, such as mom or dad's face, are often close enough to the infant to be recognizable despite their low acuity. Measurements indicate that human visual acuity reaches adult values by about five years of age.

Take off your glasses

If you are shortsighted (myopic) and take off your glasses, distant objects will appear blurry and your distance acuity will be reduced. Similarly, if you are hyperopic (farsighted) and you take off your glasses, print in books or other near objects will be blurry and your near acuity will be reduced. The degree of acuity loss in these two cases depends on the severity of your refractive error and also the size of your pupils. In a 1987 study conducted with my colleagues Kathy Mullen, George Woo, and Fergus Campbell while I was a visitor at Cambridge University, we measured the relationship between reduced acuity and the extent of defocus associated with different levels of refractive error. For example, we found that for someone with four diopters of uncorrected myopia (and dilated pupils), distance acuity is reduced to approximately 20/200.

If you are a normally sighted person, is taking off your glasses a good simulation of low vision? Your temporary reduction of acuity for distant objects (if you are myopic) or nearby objects (if you are hyperopic) does give you some idea of objects that are difficult to see for a low-vision person with the corresponding reduction in acuity. But the simulation is inadequate in two major ways. First, most people with long-standing low vision, either congenital or acquired, do not describe their reduced-acuity world as being blurry. Yes, objects beyond the acuity limit cannot be seen, but not because they appear blurry. Apparently, the visual system adapts so that objects within the acuity limit continue to look sharp, despite reduced acuity. Second, in most cases of low vision, a full description of visual impairment requires consideration of factors in addition to reduced acuity. Most important are reduced contrast sensitivity and visual-field loss. We will consider these two aspects of low vision in the following chapters. Removing glasses will not provide a good simulation of these two additional aspects of impaired vision.

3

Contrast and Color

We see a cup on the table, a cat on the floor, or an apple in the tree because they contrast in some way with the background. Difficulty in perceiving these contrasts can be a major problem for people with low vision. Contrast sensitivity is one of the big three clinical measures of low vision, along with acuity and visual-field status. Color perception has been harder to evaluate in low vision, but it is also important. We'll consider the roles of both contrast and color in this chapter.

•••••

What is contrast sensitivity?

Contrast sensitivity refers to the eye's ability to distinguish between an object and its background based on light-dark differences, such as a white piece of paper visible on a gray wall. The light-dark dimension is often referred to as grayscale, with the white paper having a high grayscale value and the dark wall a lower grayscale value. Colored objects also have grayscale values. For instance, a bright red paper on a dark gray wall might be visible to someone with no color vision because of the difference in grayscale values between the paper and the wall. Later in this chapter, we'll consider the value of color cues per se (red, green, blue, etc.) in low vision, but we'll begin by focusing on contrast due to differences in grayscale.

Low contrast can limit visibility, even for objects that are well within the viewer's acuity range. The object need not be small or far away. Think about trying to see a nearby white rabbit in the snow. If the rabbit is still and its fur is almost the same shade of white as the snow, it will be very difficult to see because the contrast is low. If you have good vision, you may be able to distinguish the rabbit from its background based on the difference in texture between the rabbit's fur and snow. If you have low vision and this texture difference is not visible, you will probably not see the rabbit.

With my very low vision, I rarely see rabbits under any condition. Of more immediate importance to me, my low contrast sensitivity means that

Low Vision. Gordon E. Legge, Oxford University Press. © Oxford University Press (2026).
DOI: 10.1093/9780198946960.003.0004

I may fail to see our black cat, named Hudson, on the black slate floor in our entrance hall at home (Figure 3.1, left panel). On occasion, I've accidentally stepped on a cat's tail or a cat, not a happy or safe event for me or the cat. When Hudson is lying on the white bedspread, he is easily visible to me (Figure 3.1, right panel).

Unlike acuity reduction and visual-field loss, reduced contrast sensitivity is not usually included in statutory definitions of low vision. Reduced contrast sensitivity is not widely recognized by the general public as a problem for people with low vision. Nevertheless, in many situations, reduced contrast sensitivity hampers low vision more than acuity. Research has shown that difficulties in reading, mobility, face recognition, and many everyday activities are caused by reduced contrast sensitivity. In this chapter, we'll discuss the meaning and measurement of contrast sensitivity and the consequences for low vision. We'll also discuss the value of color information in low vision. In later chapters, we'll consider how contrast and color affect reading and mobility.

Normal human vision is capable of detecting very small grayscale differences between objects and their backgrounds; we say that human vision has high contrast sensitivity. Grayscale differences refer to differences in light intensity between an object and its background. Black print on a white page has high contrast, but light gray print on the same white page has much lower contrast. Researchers have found that the human retina and visual cortex of the brain are specialized for detecting very small contrasts. Under some conditions, healthy adult vision can detect less than a 1% difference between the light intensity reaching the eye from a target and its background.

There are two attributes of contrast: magnitude and polarity, both illustrated in Figure 3.2. The *contrast magnitude* of text letters refers to a measure

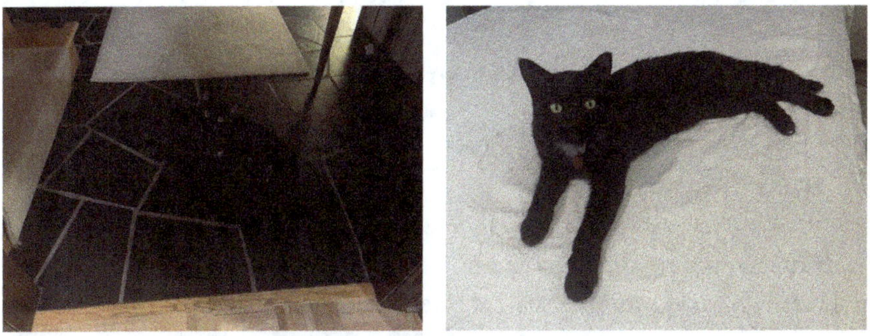

Figure 3.1 Photos of a black cat on a black slate floor (left) and on a white bedspread (right), illustrating the importance of contrast in determining visibility.

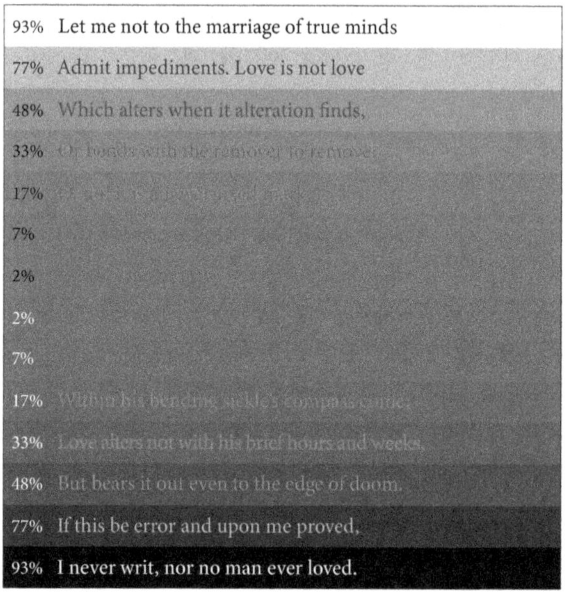

Figure 3.2 Illustration of two attributes of contrast—magnitude and polarity. The 14 lines of Shakespeare's Sonnet CXVI are rendered with seven contrast levels (magnitudes) for each of the two contrast polarities.

of the difference in light intensities reaching the eye between the strokes of the letters and the page. Contrast magnitude ranges from a low value of 0 (white letters, identical to the white of the page, and therefore invisible to anyone) to a maximum of 100% which would occur for the blackest black letters on a white background.

The *contrast polarity* of text refers to the difference between the typical rendering of dark letters on a white background and the more unusual rendering of white letters on a dark background. Sometimes, text with white letters on a dark background is said to have "reverse contrast" to distinguish it from the more common rendering of black on white.

Contrast magnitude

Contrast magnitude refers to the difference in light intensity between any target and its background. The light intensity reaching the eye from a surface region is referred to as the *luminance* of the region and can be measured by a photometer, an instrument capable of focusing selectively on the region. More specifically, the luminance of a surface is determined by the product of two factors—the intensity of the light incident on it and its reflectance. A surface's reflectance is the fraction of the incident light that bounces off it and is not absorbed. A white piece of paper has high reflectance while a gray or black piece of paper has lower reflectance. More details are given in Box 7.2, Light Measurement, in Chapter 7.

There are several different units of measurement for luminance, but the most common metric unit is candelas per square meter, written cd/m^2. A conventional standard for the luminance of the white background on an eye chart is 100 cd/m^2.

One definition of the contrast at the boundary between an object and its background is called Weber contrast and is defined as the difference in luminance between the object and the background divided by the luminance of the background. For example, if a light gray letter has a luminance of 90 cd/m^2 on a white background of 100 cd/m^2, the Weber contrast would be 10/100 or 0.10. Expressing this ratio as a percentage, we would say that the letter has 10% contrast. People with normal vision are able to read text with 10% contrast—light gray text on a white background—although they would describe the text as having poor quality. Many people with low vision would not be able to read such low-contrast text. We will return to the issue of text contrast and low-vision reading in Chapter 6.

The darker the letter on a white page, the higher its contrast, with a maximum value of 100% for the blackest letter having zero luminance. Some electronic displays can achieve contrast of text near 100%. Typical high-quality black print in hardcopy text is less than 100% contrast. Although the print looks black, it is still reflective of a portion of the incident light, so the contrast is less than 100%. If you print your resume on white bond paper (90% reflectance) with high-quality laser black toner (reflectance 5%), the Weber contrast of the text will be 94%.

Weber contrast is named for the 19th-century German physician Ernst Weber. A second definition of contrast, yielding somewhat different numerical values, is called the Michelson contrast, named for the American physicist Albert Michelson, famous for measuring the speed of light. The Michelson contrast at a boundary between an object and its background is the difference in luminance values between the object and the background divided by the sum of luminance values for the object and the background. Yet another measure is the contrast ratio, often used to describe the range of light intensities for visual displays. It is the ratio of the highest to lowest intensities (luminance values) that can be produced by the display. For example, a computer liquid crystal display might have a contrast ratio of 1000:1, representing the luminance ratio of its brightest to dimmest pixels.

Measuring contrast sensitivity

A person's contrast sensitivity refers to the smallest grayscale difference (smallest contrast) they can detect. Several tests have been developed for measuring contrast sensitivity. Figure 3.3 is a picture of the Pelli–Robson chart.

This chart was designed by Denis Pelli, now at New York University, and John Robson at Cambridge University and originally described by Pelli, Robson, and Wilkins (1988). Like the letter acuity chart, the Pelli–Robson chart consists of test letters to be named by the subject. But, in this case, the letters

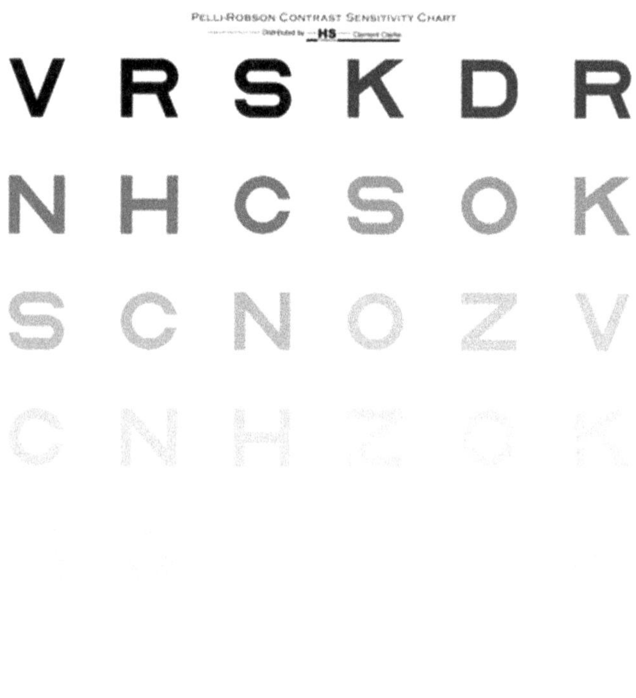

Figure 3.3 The Pelli-Robson chart for measuring contrast sensitivity.

all have the same large size. The chart is organized into sets of three letters with the same contrast. The contrast of the letters decreases from left to right and down the chart. At the top left, the contrast is very high, near 100%. For each succeeding set, the contrast decreases to about 71% of the preceding set. With this progression, the eighth set of three letters has contrast less than 10%. Similar to the letter acuity chart, the farther down the chart you go, the better is your contrast sensitivity. Box 3.1 describes the scoring used with the Pelli–Robson chart.

Box 3.1 Units for measuring contrast sensitivity

Pelli–Robson contrast sensitivity ranges from 0 (poorest) to 2.25 (best). The score is calculated by finding the reciprocal of the lowest contrast that can be read and by taking the logarithm (base 10) of that value. For instance, the Weber contrast of the eighth set of three letters on the Pelli–Robson chart is 0.089, its reciprocal is 1/0.089 = 11.12, and the $\log_{10}(11.12)$ is 1.05. A person who reads all the letters through the eighth set and not further has a Pelli–Robson contrast sensitivity score of 1.05. A young adult with very good vision who completes the 14th set, having a contrast of 1.12%, but can't read further will have a Pelli–Robson score of 1.95. Someone who can correctly identify the 16th set, having the lowest contrast on the chart, has a Pelli–Robson contrast sensitivity of 2.25. Averaging across the population of people with healthy vision, contrast sensitivity declines very slightly with age, even with healthy vision. A 70-year-old with healthy eyesight might only read through the 12th contrast level on the chart where the letters have a contrast of about 2% (Pelli–Robson score of 1.70). A higher Pelli–Robson score means better contrast sensitivity.

A customary viewing distance for the test is 3 meters. For people with low vision, testing is frequently done at a nearer distance of 1 meter so that the angular size of the letters is larger than the acuity limit for most people.

A chart that also measures contrast sensitivity, the Mars Contrast Sensitivity Test, is intended for testing at a near distance of 16 inches (40 cm). It was designed by Aries Arditi (2005). Mars is the Roman god of war, known to the ancient Greeks as Ares. The Mars test is widely used in low-vision clinics because of its convenience for testing.

People with low vision usually have reduced contrast sensitivity, with the reduction being more extensive for people with lower acuity. Data assembled from several studies by Ying-Zi Xiong (2020) and colleagues at the University of Minnesota have shown how reduced contrast sensitivity is associated with reduced acuity and how this relationship depends on the cause of vision impairment. Their review indicates that a typical person with age-related macular degeneration and 20/200 acuity might be able to read through the seventh contrast step on the Pelli–Robson chart, corresponding to letters with about 13% contrast. People with retinitis pigmentosa (RP) and the same 20/200 acuity tend to have lower contrast sensitivity and might only read through the fourth or fifth step on the chart. People with cataract and the same 20/200 acuity tend to have higher contrast sensitivity and might read through the ninth or tenth step on the chart.

As with acuity, a person's contrast sensitivity places a boundary on visual performance in the real world. In most everyday contexts, good visual function will require contrasts substantially higher than the thresholds measured with the test charts. The difference between the threshold contrast and the contrast required for good, everyday performance is sometimes referred to as the *contrast reserve* required for the task. For some visual tasks, the contrast reserve may be substantial; contrasts 5 or 10 times higher than the chart threshold may be required for best performance. A person with low vision who has a high contrast threshold may not have an adequate contrast reserve, even at 100% contrast. For example, some low-vision readers with reduced contrast sensitivity are fundamentally limited by the inability to achieve adequate contrast, even with sufficient magnification of letter size. We'll return to this topic in connection with reading in Chapter 6.

Contrast polarity

Text can be rendered as black letters on a white background or in "reverse contrast" as white letters on a black background. We refer to these alternatives as the *contrast polarity* of the text.

Contrast polarity plays a role in determining whether a target appears to be light or dark. The same target viewed against a dimmer (lower-luminance) background will appear to be light in color, but if placed against a brighter (higher-luminance) background, it will appear to be dark. For example, a square of low-luminance black ink on a white page appears dark. But, if the white surrounding portion of the page is replaced with an entirely dark background, the illuminated square of ink will appear to be white. The appearance of a target as light or dark, depending on its background, is a perceptual phenomenon termed *simultaneous contrast*, not to be confused with the physical measurement of contrast between a target and its background.

Most electronic displays designed for low vision include a contrast-polarity option. Many people with low vision read better with white text on a dark background than with conventional black-on-white text. Mainstream electronic platforms, such as web browsers, the Amazon Kindle, and Apple and Android mobile devices also provide options for contrast reversal. These options go by names such as "color invert," "dark mode," or "dark theme." In addition to potential benefits for low vision, reverse contrast is thought to reduce power consumption in electronic displays, to be more comfortable for reading in the dark, and sometimes to reduce eye strain. If we consider a typical white page containing single-spaced black text, more than 80% of the page is white space and less than 20% is black print. Reversing the contrast so that more than 80% of the page is dark, the average illumination at the eye would be substantially reduced, perhaps contributing to visual comfort. Some of my normally sighted students have reported that they use reverse-contrast displays for computer programming, a task requiring lengthy and meticulous scrutiny of alphanumeric characters. Perhaps, programming is an activity in which the overall lower light level of reverse-contrast is more comfortable for the eyes.

When text legibility and visual acuity are compared for black-on-white and white-on-black letters for normally sighted subjects, the differences are small or absent. For some categories of low vision, there are substantial benefits for reading reverse-contrast (white-on-black) text. Advanced cataract is one such category. High-acuity vision requires clarity of the optical image-forming elements of the eye, particularly the cornea and crystalline lens. In cases of advanced cataract, all or part of the crystalline lens can become cloudy, reducing acuity and resulting in substantial light scatter within the eye. The cloudiness of the crystalline lens in advanced cataract is sometimes said to be like smearing Vaseline on your glasses. There are also eye disorders in which the cornea becomes cloudy or translucent. In instances of cloudiness of the optics of the eye, abnormal light scatter from the abundant white space on a hardcopy page or computer display can reduce the retinal-image contrast of letters or other objects being viewed. If the contrast is reversed, the background becomes dark, and the contrast-reducing impact of light scatter diminishes.

Low vision associated with albinism is another vision condition in which reversed contrast is sometimes helpful. Albinism is a genetic disorder, characterized by the inability of the person's body to produce the pigment melanin. Many people with albinism have snow-white hair, due to the lack of pigment. In the eyes, pigmentation is missing, including iris coloration. The lack of light-absorbing pigmentation in the iris results in abnormal leakage of extra light into the eye which dilutes retinal-image contrast. Reversed contrast helps in reducing the impact of this light leakage. I'll return to albinism in Chapter 9 when I discuss childhood low vision.

According to findings by Michael Sandberg (2006) and colleagues at the Massachusetts Eye and Ear Infirmary, some people with RP, especially those with lower contrast sensitivity, read better with reversed contrast. RP refers to several types of inherited retinal degeneration, which affect the retina rather than the optics of the eye. It remains unknown why reversed contrast is often helpful to people with RP. Macular degeneration is also a prevalent form of retinal disease, but there is no clear evidence that people with this disorder benefit significantly from reverse contrast.

Contrast challenges in everyday life

When does low contrast in our everyday environment challenge the contrast sensitivity of normal healthy vision? Both acuity and contrast sensitivity decline in very dim illumination. If you are reading a book or newspaper outdoors after sunset, the print may seem to fade in contrast. Ultimately, the print becomes unreadable as darkness descends. Nighttime sensitivity for dim points of light such as stars in the sky can be very high, but the ability to resolve differences in grayscale declines. The cone photoreceptors, which are the retinal cells responsible for high-acuity central vision, are active in daylight. Light levels at night are too low for the cones, and our vision relies on the rod photoreceptors.

Nighttime drivers may need to deal with low-contrast hazards. Even if headlights illuminate the road ahead, low-contrast objects such as a deer or a pedestrian in dark clothing at the side of the road, viewed against a dark background, may be hard to see because of low contrast.

The history of the white cane provides an example of the importance of contrast. The white cane is widely used by both blind and low-vision individuals for two purposes. The white cane alerts drivers and others that a pedestrian with the cane is visually impaired. Of course, the cane can also be used by the pedestrian to explore the terrain ahead. According to the history of the white cane,[1] compiled by Philip Strong (n.d.), visually impaired individuals have been using canes and sticks to explore ahead since ancient times. But, only in the first half of the 20th century was it appreciated that painting a cane white would make it more visible for drivers by enhancing its

[1] https://www.njcounciloftheblind.org/brochures/history_of_white_cane.htm#:~:text=The%20following%20short%20history%20of,ACB%20office%20for%20pedestrian%20safety.text=This%20new%20role%20for%20the,then%20spreading%20to%20North%20America.

contrast, thereby providing greater safety for visually impaired pedestrians. The widespread adoption of the white cane by people with vision impairment came about in the 1930s.

People with impaired vision often choose brightly colored jackets or other clothing to enhance their visibility for drivers. Brightly colored clothing worn by others can also serve as visual cues for people with low vision. When my wife wears a brightly colored coat, it makes it easier for me to spot her in a crowd.

Fog and snow provide other examples in which objects may disappear because of low contrast. As sailors know well, distant objects that are easy to see under most daylight conditions can grow faint and disappear when the fog rolls in.

Even a light coating of snow can reduce the contrast of important environmental features. Figure 3.4 is a photograph illustrating the reduced visibility of a sidewalk curb during a light dusting of snow in Minneapolis. Can you see the curb?

While low contrast rarely causes problems for normally sighted people, low contrast often causes problems for people with low vision. When a person's

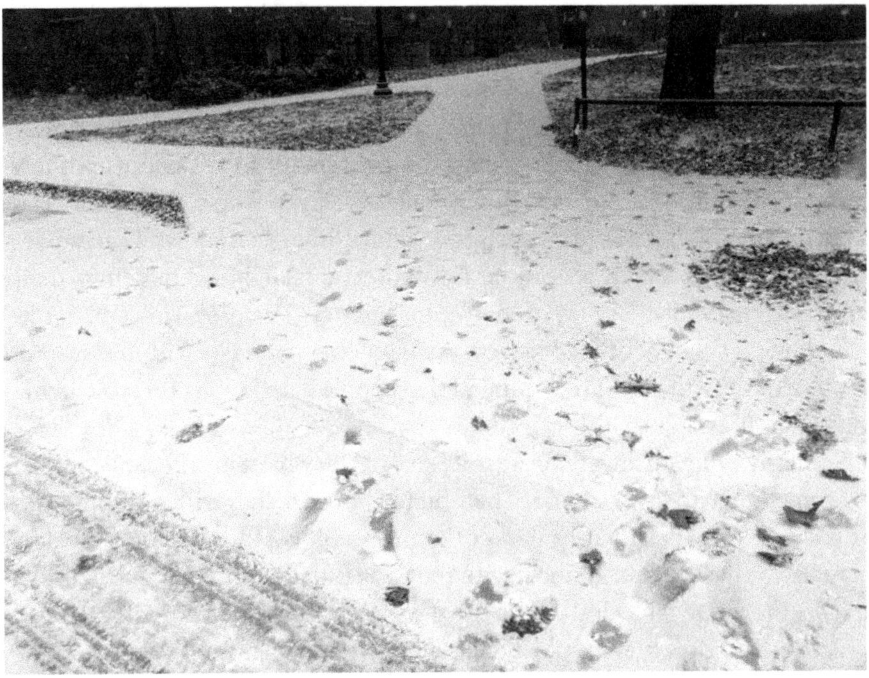

Figure 3.4 A photo of a low-contrast curb in snow.

contrast sensitivity is reduced, many subtle features of the environment become invisible. I live in Minnesota where we encounter snow from November to April. After the snow has fallen, steps and curbs become hard to see. White cars disappear next to snow banks. Sidewalks are white and so is the adjacent street or grass. Often, the edges of the sidewalk are below my contrast threshold, so there is no visible path. If there are piles of snow beside the sidewalks, I can make course corrections when I bump into the snow banks. If the sidewalks are shoveled, they may appear dark next to the white snow on the ground, forming a visible, high-contrast boundary. In the early spring, after the snow has melted but before the grass has turned green, the neighborhood sidewalks are a brownish gray against the brownish soil. Once again, the contrast is low and the sidewalks are difficult to follow. But, then in May, the grass turns lush green, darker than the lighter-colored pavement; visible contrast returns. The same city landscape has transformed from high to low contrast and back again with the change of seasons.

Rain can also make wet surfaces less distinct. Walkways become darker when wet, sometimes making them harder to see next to dark soil. I had a potentially dangerous experience when rain reduced the contrast of my environment. We had a wooden pier at our lakeside cabin. When the pier was wet from rain, the light-colored wooden planks of the pier darkened, taking on the color of the surrounding water. On one occasion, I lost sight of the boundary between the pier and the lake and I fell into the water. Fortunately, the water wasn't deep, and I do know how to swim. I climbed out, drenched but unhurt. It did take a long time for the contents of my wallet to dry.

Household furnishings can sometimes be difficult to see because of low contrast. Imagine a white table on a white floor. Even worse, imagine a glass table on any floor. Clear glass surfaces—tables, doors, windows—can sometimes be made visible by reflections from directional lighting, but often, their contrast is very low because of their transparency. The problem can be mitigated by placing a visible object on the glass that contrasts with the surface behind it. Nevertheless, I recommend that people with low vision avoid living in glass houses.

Similarly, white dishware on a white surface may have insufficient contrast for someone with low vision. It's helpful to choose dishes with a colored rim or dishware that is lighter or darker than the table top. An empty wine glass may also be hard to see. Filling it with red wine usually helps, making it visible against the white tablecloth. Do people with low vision prefer red or white?

People with low vision may deliberately choose dishware, furniture, carpets, and other household articles to enhance visual contrast in their own homes.

In Chapter 2, I pointed out that face recognition is a major challenge for people with low vision. Some people with low vision, like me, are unable to recognize faces at all. For others, acuity imposes a limitation: The poorer a person's acuity, the nearer they must be in order to recognize someone. Face recognition makes use of subtle differences in the appearance and configuration of facial features such as eyes, eye brows, nose, and mouth. Visualization of these features requires luminance contrast or color differences between these features and the skin on the face. In 2017, a team led by Aurélie Porcheron at Chanel PB in France showed that, on average, the contrast of facial features declines with age and is lower for males than females. The use of cosmetics, such as lipstick, enhances the contrast of facial features.

It stands to reason that people with low vision who have reduced contrast sensitivity will have difficulty discerning facial features and thereby difficulty in recognizing faces or facial expressions. Several studies have demonstrated a correlation between reduced contrast sensitivity and poorer face recognition in groups of people with low vision. A summary of these studies and additional data were provided by Venugopal et al. (2023). Most laboratory studies of face-recognition ability are done with static photos or screen displays of good images of faces. In everyday environments, variations in lighting or shadows and the motion of individuals can make face recognition more challenging. These variations, in addition to limitations due to acuity and contrast sensitivity, help explain why face recognition is so difficult for many people with low vision.

People with vision impairment often have difficulty following and recognizing characters in movies, TV shows, and live theater. Audio description (AD) is a service in which narration is added to identify characters and to provide information about visual details of action or scenes in the show. Many contemporary movies and TV shows have an option for AD. Some live theaters have AD for selected performances. I'm a fan of AD: It enhances my enjoyment of entertainment events. For more information and examples of AD, see the homepage of the Audio Description Project.[2]

The importance of contrast

Acuity is the best known attribute of vision. Your acuity puts a limit on the size and distance at which you can recognize letters, faces, and other objects. But, even if an object is large enough and close enough to be within your

[2] https://adp.acb.org/index.html.

acuity limit, you won't be able to see it unless it has sufficient contrast with its background. Large, nearby objects can go unseen because they fall below a person's contrast threshold. Most people with low vision have reduced contrast sensitivity. They may fail to see a step, a cup on the table, or a cat on the floor, not because the object is too small or too far away but because it has low contrast.

We have focused on contrast conveyed by grayscale levels, that is, differences in light intensity reaching the eye between an object and its background. We refer to such differences as *luminance contrast.* Sometimes, objects can be made visible by other visual features. For example, the motion of an object against a stationary background can sometimes provide a cue to its visibility. Imagine a spotted Dalmatian standing still against a spotted background. If the animal moves and you can discern the pattern of moving spots, you will see the dog. Motion cues are often helpful for people with low vision. We will return to the role of motion when we discuss mobility in Chapter 7. At the beginning of this chapter, I mentioned that the texture of a white rabbit's fur might enable someone to see the rabbit in snow. Texture differences provide another type of contrast useful to vision. But, texture differences often rely on acuity for fine details and may be unseen by many people with low vision. Differences in color between an object and its background provide another form of contrast. We'll turn to color and low vision in the next section of this chapter.

Adequate contrast between an object and its background is a necessary condition for visual object recognition. This is why contrast sensitivity is important to understand and why it is so important for people with low vision.

How useful is color for people with low vision?

In everyday language, *color* refers to hues of the rainbow and their mixtures—red, yellow, green, blue, purple, and many others. Colors can be used to distinguish objects from one another and from their backgrounds. Colors can be important for people with low vision. I use color to sort the laundry, match socks, and pick out clothing. People with low vision vary widely in their ability to distinguish and make use of colors. How important is color for people with low vision?

An enterprising undergraduate student of mine, Lee Wurm was looking for an honors research project. He was interested in both color vision and low vision. We knew that eye diseases sometimes impair color vision. We decided to address two major questions: Would the presence of color help people with low vision to recognize objects? And, would color also be helpful for people with normal vision to recognize objects? We asked the latter question because normally sighted people can easily recognize objects in black-and-white photos and have no trouble following black-and-white movies.

We planned an experiment in which we would compare the speed and accuracy of subjects to recognize pictures of objects in color and grayscale. What type of objects should we use? The famous neuroanatomist Stephen Polyak (1889–1955) had an influential photograph in his 1957 book, published posthumously, showing that red berries are easily seen against a background of green leaves, whereas the unripe green berries are much harder to see. In Polyak's view, color vision evolved to facilitate food gathering. Motivated by Polyak's view, we decided to use food objects as our stimuli because of their ecological importance. We made video images of 21 food types varying widely in color and shape: apple, banana, bread, cantaloupe, carrot, celery, cookie, grape, lemon, olive, orange, pea, peanut, pear, pepper, pickle, pineapple, potato, pretzel, tomato, and watermelon. For each of the 21 foods, we had four examples showing distinctly different versions; for bananas the four images showed a single banana, a peeled banana, a bunch of bananas, and a sliced banana. For each of the 21 times 4 images, we made both full color and grayscale video images, being careful to match the color and grayscale images pixel by pixel for screen brightness. We also made blurred versions of all of the food images to see if normally sighted subjects would show greater benefits of color with blurry images, artificially simulating reduced acuity. In total, we had four versions of each of the 84 food images. Figure 3.5 shows the four images for an apple, a slice of pineapple, and a piece of watermelon.

Our study (Wurm et al., 1993) had 48 normally sighted subjects and 16 low-vision subjects, all screened to have good color vision. Our low-vision subjects had a variety of eye conditions including macular degeneration, glaucoma, congenital cataract, and diabetic retinopathy. Before beginning the experiments, the subjects were shown a list of the 21 possible food categories. Their task was to name the food category as quickly and accurately as possible when an image was shown on the video screen. We used a voice-activated switch to measure the time in seconds (reaction time) to name the food category. We also measured accuracy (percent of correct identifications across all of the trials for a given condition). Each subject was tested on the

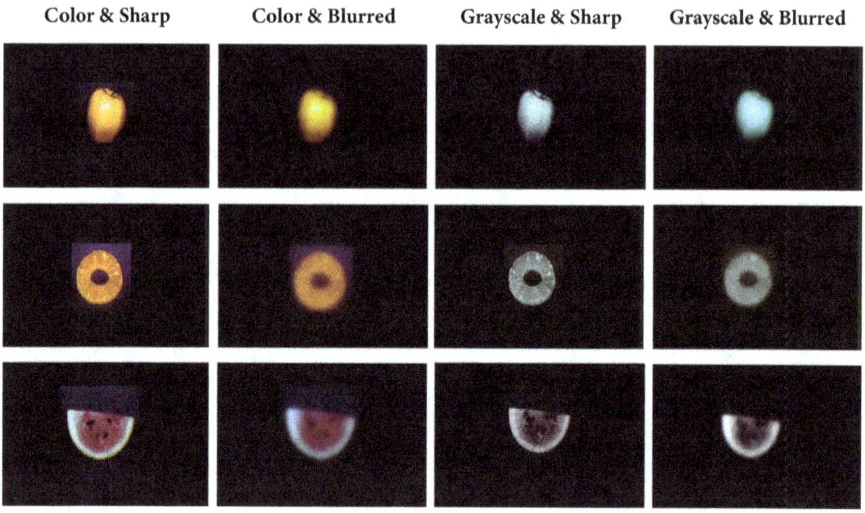

Figure. 3.5 The three rows show examples of apple, pineapple, and watermelon images used in the Wurm et al. (1993) study. Each row has the same image shown in color and grayscale, with sharp and blurred versions. Imagine seeing one of these images, at a larger scale on a video screen, and being asked to identify the type of food item. Would the color versions be easier than the grayscale versions? Would the sharp images be easier than the blurry images?

full set of color and grayscale images, and the normally sighted subjects were also tested with the blurred versions.

Both the normally sighted and low-vision subjects were faster and more accurate in naming foods in the color images than in the corresponding grayscale images. The differences were statistically significant. Not surprisingly, low-vision subjects with lower acuity took longer and made more errors than those with better acuity. Similarly, normally sighted subjects took longer and made more errors when naming blurry images compared with the sharp images. We concluded from our results that color can be beneficial to people with low vision in recognizing food objects. The results also showed that normally sighted subjects benefit from color.

This study motivated us to adopt the carrot for our lab mascot (see Figure 3.6).

Why carrots rather than one of the other food categories in our study? Carrots are good for vision, especially night vision! Carrots and other foods with beta carotene are used by the body to produce Vitamin A. Vitamin A plays a role in the conversion of photons absorbed by pigment molecules in the retinal rod cells into neural signals.

Figure 3.6 Our lab mascot is a carrot.

Human color vision is trichromatic

Now that we've established that color can be useful in low vision, let's look a little more deeply into the properties of human color vision. First, recall that the light-sensitive cells in the retina, the photoreceptors, come in two major categories—rods and cones. Refer to the appendix for a brief anatomical summary. The rods function at night under very low illumination and do not convey information about color. Rod vision accounts for the expression "at night, all cats are gray." The retinal cones operate in daylight vision. The cones convey color information and are responsible for high-acuity central vision.

Humans with normal color vision have three types of cones containing pigments that are sensitive to different ranges of wavelength. The S cones are sensitive to short-wavelength light at the blue end of the visible spectrum. The M cones are sensitive to a range of medium wavelengths (yellows and greens) and the L cones to longer wavelengths toward the red end of the visible spectrum. Differences in the responses of L and M cones (L-M) code for differences between reds and greens. Differences in the responses of the S cones compared with the sum of L and M cones (S – (L + M)) code for information in the blue-yellow direction in color space. The differencing operations involving the cone photoreceptors are termed opponent processes and play a crucial role in conveying color information to the brain.

Because normal human color vision relies on three types of wavelength-selective cells, it is said to be trichromatic. The trichromacy of human color vision explains why most colors can be reproduced by combinations of three primary colors. For example, televisions and computer displays produce a wide gamut of colors with mixtures of only three color signals with different intensities.

The common forms of inherited color deficiency are due to genetically determined variations in the light-absorbing pigments in the three types of cones. Some humans and many mammals are dichromatic, that is, they have only two cone pigments, typically missing either the L or M pigments. They perceive fewer distinctions among colors. It has been estimated that human dichromats perceive only about 1% of the shades of color discriminable by people with normal trichromatic vision (Perales et al., 2010). Some humans have three cone pigments but unusually extensive overlap in the wavelength ranges covered by the M and L cones. This greater overlap results in a decreased ability to distinguish some colors, especially among the reds and greens. These individuals are called anomalous trichromats.

Many tests of color vision have been developed to distinguish among inherited deficits in color vision. One type uses patterns of dots with different colors. An example is the Ishihara test, developed by a professor at the University of Tokyo in the early 20th century. You may have been asked to look at a picture composed of colored dots and report a number. The Ishihara test consists of pictures with color combinations chosen to make the numbers difficult to see for people with specific types of inherited color defects. This type of test may not be appropriate for many people with low vision because of the acuity requirement for distinguishing the small, colored dots.

A second type of color vision test—called an arrangement test—requires the subject to arrange colored caps in order of color similarity. The best known of these is the Farnsworth–Munsell 100 Hue Test (FM-100). The test is subdivided into four sets of caps covering different ranges of color. Imagine, for example, trying to arrange 25 coin-size caps in a row with very small color steps from yellow to green. The test is scored by counting the number of caps out of order and the size of the displacements. This test originated with physical caps but now comes in digital versions for on-screen testing. For people with low vision, the small caps may be difficult to work with. A shorter version called D15, including only 15 caps, can be used and is effective in identifying major color deficits. In the Wurm et al. study described earlier in this chapter, we tested subjects with low vision using a variant we call the enlarged D15; it uses extra-large colored caps.

Dichromats and anomalous trichromats are sometimes said to be "color blind," but this is a misnomer. They can see objects and perceive color; but the colors are simply less distinctive and have fewer variations. They can see the red and green apples but may have trouble distinguishing their colors. They retain normal high acuity and are not considered to have low vision. Undoubtedly, they encounter challenges in their daily lives. When PowerPoint and other graphics software first became popular, conference presenters and classroom teachers would sometimes show off their artistic creativity by creating slides with ill-chosen color combinations. I recall attending a major research conference on vision and ophthalmology and hearing attendees with inherited color defects complain about the illegible color combinations on the slides of some of the presenters. Since those early days, presenters have usually learned to select color combinations that are accessible to people with inherited color defects. Many websites make recommendations about how to avoid choosing bad color combinations.

Color deficits in low vision

Inherited achromatopsia is a recessive autosomal disorder, characterized by a complete loss of color vision. (A recessive autosomal disorder can result when a child inherits two recessive gene variants, one from each parent. The parents may be carriers without the disorder.) People with achromatopsia also have low vision. The specific gene variant renders the retinal cones ineffective, so the individual has only rod vision. Sometimes, people with this disorder are called rod monochromats. Knut Nordby (1942–2005), a Norwegian colleague of mine and fellow vision scientist, was a rod monochromat and played a prominent role in enhancing understanding of achromatopsia. In a highly readable and informative article, entitled *Vision in a Complete Achromat: A Personal Account* (Nordby, 1990), he described his life experiences with low vision and without color vision. He said his lack of color perception resembled a normally sighted person's perception of black and white film or photography. He recalled his childhood experience drawing pictures:

> When using colouring pencils or crayons, I am told, I always confused the colours, breaking all the conventions and "rules" about what were the "correct" colours to use: I would happily colour the sky light green, yellow or pink; the grass and leaves orange or dark blue; the sun white or light blue, and so on. I was always corrected in my choice of colours by those who knew better, and, eventually, I gave up painting and colouring my drawings.

Knut's acuity was 20/200, a typical boundary for legal blindness. He experienced challenges with print reading, mobility, and social interaction like others with reduced acuity. But, despite his lack of color vision and reduced acuity, he said that his greatest disability was his hypersensitivity to bright light, often termed photophobia. Because the retinal rods only function well in dim illumination, typical daylight was uncomfortable for him. He wrote:

> I am easily dazzled and, in effect, blinded if I expose my eyes to bright light. If I open my eyes fully for more than one or two seconds under such conditions . . . the scene I am gazing at is quickly washed out, turned into a bright haze and all structured vision is lost. It can be very distressing for me, and sometimes even painful, to perform demanding visual tasks in very bright light.

Like others with achromatopsia, he dealt with his photophobia in brightly lit situations with a variety of strategies including squinting, blinking, and using sunglasses and a visor.

Once, Knut and I and my wife Wendy and others were hiking together, taking an afternoon break from an ongoing conference. We were climbing a hill in the English Lake District on an overcast day. Wendy asked Knut about his vision. Smiling, he replied: "My vision is like a cat. I have lower acuity than you and no color vision. I prefer dimly lit places." But, in reality, Knut was giving his vision a little too much credit. Cats have better than 20/200 acuity and at least rudimentary color vision.

Knut Nordby traveled to the South Pacific island of Pingelap with the famous neurologist and author Oliver Sacks. The island has a high prevalence of achromatopsia. Together, they explored the lives and adaptations of the community of people there lacking color vision. Their intriguing insights into achromatopsia are described in Oliver Sacks's book *Island of the Colorblind* (1996) and in a BBC video documentary with the same name.

What about the impact of more common types of eye disorders on color perception? Cataracts result when part or all of the crystalline lens in the eye loses its optical clarity. In advanced forms, acuity is reduced and low vision results. The crystalline lens becomes yellowish in appearance. Think of the yellowing of the crystalline lens as being similar to looking through a yellow filter. The short-wavelength blues and greens are reduced in intensity in retinal images. The filtering out of blue light through cataracts can be demonstrated with careful measurements. One study compared the wavelength composition of a test light that appeared white to patients before and after cataracts were surgically removed and replaced by a clear interocular lens (Delahunt et al., 2004). Following the surgery, the patients required more yellow in the test light to balance their increased sensitivity to short-wavelength blue light in order for the test light to appear white.

Despite the yellowing of the crystalline lens, people with cataracts don't usually notice distortions in the colors of things around them. The human visual system flexibly adapts to changes in the overall wavelength spectrum of light reaching the eye. A similar adaptation occurs on a temporary basis when people with normal vision observe scenery through the tinted windows of a tourist bus; objects outside the bus retain their color appearance. But, after cataract surgery, people may notice a change. Sometimes, they report on the vividness of some colors, especially blues, as well as an improvement in their acuity. In a 1990 article, Walter Granville described the difference in color appearance through his "new eye" following cataract surgery compared with colors seen by his "old eye," which still had cataract. He wrote,

> Flowers presented lovely shifts. Lilacs went from a dirty maroon to a clear purple. Jacaranda (in Mexico) shifted from a reddish purple to a purplish blue with the new eye. ... Another example was the color of the sky at dawn. While still in bed I often viewed a patch of sky. With the new eye it was a more saturated violet-blue. To the old eye it was a grayish blue-green. I had no idea the early morning sky could look so lovely.

These differences in color appearance make sense because the cataract in his "old eye" filtered out light in the short-wavelength (blue) end of the visible spectrum.

In Chapter 5, we'll discuss the loss of central vision that can occur in advanced forms of macular degeneration and other maculopathies. People who lose their central vision must rely on their peripheral vision which has lower acuity. What is known about color perception in normal peripheral vision? It has long been known that the density of cone photoreceptors declines in peripheral vision. So, it may not be surprising that it is often reported that color vision also declines severely in peripheral vision. In a 2009 study, Thorsten Hansen and colleagues at Justus Liebig University Giessen in Germany found that both red-green and blue-yellow color mechanisms are present throughout the visual field to at least 50 degrees from central fixation, but with diminishing sensitivity. In a 2015 publication, Christopher Tyler at the City University of London demonstrated that objects viewed in peripheral vision can have strong color percepts. He showed that if colored disks are suitably scaled up in size to compensate for decreasing acuity in peripheral vision, their colors remain as vivid as disks seen with central vision.

Tyler's observations imply that the seemingly diminished salience of color percepts in peripheral vision is related to reduced acuity. Similarly, some reports of poorer color perception in low vision may be associated with reduced acuity. My own case may be an example. I have normal color vision based on results from the enlarged D15 arrangement test. Colors are distinct for me as long as the color features are large enough so that I can see them with my very low acuity. If a friend is wearing a shirt with colorful stripes, I will usually not be able to see the individual stripes. Instead, I'll see the shirt as a uniform, washed-out color. It may seem as if my color vision is weak, but my reduced acuity explains why I'm not appreciative of my friend's distinctive striped shirt. Even though I score well on the enlarged D15 test, I fail to see many salient colors in the everyday world because the objects or features in question lie outside my range of acuity.

Given these observations, it is to be expected that people with central-field loss will sometimes experience a decrease in their ability to distinguish colors, with the severity increasing as the extent of central loss increases. At least a portion of the deficit is likely due to reduced acuity in peripheral vision. It is possible that the disease process underlying the central-field loss may also contribute to a deficit in color vision. As reviewed by Lovie-Kitchin and Feigl in a 2005 article, several studies have demonstrated subtle disease-related deficits in the color vision of people with early forms of AMD. The deficits seem to be greater in blue-yellow discrimination, possibly because of selective damage to the short-wavelength-sensitive S cones. One complicating issue is that people with normal vision also demonstrate some age-related decline in color vision as measured using sensitive tests such as the FM-100, so age-matched controls need to be included in studies of people with AMD.

Do color deficits in AMD play a role in everyday vision? The Wurm et al. study of the role of color in food recognition included a few subjects with macular degeneration, but we were not primarily focused on AMD. A 2008 study led by Muriel Boucart at the University of Lille in France tested 15 AMD subjects with moderate-to-severe loss of acuity. As in the Wurm et al. study, the subjects were shown images in color or in grayscale. The subjects' task was to decide whether the image contained a face or an animal. In one condition, isolated objects were shown on the screen, but, in another condition, the face or animal was presented in the context of a natural scene. In both conditions, the AMD subjects were faster in responding to the colored versions of the images. The results of this study indicate that although people with AMD may exhibit deficits in color vision measured using standardized tests, color is still beneficial in object recognition and scene interpretation.

Making use of color cues

The variation in eye conditions causes a wide range of color-vision disabilities in people with low vision. Unlike the inherited forms of color deficiency that have well-defined characteristics, it is not feasible to make generalizations about the color capabilities of people with low vision. Some of them will make much better use of color than others.

My recommendation is this: When considering the visibility of text or other features on screens or pages, or the visibility of hazards or other key features in the environment, for people with low vision, first, be sure there is good luminance contrast (a good light-dark difference between the target of interest and its background). Next, take into account the potential value of color in providing useful information, keeping in mind the variability in color perception across the population of people with low vision. Aries Arditi (n.d.) has provided useful guidance in selecting effective color contrast for people with low vision.[3] Three guidelines adapted from Arditi's recommendations are mentioned below:

- Maximize the luminance contrast between a target of interest and its background.
- For contrasting colors between a target and its background, choose the light color of the pair to be white or predominantly from the middle of the visible band of wavelengths (green or yellow). Choose the dark color of the pair to be black or predominantly from the ends of the visible spectrum (red, blue, or purple). The logic is that eye diseases or congenital color defects are more likely to depress sensitivity at the ends of the visible spectrum, so it is best to use these for the darker color component of the contrasting pair.
- Choose the hues of the target and background to be far apart in color space, that is, use high chromatic contrast.

We've already seen that color may be useful in low vision for object recognition. In what other situations might color cues be beneficial, keeping in mind that some people will benefit more from color cues than others? Color can be useful in two general ways—in distinguishing a target object from its background (panels A and B in Figure 3.7) and in conveying specific meanings (semantic information) about a target object (panels C and D).

[3] https://pages.mtu.edu/~nilufer/classes/cs3611/interesting-stuff/designing-with-colors-1/color_contrast.htm.

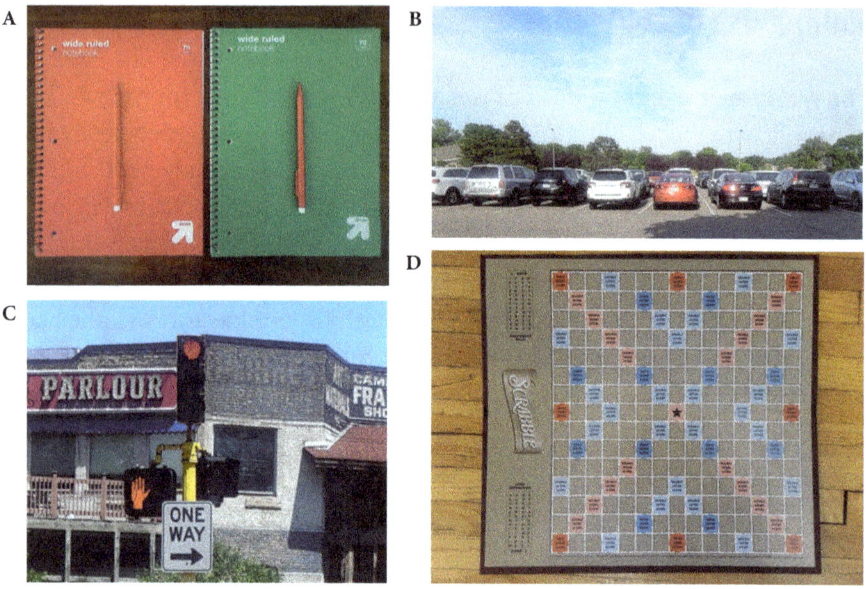

Figure 3.7 Examples of the usefulness of color cues. A. A red pencil is easier to see on a green notebook than on a red notebook. B. Color can be used to locate a familiar object in a crowded scene, such as a red car in a parking lot. C. A red stoplight is a well-understood signal to stop. D. Color coding on a scrabble board designates squares with special scoring rules: pink for Double Word scores, dark red for Triple Word, light blue for Double Letter, and dark blue for Triple Letter.

I've been emphasizing that the most important way to make an object stand out from its background is with high luminance contrast, that is, with a large light-dark difference. For instance, a black cup is easier to see on a white counter than a white cup on a white counter. It is also possible to use contrasting hues to distinguish an object from its background; for instance, a red pencil is easier to see on a green notebook than on a red notebook (Figure 3.7A). Conversely, similar colors of objects and background may make them difficult to see, such as green vegetables on a green plate. In a situation like this, there may still be adequate luminance contrast for good visibility; perhaps, the vegetables are a darker shade of green than the plate.

Color differences can also be useful in finding familiar objects when visual acuity is not good enough to recognize the object by shape or texture. This may be the most important use of color for me, given my very low vision. I'm looking for my red sweater; where did I leave it? I see a black thing on the bed. No, that's not my sweater; maybe, it's my cat, Hudson, taking a nap. But, there's a red thing on the floor. I bet it's my sweater! Sometimes, I will use color to "recognize" people at a distance. My wife has a bright pink windbreaker. I may look for the pink jacket when I try to find her in a crowd. Similarly, color may help you find your distinctively red car in a crowded parking lot (Figure 3.7B).

Color can also convey specific meanings about visual targets. For instance, red means stop and green means go in traffic signals (Figure 3.7C). A yellow stripe often means a curb or, sometimes, a crime scene. Red, green, and yellow are often adapted from traffic signals to code buttons or other features in apps and websites. Many people with low vision with adequate color perception do make use of stoplights and other meaningful environmental colors.

Similarly, color assignment can also be used to highlight specific items in a group of otherwise similar looking items, such as the colored squares on a Scrabble board (Figure 3.7D). Another example might be a collection of buttons on a device, such as a TV remote. Perhaps all the buttons have good luminance contrast, so at least they can be seen against their background. But even so, the buttons with their separate functions may be hard to distinguish. Color can be used to highlight important buttons. Maybe, the Power button is red, and the 5 button on the number pad has a different unique color. The special case of TV remotes is one that can perplex people with normal vision and also those who have low vision or who are blind. A good universal design would include tactile coding as well as color. People are often handling their remotes while looking at the TV screen, sometimes in dim lighting. Good tactile cues would often be helpful and more compliant with the principle of universal design.

Art and aesthetics

The low-vision requirement for high-contrast features may sometimes conflict with aesthetic judgments favoring subtle color variations such as pastels. An architect friend of mine was consulted about a design to remodel one floor of a public building. The remodeled floor would be used frequently by people with visual impairment. The interior designer planned to include low-contrast furnishings to match the color scheme of furnishings on other floors of the building. My friend explained to the designer that some visually impaired users of the remodeled space would not be able to see the low-contrast furnishings. He met with resistance on aesthetic grounds but ultimately prevailed in convincing the designer that the plan should be modified to include higher-contrast furnishings.

Low vision can compromise appreciation of the visual arts. Given my low acuity and severely reduced contrast sensitivity, I favor bold colors, high contrast, and large geometrical shapes in art. On a trip to the Netherlands, I had especially good luck in visiting art museums. I took pleasure in Rembrandt's paintings in the Rijksmuseum in Amsterdam. Rembrandt was a master of light and shadow. I especially liked his most famous painting, *The Night Watch*. It is enormous in scale (roughly 12 feet by 14 feet) and features high-contrast white images (faces and lace) on a dark background. (Remember the advantages of reverse contrast for low vision.) At the Gemeentemuseum in The Hague, I visited a special exhibit by Piet Mondrian (1872–1944). I enjoyed seeing the patchworks of colored, large, and irregular rectangles making up many of Mondrian's later paintings. The visit was also intriguing for me because Mondrian's works have had an influence in vision science and were used by Edwin Land (of Polaroid Camera fame) in his theory of lightness perception.

Of course, I can't claim that my preferences in art are shared by others with low vision. But, I do suspect that large paintings with big, bold features will be easier to see than paintings containing only fine details and subtle colors.

For me, stained glass is often more accessible than paintings. In dark interior spaces such as cathedrals, daylight shining through the stained glass yields high contrast and vivid colors. I'm a fan of the glass sculptor Dale Chihuly (1941–). On a visit to the Chihuly Garden and Glass Museum in Seattle, I enjoyed seeing the large-scale blown-glass sculptures. There were colored glass flowers that shone vividly in the sun in the outdoor garden. In a darkened interior room, I inspected colorful glass flowers, vines, and balls that were brilliantly illuminated and clustered on a large, rectangular platform. The combination of scale, color, and contrast meant that many of the glass sculptures were beautiful and salient for me despite my very low vision.

Some famous artists have acquired vision impairment later in life but continued to paint. How did the changes in their visual world affect their art? Several scholars have addressed this intriguing question at the boundary of art history and vision science. In 2006, Michael Marmor from Stanford University wrote about the case of Claude Monet (1840–1926). Monet suffered from increasingly severe cataracts from 1912 to 1922, while continuing to paint. (He underwent a successful cataract surgery in 1923.) How might an artist respond to such perceptual changes in composing works of art? Of course, the onset of vision impairment might affect the choice of topics and the emotional content of composition. But what about the visual content of the work? Marmor used digital filtering to modify photographic images to simulate the effects of severe cataract. The filtering included blurring which

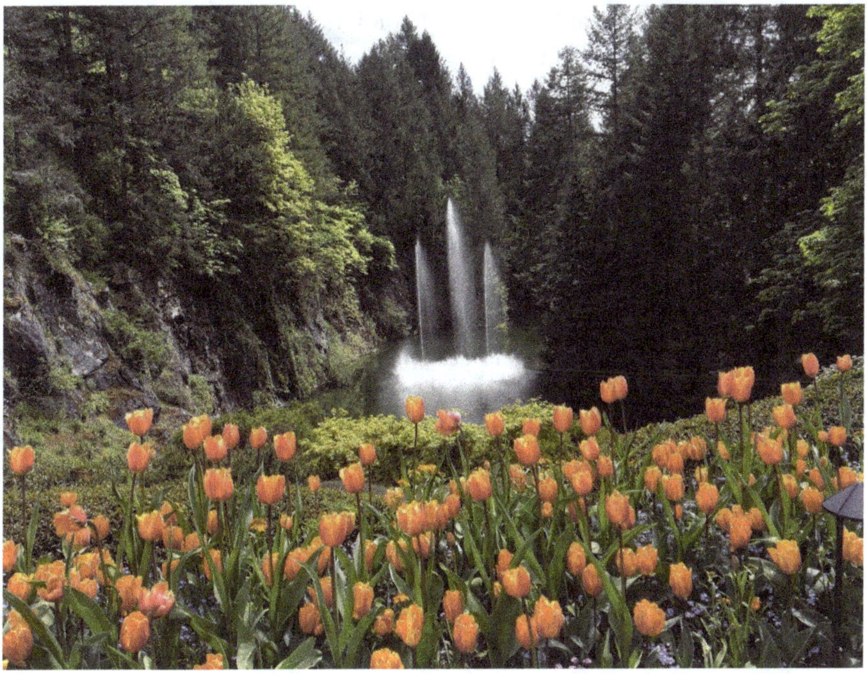

Figure 3.8 A photo of a large bed of orange tulips in front of a fountain in Butchart Gardens, Brentwood Bay, British Columbia.

reduced resolution equivalent to an acuity of 20/200. Color filtering simulated how cataract selectively reduces short-wavelength blue light entering the eye, while leaving the longer-wavelength oranges and reds less affected. The impact of color filtering is similar to wearing yellow-tinted sunglasses. Marmor's article included an original photograph of the lily pond in Monet's garden at Giverny, France, and a version of the photograph modified by the cataract simulation.

Monet's cataract undoubtedly had a significant impact on the sharpness and color content of images falling on his retina. These changes would have reduced his ability to make fine color discrimination and to visualize small pattern features on his canvases. But, would his impaired vision have biased him to choose blurry contours or more yellows and reds in his color schemes? Several factors may have helped Monet to compensate for his vision disability. His severe cataract likely resulted in blurry images on his retina, but, as I mentioned in the previous chapter, most people with low vision adapt to blur and describe their visual percepts as sharp. Monet may also have adapted to the yellowing of retinal imagery due to his cataract. People with healthy vision readily adapt to wearing color-tinted sunglasses; after wearing yellow-tinted or green-tinted sunglasses for a short period of time, colors appear natural and unaffected. Marmor also pointed out that Monet probably relied on his accumulated experience in the choice of paint colors to represent sky, grass, or other natural objects. In short, memory and lifetime expertise help in compensating for vision impairment. Marmor pointed out, however, that Monet's depictions of the lily pond did change. "These late paintings are almost abstract in the applications of paint and show a predominant red-orange or green-blue tone that is quite different from the subtle color shading that characterizes Monet's earlier Impressionistic work."

I enjoy expansive splashes of natural color. Figure 3.8 is a photo of a large bed of brilliant-orange tulips, taken by my wife during our visit to Butchart Gardens. The famous gardens are located near the city of Victoria on Vancouver Island in British Columbia, Canada. We visited in early May when the kaleidoscope of colorful tulips in bloom was an amazing sight, even for someone with very low vision.

4
The Peripheral Visual Field

Parts and Wholes

While low vision is often characterized by a loss of acuity and sometimes a loss of contrast sensitivity, the everyday challenges of many people with visual impairment come about because of visual-field loss. In this chapter, we will consider important properties of the normal visual field, how visual fields are measured, and peripheral-field loss in low vision. We will also touch on vision impairment due to loss of vision in one eye or in one half of the visual field. In the next chapter, we will focus on the loss of central vision.

• • • • •

The many patterns of visual-field loss

A person with a loss of vision in the central field from macular degeneration may encounter serious difficulty with reading, even if the print is magnified to compensate for reduced acuity. Another person with peripheral field loss from retinitis pigmentosa (RP) may retain high acuity and be able to read regular print but may bump into people in the corridor or miss seeing steps. Most people with low vision have some form of field loss, in addition to reduced acuity and reduced contrast sensitivity.

Visual-field loss can refer to either a total loss of vision or a reduction of visual function in a portion of the visual field. A complete loss of vision in a region of the field is called an absolute scotoma or informally a blind spot, and a reduction of vision without total loss in a region is called a relative scotoma. There are different patterns of field loss associated with particular eye diseases.

The Scottish ophthalmologist Harry Moss Traquair (1927) (1875–1954) portrayed the normal visual field of each eye as "an island of vision or hill of vision surrounded by a sea of blindness." In his metaphor, the island represents the field of view with the hill representing acuity which rises to a peak near the center. The "sea of blindness" refers to the region of space out of

Low Vision. Gordon E. Legge, Oxford University Press. © Oxford University Press (2026).
DOI: 10.1093/9780198946960.003.0005

sight behind us. Traquair used this metaphor to represent different patterns of field loss as geological distortions of the island of vision.

Figure 4.1 depicts visual-field maps from white to black. The bright areas represent high acuity, and the gray areas represent reduced acuity, with black representing Traquair's "sea of blindness" outside the boundary of the visual field. The three panels in the left column represent the normal visual fields of the left eye, the right eye, and binocular vision (the two eyes together). The bright areas near the center represent the region of high acuity in central vision. The small black holes near the center of the left- and right-eye maps represent the naturally occurring blind spot in each eye (which is where the optic nerve exits the retina). The binocular map does not show the blind spots. Blind spots will be discussed later in this chapter.

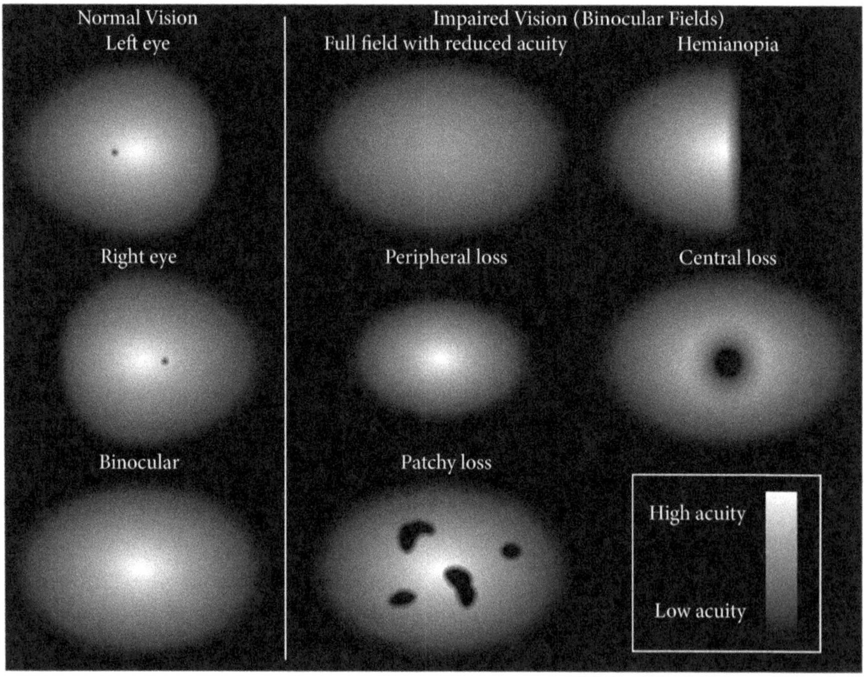

Figure 4.1 Visual-field maps depicted with grayscale from high acuity (white) to blindness (black). The left column depicts maps of the normal visual field for the left eye, right eye, and binocular viewing (both eyes together). The right side of the figure shows binocular visual-field maps depicting five general patterns of impaired vision—full field with reduced acuity, hemianopia, peripheral loss, central loss, and patchy loss. These are qualitative renderings intended to convey general patterns only and not the exact pattern for any specific individual.

The five panels on the right side of Figure 4.1 depict major categories of visual impairment. These include:

- Full field with reduced acuity (widespread or diffuse loss): The extent of the visual field is normal, but central acuity is reduced. An example is advanced cataract in which central acuity is low, but there is visual function across the entire visual field.
- Hemianopia: This is a condition in which half of the visual field is lost in both eyes, typically resulting from a stroke.
- Peripheral loss (visual-field constriction): This refers to loss of vision outside the central region. In advanced cases of RP or glaucoma, most of the peripheral vision may be lost, leaving a small zone of functioning central vision, sometimes termed *tunnel vision.*
- Central loss: This is termed either *central-vision loss* or *central-field loss,* and it refers to a partial or complete loss of vision in the center of the visual field. It is usually due to damage to the central retina containing the macula and fovea. Advanced age-related macular degeneration (AMD) is the most common cause of central-field loss. Central loss is often depicted as a perfectly circular scotoma, but, as shown in the figure, its shape often departs from circularity.
- Patchy loss: Some retinal diseases including diabetic retinopathy and dry AMD can result in patches of vision loss (small scotomas) scattered across the visual field.

The normal visual field

The field of vision refers to the wide panorama of vision simultaneously in view at any one time. Try this simple experiment. While looking straight ahead fixedly at a small target several feet away such as a light switch, extend your arms. First move your right arm out to the right at shoulder level with your palm up, and make a fist. Open and close your fist to generate a motion cue. Note whether you can see the motion while keeping your eyes locked on the fixation target. How far out to the right can you see the motion of your fist? Now repeat with the left arm, moving it out to the left with your palm up. How far out can you detect motion in that direction?

If you are a person with normal, healthy vision, you will probably be able to see the fist motion on both sides almost to the point where your arms are extended directly to the right or left.

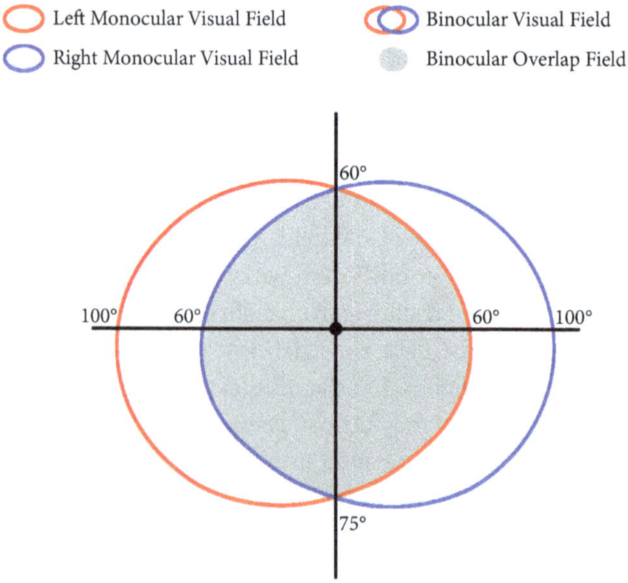

Figure 4.2 Illustration of the monocular fields of view (red and blue circles, the binocular field, and the region of binocular overlap [gray shading]). The fields are superimposed on a grid showing angular dimensions, and the two eyes are assumed to be fixated on the plus sign at zero degrees in each eye. Notice that the monocular fields are not perfectly circular. Each monocular field has a crescent-shaped region lying outside the region of binocular overlap.

Figure 4.2 is a drawing that illustrates the fields of view of the two eyes separately (the monocular fields), the overall combined field of the two eyes (the binocular field), and the region of binocular overlap. Each eye has a horizontal field of about 160 degrees—roughly divided into 60 degrees on the nasal side (between central fixation and the nose) and 100 degrees on the temporal side (between central fixation and the outward or "temple" side). There is a large region of binocular overlap, that is, a region of visual space covered by both eyes. It extends about 120 degrees horizontally and 135 degrees vertically. This binocular region is used in stereoscopic depth perception. The binocular visual field refers to the total extent of vision from the farthest right point (only visible to the right eye) to the farthest left point (only visible to the left eye) and covers about 200 degrees of the full 360 degrees. Despite this wide field of view, there is a region of about 160 degrees behind us that is out of sight; no, we don't have eyes in the back of our heads. Some animals, such as rabbits, with eyes placed laterally on the sides of the head have a binocular field that covers all or nearly all 360 degrees of view in the horizontal plane. It has been hypothesized that predator animals, such as humans and wolves, have evolved to have eye placement more forward on the head to take advantage of binocular overlap for use in stereoscopic depth perception, while prey animals such as rabbits have evolved to have more laterally placed eyes to emphasize extending the overall field of view (what's coming behind me?).

The optical elements of the eye (cornea and crystalline lens) create an image on the retina at the back of the eye (Appendix Figure A1). We can think of the process of optical image formation as mapping the visual field into a retinal image. Regions of the scene near the line of sight are represented by image features on the macula in the center of the retina. The portion of the scene in peripheral vision forms image features on peripheral retina outside the macula. The appendix provides some additional details on the structure of the retina.

The wide visual field is not uniform in acuity or light sensitivity. There are two major properties of the visual field that are important for understanding low vision. Both are related to the anatomy of the retina. First, visual acuity and contrast sensitivity decline in peripheral vision; the farther out, the worse vision gets. If you fixate on a point straight ahead and try to recognize letters in your peripheral vision, the letters will need to be larger for you to be able to read them. For example, in normal peripheral vision, letter acuity 30 degrees away from the line of sight is poorer than 20/200.

For those who prefer a more technical description, a simple formula describing the decline of acuity in peripheral vision is: $F = 1 + E/3$, where E is the number of degrees away from the line of sight and F is the factor by which acuity letters in central vision must be enlarged. For example, when $E = 30$ degrees, $F = 1 + 30/3 = 11$. For someone with central acuity of 20/20, we would estimate acuity letters at 30 degrees in peripheral vision to be 11 times larger than in central vision resulting in a Snellen ratio of 20/220. Since there is substantial individual variability for acuity in peripheral vision, the formula and example here are only approximate. Detailed formulas and data for the change of size thresholds for characters in peripheral vision, including the effect of contrast reduction, are given in a comprehensive review article by Strasburger et al. (2011).

The decline in acuity in peripheral vision is related to the decreasing density of cone photoreceptors. The highest acuity in the normal human eye is in the foveal region at the center of the macula where the density of cones is at its maximum, about 160,000 cones per square millimeter. The density of cones at 30 degrees in peripheral vision is only about 6,000 per square millimeter (Wells-Gray et al., 2016).

The second important property of the visual field is due to the rod photoreceptors that dominate peripheral vision. The rods are responsible for night vision. They do not convey color information. The lack of color vision in dim illumination when only the rods are active underlies the old expression "At night, all cats are gray."

Together, these two major properties of the visual field motivate the analogy posed in the 19th century by the famous German physician-physicist Hermann von Helmholtz (1821–1894). The visual field is like a painting where most of the paint has been devoted to a small region at the center—with fine details and lots of color. There is progressively less detail and color toward the edges, until there is only a very coarse representation of shape and little color at the outer boundary. This metaphor will help us to understand the differences in vision experienced by people with peripheral visual-field loss and those with central-field loss.

As an aside, Helmholtz is widely considered to be the father figure of vision science. Among many other discoveries, in 1850, at the age of 29, he invented the ophthalmoscope (Ravin, 1999), which allowed visualization of the back of the eye. This was a foundational contribution to ophthalmology and the science of vision.

Each eye has a naturally occurring blind spot, that is, a patch of the visual field without sight. In Figure 4.1, the blind spots are shown by the small black holes near the centers of the visual-field maps for the left and right eyes. Each blind spot corresponds to a gap in the retina, called the optic disc, through which the optic nerve fibers pass out of the eye on their way to the brain. The blind spot is located about 15 degrees away from the line of sight in each eye on the opposite side from your nose. It is elliptical in shape and surprisingly large, about 8 degrees high and 6 degrees wide, roughly equivalent to the angular size of a 3 × 5 inch index card held at a distance of 30 inches. Helmholtz described the size of the natural blind spot graphically as the width of 11 moons side by side. You can easily demonstrate the presence of your blind spots. Place a blank sheet of paper on the table in front of you, and put a fixation dot on it. Cover one eye. Fixate on the dot with your open eye. Use your finger to slide a small coin or button horizontally away from your fixation point in the direction opposite from your nose. When the coin is 4 inches or so from the fixation mark, pull your finger away. The coin may have disappeared into your blind spot. If not, slide it a bit further until it disappears. This should work for both eyes, provided you move the coin in a direction opposite from your nose. Notice that the coin just disappears; nothing seems to be hiding it.

Why don't we routinely notice things disappearing into such a large hole in our visual field? When both eyes are open, the portion of the visual field with a blind spot in one eye usually has sighted coverage from the other eye, so objects don't disappear from view in binocular vision. This is why the binocular field map for normal vision in Figure 4.1 does not show the blind spots. Even if you cover one eye, the blind spot in your open eye is not noticeable. It is thought that the brain "fills in" a perceptual representation based on what is visible surrounding the blind spot. For example, if a grassy area is present in your peripheral vision as you stroll along a sidewalk with one eye closed, the portion of the visual field occupied by your blind spot in the open eye will appear as a grassy texture.

The existence of a blind region in the visual fields of normal eyes was unknown until it was reported in 1668 by the French priest and scientist Edme Mariotte. He realized that the blind spot was associated with the optic disc. Chris Johnson and colleagues in their 2011 article on the history of visual-field testing described how Mariotte enjoyed "beheading" a person optically by closing one of his eyes and arranging fixation so that the person's head would fall in the blind spot of the open eye.

If an area of the visual field without sight, having the size of the natural blind spot, were to be present in your central vision in both eyes, you would have a serious visual impairment. Some people with advanced forms of macular degeneration have blind spots of this size or larger in their central vision. We'll discuss the consequences for their vision in the next chapter.

Vision with one or two eyes

Having two eyes increases the binocular field of view, but are there other benefits of binocular vision? The binocular overlap region means that the two eyes have slightly different views of objects in the overlap field. The different views mean that objects, as seen by the two eyes, appear to lie in slightly different directions. These offsets are referred to as disparity and provide the geometrical basis for stereoscopic depth perception. (The small separation between the two eyes means that stereo vision is less and less effective for judging the depth of objects at greater and greater distances.) It is remarkable that our visual brains can combine the two laterally offset views of the scene from the two eyes into a singular view with the perception of depth. In 1838, Charles Wheatstone (1802–1875), an English scientist and inventor, built a mirror stereoscope that delivered slightly offset pictures of the same scene to the two eyes. People looking into the stereoscope saw depth in the scenes and were amazed. Subsequently, several techniques have been used to simulate stereo depth from separate monocular views of slightly disparate images. Many people may recall having a View-Master as a child, a toy that projected pairs of stereo images to the two eyes providing a sense of depth. In the anaglyph method for simulating stereoscopic depth, separate color filters are placed in front of the two eyes, for instance, a red filter in front of the right eye and a blue filter in front of the left eye. By arranging the colors in an image viewed on a flat display, the color filters transmit spatially offset images to the observer's two eyes yielding a sense of depth.

I need to emphasize that there are many cues to depth other than stereo depth. Artists are trained in using perspective, occlusion, familiar size, and many other cues to convey depth in their paintings. These cues are sometimes referred to as pictorial depth cues and don't require two eyes; you can see the depth from pictorial cues with one eye. I'll have more to say about the usefulness of depth cues for low vision in Chapter 7.

There is also evidence that two eyes can be better than one in performing everyday tasks even when disparity cues are minimal or absent. Rebecca Jones (1981) and David Lee at the University of Edinburgh in Scotland tested 10 normally sighted adults in 10 visual tasks comparing performance with monocular and binocular vision. The tasks ranged from picture perception (such as the time taken to find a camouflaged octopus in a photograph), to postural stability (measurement of body sway while standing in an awkward position), to hand-eye coordination (accuracy for pouring water from one container into another). In all cases, they found faster or more accurate performance with binocular viewing compared with monocular viewing. They concluded that there is an ecological advantage of using two eyes from the concordance or redundancy of information provided by two views of the same scene.

Having two eyes also provides a small benefit in acuity and contrast sensitivity. If you are a person with two healthy eyes and up-to-date refractive correction, you will do a tiny bit better with binocular viewing in tasks requiring high acuity or very good contrast sensitivity compared with monocular viewing. For example, a study by Ying-Zi Xiong (2020) at the University of Minnesota showed that the average binocular acuity of a group of normally sighted subjects was 4.7% better than their best monocular acuity. A 5% difference in the size of acuity letters is much smaller than the size difference between adjacent lines on the Early Treatment Diabetic Retinopathy Study chart (Figure 2.2).

The biggest advantage of having two eyes is having a spare. There are many people who have normal, healthy vision in only one eye. Vision in the other eye may have been compromised due to injury, disease, or a deficit in early visual development. Impairment of vision in one eye due to some form of deprivation early in life is termed *amblyopia*. The most common cause is strabismus. In normal binocular vision, people converge (rotate) their two eyes in order to fixate on visual objects so that images of the same object are formed at the center of both retinas. For instance, in reading, the two eyes will converge on the same word in the text. In strabismus, sometimes called squint, an imbalance in the extraocular muscles means that this proper binocular coordination cannot be achieved. While one of the eyes fixates on the object of interest, the other eye may deviate inward ("esotropia" or "crossed eyed") or outward ("exotropia" or "wall-eyed"). While the fixating eye forms an image of the object of interest in central vision, the deviating eye is looking elsewhere and forms an image of something else in its central vision. The two eyes are looking at different things. There is now a competition in central vision between the two eyes. Diplopia (double images) causes perceptual confusion and annoyance. Figure 4.3 illustrates the confusion that might result if the two eyes have significant misalignment during reading. In this example, the left eye and the right eye are fixated on different words in the text, resulting in a jumble of letters in the region of binocular overlap.

After a prolonged period of misalignment of the two eyes, the brain solves its interocular conflict by suppressing information that enters through the deviating eye. If this suppression persists over a long time in childhood, the acuity and contrast sensitivity in the suppressed eye decline. The condition is termed amblyopia or "lazy eye." If not addressed through surgical correction of the strabismus and/or appropriate eye therapy, the person experiences a permanent reduction of acuity in the amblyopic eye and must rely primarily on vision in their remaining good eye.

Accidents or disease, such as a malignant tumor of the eye, can lead to the surgical removal (enucleation) of an eye. Patients are then often fitted with a prosthetic eye. People who have one eye enucleated or have reduced acuity in

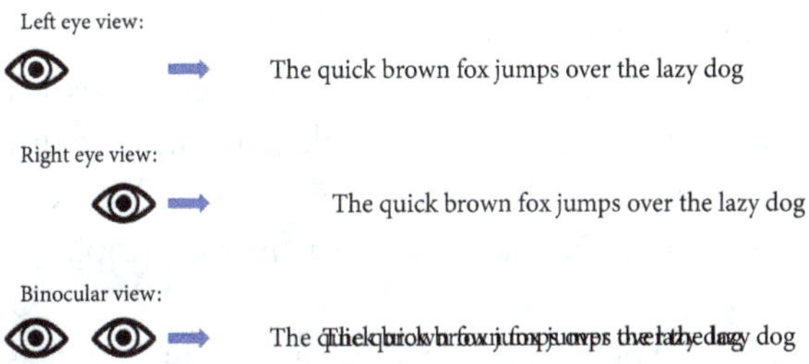

Figure 4.3 Simulation of misalignment of the two eyes in reading. If the left and right eyes are fixating on different words in a line of text, central vision will be confronted with a confusing jumble. The problem may be solved by suppressing the input from one of the eyes.

an eye due to amblyopia are not classified as having low vision. If they retain good vision in one eye, their acuity and contrast sensitivity fall in the normal range. They are usually able to function effectively in everyday life. Jay Adkisson hosts the LostEye[1] website to support and provide advice to people experiencing loss of an eye. He lost an eye to choroidal melanoma, a cancer of the eye; he was back at work at his law practice five days after the enucleation. A short and insightful book by Frank Brady (2004) entitled *A Singular View* describes the experiences of a pilot who lost an eye in a flying accident. Brady acknowledged that loss of an eye can be traumatic but stressed the ability to carry on life's activities with minimal disruption. He described some difficulties he had with depth perception, such as reaching appropriately to shake hands or pour liquid into a glass. He acknowledged a small reduction in the field of view on the side with the lost eye but commented that many two-eyed people willfully inflict even greater field restriction on themselves with the use of wide-rimmed glasses.

Brady listed numerous examples of well-known people who have succeeded in life with just one seeing eye. A famous example is Lord Horatio Nelson (1758–1805), Vice Admiral of the British Navy. He led the fleet to victory in the Battle of Trafalgar against the French and Spanish. He lost vision in his right eye at the age of 36. In the Battle of Copenhagen (1801), Nelson is said to have defied a visual signal from his commander to withdraw by raising a telescope to his blind eye and saying "I really do not see the signal."

Many people with low vision have differences in the vision status of the two eyes. Often, vision is much better in one eye than in the other. In such cases, performance in tests of acuity and contrast sensitivity is dominated by the better eye, even when testing is binocular (both eyes open).

When acuity is low or when one eye has much better vision than the other eye, stereoscopic depth cues are not effective. The well-known neurologist and writer Oliver Sacks bemoaned the loss of stereoscopic depth perception when he lost vision in one eye. He claimed that 3-D depth from stereo is qualitatively different from 3-D information acquired from other depth cues. But, despite the absence of stereopsis, people with one eye or people with a large difference in vision status between the two eyes still have access to depth information through pictorial cues. We'll return to this topic in Chapter 7 on mobility.

I've had personal experience in using one of my eyes as a spare. As I described in the Introduction, the life-threatening disorder that caused my

[1] https://losteye.com/.

low vision occurred when I was six years old. From then on, the vision in my right eye was much better than the vision in my left eye. I relied on my right eye for my everyday visual function. In adulthood, I felt that if any high-risk treatments or surgeries for restoring vision were to emerge, I could gamble with my left eye since I didn't rely on it for my daily functioning. And then, in my early 50s, a new, high-risk treatment did emerge. It involved a limbal stem cell transplant to be followed by a corneal transplant. (The eye's limbus is the boundary between the cornea and the white of the eye [the sclera]. The limbus contains stem cells that are important for replenishing cells in the corneal surface.) I thought to myself: I'm getting older. I have one eye that does not provide me with useful vision. This is my chance to take a high-risk shot at vision restoration. I had an accomplished corneal specialist who would do the surgery. I underwent what turned out to be a series of surgeries. The day after the critical corneal transplant, the bandage was taken off my surgically treated left eye. Would there be a miraculous recovery of vision? Sadly not. The new corneal tissue was cloudy. The miracle of restored vision had not occurred for me. Subsequently, increasing pressure in that eye following the surgery resulted in glaucoma. More surgeries sought to reduce the pressure, but eventually, all vision was lost in that eye due to the glaucoma. How did I feel about this lost opportunity? Of course, dealing with a series of surgeries over five years, with hopes raised and dashed, was difficult. But ultimately, I had understood that the effort was of high risk. And although I entirely lost the vision in my "spare" left eye, I retained functional low vision in my right eye. So, I have no regrets. Like many things in life, we try and aspire. And sometimes, that's all we can do.

Hemianopia

Hemianopia (sometimes spelled hemianopsia) refers to the loss of vision in half of the visual field. The most common form, termed *homonymous hemianopia* (HH), refers to the loss of either the left half of the visual field or the right half of the visual field. (A half of the visual field is known as a "hemifield.") Imagine, for example, fixating on a target such as a light switch or the nose of a friend, and suddenly, all vision to the right (or left) of your line of sight disappears. By some estimates, HH is quite common, with as many as 500,000 to 1 million Americans afflicted (Costela et al., 2018). Most vision impairment results from a problem in the eye itself. In HH, the eye is healthy but vision impairment results from a stroke or tumor that damages the visual areas in one hemisphere of the brain. We usually think of the left hemisphere of the brain as representing function on the right side of the body and the right hemisphere as handling the left side. You might think that the right eye would send its signals to the left hemisphere and the left eye to the right hemisphere. Not so! The neural projections from eye to brain are such that the right visual fields of both eyes are represented in the left hemisphere, and the left visual fields of both eyes are represented in the right hemisphere. This arrangement allows both eyes to project to both hemispheres enabling binocular functioning. Damage to the visual area in one hemisphere may lead to vision loss in the opposite (contralateral) hemifield. In some cases of HH, the dividing line between the blind and seeing half fields passes right through the center of the macula at the fovea. In rare cases, there is macular sparing, that is, the individual with HH retains some portion of their central vision beyond the midline.

Hemianopia is not classified as low vision because acuity is usually in the normal range, and the remaining half field of vision is normal in extent. But, of course, people with HH are impaired in not being able to see obstacles and other objects in their blind half field. They may bump into things or fail to see approaching pedestrians or traffic on their blind side. They may have difficulty in reading, especially with right hemianopia. Think about trying to read this text if all letters and words to the right of your point of fixation were invisible. Therapy to learn new strategies for eye movements and head rotations toward the blind field can be helpful. Useful information is available online at Hemianopsia.net.[2]

Prism glasses are sometimes prescribed for people with HH. Prisms are optical elements that shift the line of sight. If you hold a prism in front of your eye, the scene will appear to shift, with the direction of the shift (left, right, up, or down) depending on the orientation of the prism. Could prisms be used to shift part of the missing blind field into view? It is possible to build prisms into glasses to accomplish a modest horizontal shift of a person's view. But, the shift is equivalent to turning the eyes or head by a corresponding amount and it does not increase the field of view. Eli Peli and colleagues at the Schepens Eye Research Institute in Boston invented a modified prism design, called peripheral prism glasses or "Peli prisms." Instead of shifting the entire field of view, the Peli prisms, built into glasses, shift portions of the upper and lower visual fields into view but leave the central portion unshifted. As a result, the user of Peli prisms has an unshifted view of a scene

[2] http://www.hemianopsia.net/visual-fields-in-brain-injury/.

through the center of their glasses but prismatically shifted information in the upper and lower parts. An object in the blind field may then be shifted into view and noticeable in the upper or lower visual field. If an HH user can adapt to using the Peli prisms, the device can make information in the blind portion of the visual field accessible during normal viewing. Alexandra Bowers (2014) and colleagues, also at the Schepens Eye Research Institute, conducted a clinical trial which showed that the use of peripheral prism glasses was more helpful in obstacle avoidance than the use of sham control glasses.

In the early 1970s, Lawrence Weiskrantz at Oxford University made the remarkable discovery that some subjects with hemianopia retain the capacity to make visual judgments about targets presented to their blind field while having no conscious visual awareness of the targets. In a 1974 article, Weiskrantz and colleagues reported on several tests with hemianopic subject D.B. When asked to guess, D.B. was able to point to large targets presented in his blind field. When asked to guess whether a target in his blind field was an X or an O, he did much better than chance, while denying that he saw anything. Weiskrantz coined the term blindsight to describe the capacity to make better-than-chance visual judgments without conscious awareness. Typically, patients who have suffered damage to the primary visual cortex (V1) in the occipital lobe of one hemisphere of the brain have hemianopia, that is, are blind in the contralateral hemifields of both eyes. For example, D.B. had the primary visual cortex in the right hemisphere removed surgically, resulting in blindness in the left visual fields of both eyes. Nevertheless, some patients like D.B., when asked to guess about stimuli in their blind fields, are able to respond well above chance. Such patients have intact retinas and optic nerves. Weiskrantz proposed that visual information from the retina could bypass the nonfunctional primary visual cortex (area V1) and reach higher areas of the brain mediating the better-than-chance decisions. The implication is that conscious visual awareness requires processing through the primary visual cortex (area V1), but some useful visual information can be processed outside of conscious awareness. There is a growing body of evidence that even normal visual processing in area V1 divides into two streams for further processing—the dorsal and ventral streams—and that conscious perceptual awareness is associated with information processed by the ventral stream. The idea that visual processing can occur in the dorsal stream beyond conscious awareness adds credibility to the concept of blindsight. Nevertheless, the existence of blindsight has remained controversial due to possible artifacts in behavioral testing of patients with hemianopia and the possibility that they may retain some intact V1 processing. Alan Cowey, also at

Oxford University and a student and then colleague of Lawrence Weiskrantz, reviewed and addressed the controversies surrounding blindsight in a 2010 article. While acknowledging the challenges posed by possible experimental artifacts, Cowey concluded that blindsight is a real phenomenon. He raised the important question of whether blindsight might provide functional benefits for people with hemianopia. This question is yet to be answered.

In the late 1990s, there was excitement and hope concerning a new treatment for patients with hemianopia and related visual-field deficits due to lesions in the visual pathway beyond the eyeball. Bernard Sabel and Eric Kasten at the Institute of Medical Psychology, at the Otto von Guericke University in Magdeburg, Germany, introduced a new therapy called Vision Restitution Therapy (also termed Vision Restoration Therapy), VRT for short. The goal of VRT was to restore some visual function in a portion of the blind hemifields of patients near the boundary between their seeing and blind fields. The therapy involved computer-based daily training over six months or more at home. Patients would look at a fixation target on their home computer screen and attempt to see small spots of light flashed in their blind fields. Published results indicated some recovery of vision in the blind fields of many patients following the training. Sabel founded a company called NovaVision to commercialize the software and training program. This was the first vision restoration therapy available for people with hemianopia, and it generated excitement among patients and eye-care clinicians. But, skeptics quickly raised questions about possible artifacts in the method purporting to demonstrate improved vision. Could the apparent restoration of vision be due to eye movements during testing in which stimuli were actually detected by the seeing portion of the visual field? To address this issue, a team led by Susanne Trauzettel-Klosinski, at the University of Tübingen in Germany, conducted a careful study of VRT including accurate monitoring of the eye movements of patients in pre- and post-tests of the visual field. I recall a dramatic conference presentation in 2002 by Trauzettel-Klosinski in which she described the results of the study. She reported that with eye movements monitored and accounted for, there was no significant restoration of vision in the blind fields of the hemianopic patients in their study. The results were subsequently published by Reinhard and colleagues in 2005 in the *British Journal of Ophthalmology*. In an accompanying commentary, Jonathan Horton (2005) from the University of San Francisco wrote "... a proposed therapy has been retested scientifically and found to be ineffective." Subsequently, VRT has remained controversial. It is still possible that the training helps patients to develop strategies for eye scanning even if the treatment has little or no effect on restoring visual function in the blind hemifields.

Measuring the visual field

Acuity and contrast sensitivity can be measured on simple numerical scales, but visual-field loss is more complicated because of the two-dimensional variations in field loss. There are several methods for measuring the health of the visual field, collectively termed *perimetry* methods. The two main categories of visual-field testing are known as *kinetic perimetry* and *static perimetry.* Usually, in visual-field perimetry, one eye is measured at a time with the other eye covered. For a comprehensive and readable introduction to perimetry, have a look at the book by Lyne Racette (2019) and colleagues, freely available online.[3]

Kinetic perimetry is used to establish the boundary of the visual field. In the test, the patient sits facing the center of a curved display surface, either an arc of a circle or a portion of a sphere. "Kinetic" refers to the presentation of a moving target for detection. The patient is asked to look steadily at a fixation marker. In a trial, a target is moved along the curved surface into the person's field of view, starting from the far periphery and moving radially toward the point of fixation. The patient indicates when the target becomes visible by pressing a buzzer. Imagine, for example, a small bright target slowly moving into the person's view from the far left of their peripheral vision toward the point of fixation. This process is repeated several times with the test targets moving into view from different directions. After each trial, a visual-field chart is marked, indicating the field location at which the person first saw the small target, perhaps at 50 degrees to the left or 30 degrees in the upper visual field. The test maps out the boundaries of the person's visual field, determining the extent of peripheral vision in several radial directions around the clockface. For kinetic perimetry to be accurate and reproducible, it needs to use targets of a well-defined size, moving at a specified speed, and with known contrast and background luminance. A larger target will typically result in a larger estimate of the size of the visual field. It makes sense that the effective size of the visual field depends on the salience of the test object; there is a larger field for big, bright targets than for small, dim targets.

[3] https://haag-streit.com/2%20Products/Speciality%20diagnostics/Perimetry/Category%20assets/Books/HS_perimetry_br_xxx_visual_field_digest_8th_en.pdf.

The best-known version of kinetic perimetry is the Goldmann perimeter, invented by the Austrian ophthalmologist Hans Goldmann (1899–1991). During testing, a trained technician manually moves the test target along the desired radial line in the visual field. The technician selects one of the several possible Goldmann targets. For example, the Goldmann III target is 4 mm^2 in area, less than a tenth of the size of an aspirin tablet. If the test with this target indicates that the widest diameter of the patient's visual field in their better eye is less than 20 degrees, the person will meet the statutory definition of legal blindness in the United States, even if acuity is still very good in the remaining central vision.

Kinetic perimetry is helpful in establishing the boundary of the visual field, but what about the vision status within that boundary? Static perimetry can answer this question.

Static perimetry is useful for providing a detailed map of the health of the visual field and is more widely used than kinetic perimetry. Static perimetry is typically conducted using computer-based automated testing. A widely used automated perimeter is the Humphrey Field Analyzer. In this case, instead of detecting moving targets as in kinetic perimetry, the patient is asked to detect small, briefly flashed targets in their visual field. The targets are projected on a curved surface at a distance of about 30 cm from the eye at a fixed grid of locations in the visual field. The number and positioning of the grid points are determined by the selection of one of several software programs. For example, in the 30–2 test, the grid includes 76 test locations in the visual field, covering the central 60 degrees (30 degrees in each direction). The test flashes are presented against a dim background (10 cd/m^2). The flashed targets last about 0.2 seconds and are very small (the same size as the Goldmann III stimuli). If the patient sees the flash, they press a clicker. As the test proceeds, the algorithm reduces the intensity of the test flashes with the goal of estimating the threshold level at each of the 76 test locations, that is, the lowest intensity at which the patient can barely see the test flash at that location. These threshold values can then be compared with average thresholds from a large sample of age-matched normally sighted controls. If the person has field loss from glaucoma or some other disorder in a region of the visual field, the test threshold intensities will be much higher than the thresholds of normal controls.

Figure 4.4 shows field maps for a normally sighted control and a person with field loss due to glaucoma. Box 4.1 explains the basics used in scoring visual-field tests of this kind.

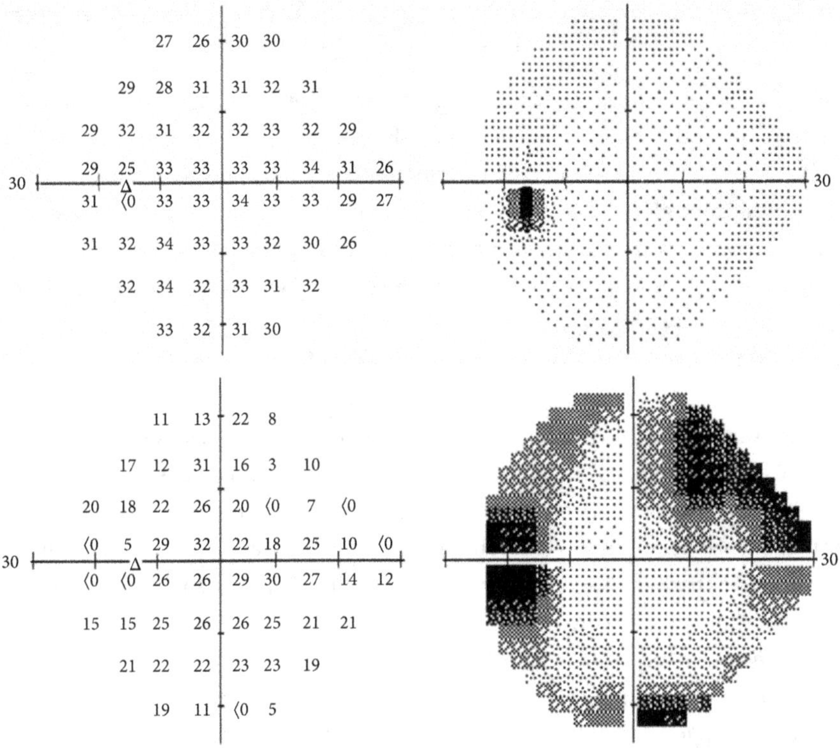

Figure 4.4 Visual-field maps are shown for the left eyes of an age-matched normally sighted control (upper) and a patient with glaucoma (lower). The maps were obtained from a Humphrey Field Analyzer using the 24–2 program which covers the central 48 degrees of the visual field with 54 test points. The horizontal and vertical axes in each panel intersect at the center of the visual field (fovea). The triangle, located about 15 degrees to the left of the fovea, represents the approximate location of the blind spot. Test flashes presented to the blind spot won't be visible if the subject is maintaining good fixation. The numbers in the maps on the left half of each panel refer to threshold light-intensity values at the corresponding field locations, with higher numbers referring to better vision (lower thresholds). Values shown as "<0" mean that the subject could not see the test flash at its highest intensity, representing total blindness at that field location. See Box 4.1 for more details of scoring. The right half of each panel replots the same maps in grayscale, with darker values meaning poorer vision (higher thresholds). The dark region in the map for the normally sighted subject (upper panel) is the location of the naturally occurring blind spot. The glaucoma patient has substantial peripheral field loss, represented by the dark ring surrounding the central region of better vision.

Box 4.1 Explaining test results from the Humphrey Field Analyzer

Figure 4.4 shows test results for the left eyes of a normally sighted control and a glaucoma patient. The numerical values on the left side of each panel represent the threshold light intensities (dimmest light intensities that can be seen reliably) at the corresponding location in the visual field. The numbers describe threshold intensities as a reduction from the brightest intensity produced by the instrument. This means that a larger number means a dimmer light and greater light sensitivity. The reduction is expressed in a logarithmic unit, the decibel (dB), where 1 dB is equal to 0.1 log unit and 10 dB is equal to 1 log unit (a factor of 10). In the field maps in Figure 4.4, a value of 10 means that the threshold light intensity at the point in question is 10 dB (1 log unit), less than the instrument's maximum light intensity. (The maximum light intensity is 10,000 apostilbs, equivalent to 3,184 cd/m^2.) A value of 30 dB means that the threshold light intensity is 3 log units (a factor of 1,000) dimmer than the maximum intensity. The numerical maps in Figure 4.4 plot these dB values. The grayscale plots represent the same data with darker areas representing poorer light sensitivity (smaller dB values).

An overall numerical score representing field loss can be computed for a patient by finding the average difference of a patient's dB scores across the map from normal controls. For instance, in Figure 4.4, the glaucoma patient (lower panel) has a threshold of 11 dB at the top left point in the map. If the normal control value at that location was 30 dB, the difference is −19 dB, that is, the patient has a deficit of 19 dB in light sensitivity compared with the control. We can compute the difference scores for all 54 points in the map and compute an average, called the mean deviation (MD) score. A patient with an MD of −6 dB might be considered as having a mild to moderate visual-field deficit. The value of −6 dB corresponds to a threshold ratio of 4:1, meaning that, on average, the threshold intensity of test flashes is about four times greater for the patient than age-matched controls. The MD value by itself may not be sufficient to give a clinician a clear understanding of the nature of the field loss. For example, the same MD value might result from a uniform loss of sensitivity across the tested field, or it might result from severe loss in a restricted portion of the field with mild or no loss of sensitivity elsewhere in the field. Other statistics are produced as output by the test and are used by clinicians in conjunction with the detailed field map to interpret the data.

What is the correspondence between the definition of legal blindness based on a 20-degree field measured with kinetic perimetry and the output of static perimetry? It has been computed that a score of MD = −22 on the Humphrey 30–2 test is equivalent to a visual field with 20-degree diameter and total blindness outside it. This means that an MD score of −22 on a Humphrey visual-field test would be considered severe vision loss.

The separate visual-field maps for the left and right eyes of an individual can be used to assess the impact of disease on the two eyes separately. It remains a challenge to understand how the patterns of monocular field loss combine in everyday binocular viewing by a person with low vision. If vision in one eye is much better than the other, then it is likely that the pattern of field loss in the better eye will be most important in determining what is seen or not seen. If both eyes contribute substantially to binocular viewing, the patterns of field loss will interact in determining the visibility of objects in the scene. Depending on the convergence of the two eyes on objects nearby or at a distance, different portions of the 3-D scene will fall into blind areas of the two eyes and go unseen. Aries Arditi, in a 1988 article, referred to the joint areas of visual space hidden by field loss in the two eyes as "volume scotomas." The geometry of the volume scotomas depends, in complex ways, on the convergence of the two eyes and the patterns of field loss in the two eyes.

Peripheral field loss

Peripheral field loss is sometimes characterized by the diameter in degrees of the remaining central vision. Recall that the normal monocular visual field has a horizontal extent of about 160 degrees (Figure 4.2).

We saw in Chapter 1 that the International Classification of Diseases (ICD-10) defines field restriction to 60 degrees as "mild" visual impairment and a field of less than 10 degrees as blindness. In the United States, a visual field of less than 20 degrees qualifies as legal blindness even if visual acuity is in the normal range.

How severe are restrictions of the field of view to 60, 20, or 10 degrees? You can get some idea of a 60-degree field of view by sitting at the dinner table and looking at the place setting in front of you—perhaps, a dinner plate with a knife, fork, spoon, and napkin neatly arranged on the left and right. For a fairly typical seating arrangement, the dinner setting will fill about 60 degrees of your visual field. If you are limited to a 60-degree field, the food on your dinner plate and the adjacent cutlery will be visible. Although this field size seems quite ample, you will not see anything further to the left or right without shifting your gaze.

What would it be like to function with a much narrower field of view, just 20 degrees or 10 degrees? Try looking through the cardboard tube at the center of a roll of toilet paper with one eye. I tried this experiment and calculated that the tube limited the field of view to about 24 degrees, close to the boundary for legal blindness in the United States. Try searching the room for your keys through a narrow field like this or finding a friend in a crowd. Try scanning your computer screen for critical links or searching through a complicated government form for the signature line. Imagine trying to catch a ball or follow the movements of a player in a soccer game.

Next, I tried looking through the longer tube at the center of a roll of paper towel. This time, I calculated that the field of view was only about 10 degrees, the boundary for blindness according to ICD-10. If you have good acuity, there will be many objects smaller than 10 degrees that are recognizable if you find them in the restricted field. But, the extremely narrow tunnel of vision makes visual search prohibitively time-consuming and the tracking of moving objects nearly impossible. Try viewing your 12-inch dinner plate with your 10-degree field of view. If you are looking at the plate from a distance of 18 inches, only about 3 inches of the 12-inch plate will be in view, hopefully enough for you to find a tasty tidbit.

To make the above field-size estimates, I measured a cardboard tube from the center of a roll of toilet paper to be 4.06 inches (103 mm) long and 1.73 inches (44 mm) in diameter. From the ratio of diameter to length, I computed the viewing angle to be about 24 degrees. I measured the tube in a roll of paper towel to be 11.1 inches (282 mm) long and 1.85 inches (47 mm) in diameter. It restricted my viewing to a field of view close to 10 degrees.

Backing away to view objects at a greater distance is one strategy to compensate for a very narrow field of view. A young woman with a very narrow field told me that her friends always teased her about why she chose to sit at the back in a movie theater. Was she antisocial? No, she just wanted to see more of the big, silver screen within her narrow field of view. People with very narrow fields often have reduced acuity and contrast sensitivity as well. If so, the strategy of adopting a greater viewing distance to fit a scene within their narrow field of view may be compromised.

Severe field restriction has a major impact on mobility. Think about trying to avoid tripping hazards as you walk with a severely restricted field of view. Unless you tilt your head down to inspect the floor immediately ahead, you will miss seeing items on the floor within the next step or two. I'll have more to say about mobility and peripheral-field loss in Chapter 7 on mobility.

Severe field restriction is neither well-recognized nor understood by the public, and sometimes, it leads to socially awkward situations. For example, a legally blind man with a severely restricted field but good acuity was carrying a white cane to aid in his mobility. He was riding on a subway in New York. Minding his business, he was reading a book with his good central vision. A fellow passenger, seeing the white cane, accused him of being a fraud for pretending to be blind.

Here's another subway story, although not related to tunnel vision. A totally blind friend of mine was seated on a subway train. He was accessing audio on his cellphone using touch gestures and the iPhone's built-in VoiceOver software. He was plugged in with earphones and had the phone's video turned off to save battery life (a distinct advantage in operating the phone nonvisually). A passenger, seated beside him, saw my friend making tactile gestures on a screen with no video. The passenger tapped my friend on the shoulder and said "Hey buddy, sorry, but your phone is broken ... Give it up!"

An important role of peripheral vision is to direct attention to salient events away from the line of sight, such as something moving, a sudden flash of color, or perhaps the appearance of a high-contrast feature. Imagine a bird suddenly emerging from foliage in your peripheral vision. People will often make rapid eye movements (termed saccades) to bring a salient feature noticed in peripheral vision to central vision. But what if you have lost your peripheral vision? You will be unaware of these salient cues that normally attract your attention. Does this mean that people with tunnel vision ignore aspects of visual scenes outside of their narrow field of view? Gang Luo (2008) and colleagues at Harvard Medical School examined the eye-movement patterns of a group of subjects with RP who had narrow visual fields. The authors tracked the eye movements of their subjects while they walked on city streets in Boston. The RP patients made many eye movements to look at details of the scene that were in their blind field prior to moving their eyes. Presumably, these eye movements to unseen locations were guided by cognitive strategies for assessing the environment. It is likely that people with very narrow fields learn to shift their eyes or turn their heads to monitor their surroundings.

Field loss in glaucoma

Glaucoma is a major cause of visual-field loss. In advanced forms, it can result in low vision, legal blindness, and even total blindness. It is the leading cause of legal blindness among African Americans and is three times more prevalent than it is among whites in the United States. A major risk factor for glaucoma is persistent elevated intraocular pressure (IOP). When you have an eye checkup, the eye doctor is likely to measure your pressure with a tonometer. Pressure is calibrated in millimeters of mercury (mmHg) with values greater than 21 considered to be elevated. Pressure in the eye is due to the production of aqueous fluid by the ciliary body which is pumped into the space between the cornea and crystalline lens. The aqueous fluid is maintained under pressure in order to keep the cornea at a proper distance from the crystalline lens. Optical image formation in the eye requires that the eye maintains its shape. Otherwise, the distance relationships between the cornea, crystalline lens, and the retina will not support focused images on the retina. New aqueous is continually being produced by the ciliary body, tending to increase the IOP. To maintain pressure at a desirable steady-state level, aqueous drains out through spongy tissue at the base of the cornea (trabecular meshwork and tubes called Schlemm's canal). Glaucoma may result when the IOP becomes excessively high for a prolonged period. Elevated pressure may occur because of some obstruction to the drainage of aqueous.

Why does elevated pressure within the eye result in visual-field loss? Imagine filling a plastic bag with water to create a firm, convex shape. Now imagine forcing more water into the bag, increasing the pressure inside. As the pressure increases, the walls of the bag begin to stretch. Similarly, pressure in the eye may cause stretching and constriction of the blood vessels nourishing the optic nerve fibers. Depending on the site at which the pressure is most acute, corresponding bundles of nerve fibers may lose function, resulting in visual-field loss. Characteristic patterns of visual-field loss are associated with glaucoma. The distinct patterns depend on which bundles of optic nerve fibers are damaged. One common pattern in advanced glaucoma is the loss of vision throughout the peripheral field as illustrated in Figure 4.4. The individual is left with a narrow central field of vision. Another well-known pattern is the "arcuate" scotoma, in which there is field loss extending from near the blind spot in an arc encircling the macula in the upper visual field.

How do people with peripheral loss from glaucoma see the world? Sometimes peripheral-field loss is pictured as a keyhole view of a scene surrounded by a black or white field, similar to a curtain occluding most of the scene. But, in practice, people with peripheral-field loss don't experience a curtain occluding their peripheral field; in many cases, they don't perceive anything beyond the boundaries of their region of central vision. This is not so surprising when we think about the perceptual experience of people with the normal visual-field maps depicted in Figure 4.1 (left column). As we saw earlier, there is a large region (at least 160 degrees) of no vision outside the boundary of the normal visual field. People with normal vision don't experience this "blind region" as perceptually black or white. Similarly, people with severe peripheral-field loss from eye disease don't experience their lost fields as black or white.

In 2013, David Crabb and colleagues at City University London reported on a study of the perceptual experience of 50 glaucoma subjects with field

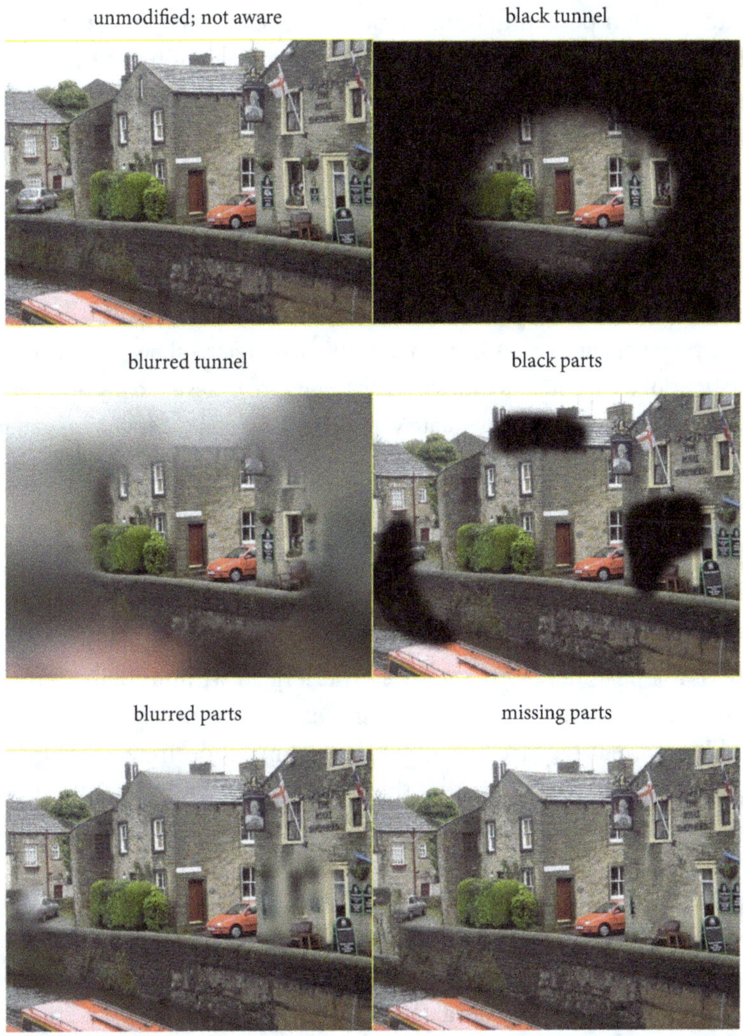

Figure 4.5 An original image and five possible representations of perception of field loss in glaucoma. Reproduced from Crabb et al. (2013). How does glaucoma look?: Patient perception of visual field loss. *Opthalmology*, *120*(6), 1120–1126.

loss but having acuity in the normal range. Each subject viewed six versions of an image of an outdoor scene shown in Figure 4.5.

The original image shows a view of cottages across a waterway. Modified versions of the picture show several possible representations of field loss with glaucoma—images with a black tunnel or a blurry tunnel, images with black or blurry patches, and an image with patchy loss filled in, similar to the natural blind spot. Each subject viewed all six images and chose the one that best matched their perceptual experience. None chose the image with a black tunnel or the image with black patches. This finding confirms that field loss in glaucoma is not perceived as a black region. Twenty-six percent of the subjects chose the original image, indicating that they did not perceive any visual-field defect. Fifty-four percent chose the image with blurry patches, 16% chose the image with missing patches, and 4% chose the tunnel image with blurry edges. The authors concluded that

> The main finding is that patients with visual symptoms do not report seeing black areas in their field of view, as is commonly (but incorrectly) shown in images and simulations of what patients with such conditions are believed to perceive. Moreover, tunnel vision does not adequately describe the visual experience of patients in this study; a combination of perceiving blur and missing areas seems to be the main visual indications of the condition.

Going Blind: Coming Out of the Dark is a 2010 film produced and narrated by Joseph Lovett. In the film, Lovett described his own journey into low vision from glaucoma. He referred to glaucoma as a "thief in the night" because of the peripheral-field loss he experienced without being aware.

When there is a lack of perceptual awareness of peripheral-field loss, people may not know that they are missing large regions of peripheral vision. They may report to their eye doctor that they have started bumping into things or failed to see merging traffic while driving. They recognize that something is wrong with their vision but don't recognize the cause.

Variations in the pattern of field loss may account for a wide range of functional deficits caused by glaucoma. In a 2009 publication, Pradeep Ramulu of Johns Hopkins University reviewed studies of the visual deficits experienced by people with advanced bilateral (both eyes) glaucoma. He found that issues with lighting are very common, especially glare from bright lights and problems adapting to sudden changes in light levels. People with glaucoma, RP, and low vision experience difficulty when emerging from a dark space, such as a movie theater, into bright daylight. Issues with walking were also commonly reported in glaucoma, including problems seeing steps, crossing the road, and bumping into things. I have seen similar problems with participants in my research. An older man with glaucoma kept bumping into the wall on the way to the elevator after completing testing in my lab. We asked him if someone was meeting him or if we could help him get a ride home. "No," he said, "I drove here." I hope he got home safely that day. We'll return to the issue of field loss and driving in Chapter 8.

We typically think of glaucoma as a problem affecting peripheral vision, sparing central vision except in the most advanced cases. But, recent findings indicate that despite normal acuity, people with mild or moderate forms of the disease may experience problems with reading and other functions of central vision. In a 2017 study by MiYoung Kwon and colleagues at the University of Alabama at Birmingham, subjects with glaucoma exhibited deficits in contrast sensitivity, stereo vision, and reading, despite having acuity in the normal range. Adding to the evidence for central-vision involvement, retinal imaging is now revealing central abnormalities in glaucoma as well. Optical coherence tomography (OCT) is a method for imaging the retina. OCT findings have revealed thinning of the retinal-nerve fiber layer supporting macular function in glaucoma, even in eyes with nearly normal perimetry in the central field (Hood et al., 2012).

All or none?

It is often convenient to think about peripheral-field loss as all or none: either you have an intact visual field or you have lost vision outside of a small circular region defining your remaining central vision. But, in reality, there are many intermediate cases. People may have reduced visual sensitivity in peripheral vision without an entire loss of vision. Reduced sensitivity may apply to certain types of visual targets and not others. For example, in glaucoma, loss of sensitivity to blue light or moving stimuli may precede other forms of vision impairment. In glaucoma, diabetic retinopathy, and some other disorders, peripheral-vision loss may be patchy. On the other hand, in RP, islands of vision may be spared in an otherwise extensive region of peripheral-field loss. Can you imagine, for example, having a central island of high-acuity vision and a separate peripheral island of low-acuity vision? How might the presence of the peripheral island influence your visual awareness and experience?

Imagine our earlier simulation of peripheral-field loss—looking at the world through a narrow tube. Your vision is good within the narrow field of view and completely absent outside it. Let's reverse the situation; you have a complete loss of vision in the central portion of your visual field but intact peripheral vision outside it. This is the situation faced by many people with advanced forms of macular degeneration. We'll discuss central-field loss in the next chapter.

5

The Central Field of Vision

Missing in Action

The loss of central vision can result from advanced forms of AMD and several other retinal disorders. AMD is the major cause of vision impairment in the United States. Central-vision loss means reliance on the remaining peripheral vision. In this chapter, we'll consider the implications of central-field loss for measures of visual function including the need for magnification and the impact on daily life. We'll also discuss a remarkable adaptation to loss of central vision: the adoption of a location in peripheral vision used for attending to objects and for controlling eye movements.

• • • • •

What is it like to lose your central vision?

Many years ago, I was a visitor at Cambridge University in England. While there, my wife and I became friends with a retired nurse who was also a musician. I'll call her Molly. Some time later, Molly wrote to me with a description of her initial experience with central-field loss from macular degeneration. Here is an excerpt from her insightful letter:

> You will be sorry to know that I have recently lost a good deal of my "useful" sight from my right eye due to macular degeneration. My left eye has always been a "lazy" eye and is quite useless for reading or crossing the road, so I am hoping that my right eye's degeneration will get no worse. Fortunately, I can still touch-type even if I cannot now read what I have typed.
>
> The first indication was a sudden distortion of the right side of people's faces, with distortion hindering my reading, especially of numbers. I went to the doctor, and he recommended a visit to an eye specialist. There I had drops in my eye (to anaesthetize and to dilate the pupil). The surgeon said then that there was no visible trouble in the retina, and he thought I might have an embolism.

Low Vision. Gordon E. Legge, Oxford University Press.
DOI: 10.1093/9780198946960.003.0006

The next morning, when the drops had worn off, I found my vision much worse. I reported this to his secretary and was seen again (for the same style exam with drops and a high-powered microscope). Alas, the following day my eyes were much worse again. Now I had a large floating object in my eye, as well as a large grey disk and much more obliteration or distortion of everything I looked at, e.g., the upright wooden window frames opposite which now appear to bend and sway out.

The eye surgeon said there had been considerable deterioration in my retina, and that this condition, called macular degeneration, was now strongly in evidence … but he said then it was small and that there was a 60% chance of improvement. But the day after that second exam under drops and high power, my eye was very much worse, and it had deteriorated even more.

So, I was wondering has it only been known since the powerful microscopes came into use in the 1950s and does exam under drops and machine tend to increase the disability in any way? I am 81 years of age, and I have had all those years of sight to be thankful for. I don't expect it to get better as of now. Is there anything to alleviate it, especially anything to counteract the distortion of words and figures, especially the latter?

If I hold a magnifying glass in a plastic frame in my hand, I have so far found that the weight of it (or the kind of grasp on it) gives me pain in the wrist, elbow and shoulder similar to the pain which comes from "repetitive small injury." I did have a severe carpal tunnel syndrome. … I do hope I am not going to incur the same problems from holding hand-held magnifiers. Do you happen to know where I can get a page-sized flat magnifier which I could place on textbooks, and so read a whole page once more as if I had slight disability? It would help me more than anything else.

I hope to do more writing. I had planned to begin this year on a volume. This means extensive reading of both words and figures. I know that there are machines, costing about 1000 pounds, which take a whole page, and these can be read on a screen, in varying sizes of print. I am hoping to find such a machine at the University Library. I have just thought that perhaps there might be flat pieces for a magnifier which stand on short legs, and so can be placed over a book, page by page. Please do comment on magnifiers.

Molly's story is an example of the challenges encountered by someone who has recently lost central vision and is facing the need to adapt to low vision.

We learn from Molly's letter that prior to the onset of macular degeneration, she had good vision in only one eye. Her left eye had reduced acuity from amblyopia (lazy eye). When she first noticed visual distortions using her right eye, she visited her family doctor. She was referred to an eye specialist who did an extensive eye exam and ultimately diagnosed macular degeneration. Molly worried that the eye exam itself might have worsened her condition, but this is unlikely. And, of course, she wondered whether some treatment could alleviate her condition. At the time, no treatments were available for macular degeneration. (Current treatments will be discussed later in this chapter.) Molly began experimenting with optical magnifiers and quickly learned about their ergonomic limitations. She also learned about screen-based electronic magnifiers (closed-circuit TV magnifiers). I admire her determination and fortitude in adapting to her new vision status. Molly's experience with macular degeneration, while unique to her personal goals and circumstances, is similar to that of many people who have acquired central-field loss in later life.

In this chapter, I will describe the special properties of central vision, the characteristics of central-field loss resulting from macular degeneration, and the nature of the resulting low vision. This form of visual impairment is distinctly different from the low vision that accompanies peripheral-field loss discussed in the previous chapter.

Central vision—The macula and fovea

Healthy vision makes use of the wide expanse of the binocular visual field, but most of the action occurs in central vision. Although the precise angular size of central vision is not well-defined, it covers 15–20 degrees of the field of view. Recall the example from the previous chapter of looking through the cardboard tube at the center of a roll of toilet paper, which limits the field of view to a little over 20 degrees. Think of the reverse situation in which the central 20 degrees of vision are missing and you must rely on your peripheral vision. This is the situation for people with advanced forms of central-field loss.

When we look at something—a face, a word in text, or a ball in flight—we shift our gaze so that the corresponding images are seen in central vision in both eyes. Acuity and contrast sensitivity are the highest in central vision, decreasing in all directions into the periphery. Color vision is best in central vision as well.

Central vision corresponds roughly to the central portion of the retina called the macula. Panel A in Figure 5.1 is a photo of a healthy human macula.

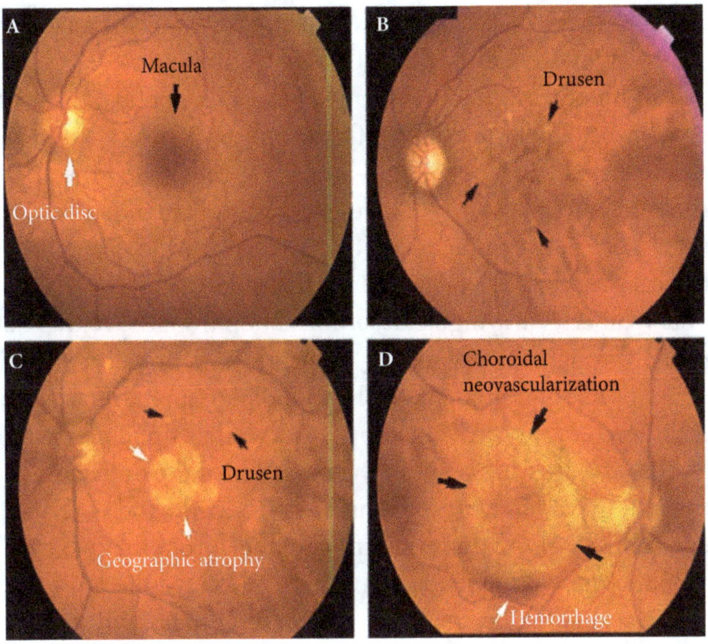

Figure 5.1 Images of the macula: A. Normal eye. B. With drusen. C. Dry AMD with geographic atrophy. D. Wet AMD with choroidal neovascularization. Adapted from Arunkumar et al. (2018). What do we know about the macular pigment in AMD: The past, the present, and the future. *Eye*, *32*, 992–1004.

I'll refer to Panels B, C, and D later in this chapter when I discuss macular degeneration.

The orange color of the macula is due to the blood vessels that provide metabolic support to the retina. The macula is about 5 mm in diameter (one fifth of an inch), corresponding to about 15 degrees of central vision. When viewed with an ophthalmoscope, the macula is yellowish in appearance compared with the rest of the retina. The color is due to pigment deposits from dietary carotenoids from leafy green vegetables and yellow and orange fruits. This pigmentation filters out some of the short-wavelength blue light, possibly reducing the risk of AMD. The term macula comes from the Latin phrase *macula lutea* meaning "yellow spot."

The fovea is a thinner part of the retina which forms a depression at the center of the macula, about 1.5 mm in diameter corresponding to 4 to 5 degrees of the visual field. The fovea is the region of the highest visual acuity. It is the retinal reference point for eye fixations and eye movements in normal vision. This means that when we look at a face or another object, we adjust our gaze so that the image of the object is formed on the macula with the point of primary interest in the fovea. For this reason, reference is often made to "foveal vision." For example, when a person looks at a face, the eyes make a series of foveal fixations near the key features of the face such as the eyes, nose, and mouth. Similarly, when we read a line of text, the eyes move from word to word, making a series of foveal fixations.

Behind the retina is a layer of light-absorbing cells called the retinal pigment epithelium (RPE). The RPE is separated from the blood vessels in the choroid (the layer between the retina and sclera) by Bruch's membrane. For an anatomical overview, see Figure A1 in the Appendix.

Optic nerve fibers, carrying neural information from the retinal network, leave the eye through the optic disc, a gap in the retina corresponding to the naturally occurring blind spot. This bundle of approximately one million fibers in each eye is termed the optic nerve. The optic nerves from the two eyes meet at a crossing point in the brain called the optic chiasm. (*Chiasm* is an anatomical term for crossing or intersection and is related to the Greek letter chi, χ.) At the optic chiasm, the fibers from the two eyes corresponding to the right visual field form a branch (termed the optic tract) that reaches the visual cortex in the left hemisphere of the brain, and the fibers from the left visual field in the two eyes form a branch that reaches the visual cortex in the right hemisphere of the brain. See Figure A2 in the Appendix for a summary of the pathways from the two eyes to the left and right hemispheres.

What is special about central vision?

The region of the brain called the primary visual cortex, also known as area V1, devotes a disproportionate amount of neural processing to foveal and central vision. Half or more of area V1 is devoted to central vision (the central 20 degrees) with the remaining wide expanse of peripheral vision occupying the rest of V1. This unequal allocation of cortical tissue across the visual field is termed *cortical magnification*. The greater allocation of cortical resources to central vision is necessary to handle the greater information flow from high-acuity vision. Unlike camera film or TV displays whose spatial resolution is uniform across the entire sensing surface, the human retina and visual cortex devote higher resolution and vastly more neuronal resources to the central part of the visual field.

For people with healthy vision, conscious attention is almost always directed to the contents of central vision. When somebody asks you what you're looking at, you'll tell them about the image formed in your central vision and not about objects in your peripheral vision. It is possible, however, to divert attention to an object in your peripheral vision. Try fixating steadily on a target ahead and at the same time shift your attention to an object in your peripheral field of view. Can you detach attention from your central vision? When people lose their central vision, they adapt by deploying attention to peripheral vision. We'll discuss more about that later.

Central and peripheral vision both play different roles in visual perception with corresponding differences in their patterns of projection to the brain. Central vision sends most of its information along the ventral pathway, from area V1 to the temporal lobe. This pathway underlies our ability to recognize what things are and is sometimes termed the *what* pathway. Peripheral vision sends most of its information along the dorsal pathway, from area V1 to the parietal lobe. This pathway plays an important role in space perception and is often termed the *where* pathway. The dorsal pathway is also thought to play an important role in visually guided motor behavior such as grasping with the hand and was termed the *how* pathway by Goodale and Milner (1992).

A primary role of central vision is to recognize things—"What is it?"—both the general category of the thing (such as person, bird, tree, or car) and the specific individual or type (such as John, a robin, a maple, or a jeep). Central vision is also used for detailed visual examination, as in reading. On the other hand, peripheral vision plays a greater role in spatial orientation, in environmental awareness, and in attracting attention—where am I and where should I look next? Because of its lower acuity, peripheral vision is less capable of conveying information about what things are and better suited to providing coarse information about the presence of large shapes, movement, or high contrast. Peripheral vision can attract attention to a salient target, resulting in eye movements that bring the salient object into central vision where the thing is recognized.

People with central-field loss must rely on their peripheral vision. How capable is peripheral vision of taking on the "what" functionality of central vision? How effective is peripheral vision in tasks typical of central vision such as reading, face recognition, or object identification? How do people with central-field loss fixate and attend to objects of interest and guide their eye movements? I'll begin addressing these questions in the remainder of this chapter. I'll return to the impact of central-field loss on reading and mobility in later chapters. Understanding the compensatory abilities of peripheral vision has been a major research focus in my lab and is important for understanding the vision abilities of people with central-field loss.

We know that acuity and contrast sensitivity decline progressively in peripheral vision. This means that people with central-field loss will require magnification and high contrast. What else is different about peripheral vision?

Visual crowding is a phenomenon that impairs pattern recognition in peripheral vision. A target, such as a letter, may be easily recognized on its own in peripheral vision (assuming it exceeds the acuity limit), but when it is flanked by nearby letters or other symbols, the target becomes difficult to recognize. An example is shown in Figure 5.2. If the "u" in Panel A is viewed in peripheral vision on its own, it is easy to recognize. But, when the "u" is viewed in peripheral vision flanked by nearby symbols, such as the x's in Panel B, it is difficult to recognize. Even in Panel C with greater separation of the flankers, the "u" is difficult to recognize. In Panel D, the separation of the flanking x's is great enough so that the "u" is no longer "crowded."

In general, a target letter in peripheral vision is much easier to identify when it is presented alone than when it is flanked by other letters. This "crowding" effect represents a difficulty in the ability to distinguish patterns from one another in peripheral vision.

Marialuisa Martelli (2005) and colleagues at New York University showed that crowding also affects face recognition in peripheral vision; faces are hard to recognize unless the facial features such as the eyes, nose, and mouth are far enough to exceed the effects of crowding. These observations show that crowding limits pattern recognition in peripheral vision for targets that are recognized based on their parts such as words or faces.

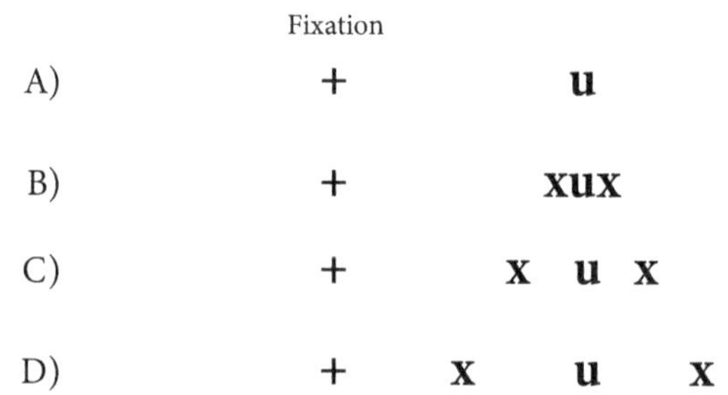

Figure 5.2 Demonstration of visual crowding. In Panel A, fixate on the +, and the isolated "u" in your right visual field is easy to recognize. In Panels B and C, when you fixate on the +, the "u" will be difficult or impossible to recognize because of the crowding effect of the flanking x's. In Panel D, the "u" should once again be easy to recognize because the flankers lie beyond the spatial extent of crowding. The crowding zone around a target refers to the region in which flankers affect the target's recognition.

While we think of crowding as a property of peripheral vision, not present in central vision, it is actually present throughout the visual field. The Dutch vision scientist Herman Bouma, at the Institute for Perception Research in Eindhoven, Netherlands, published results on crowding in 1970, which came to be known as Bouma's Law. He found that the interfering effect of adjacent symbols on letter identification extended over a surprisingly large distance, increasing for targets farther into peripheral vision. According to Bouma's Law, for a target letter (or other symbol) at any location in peripheral vision, the crowding effect influences recognition for other symbols up to half the distance to the fovea. For example, the identification of a target letter viewed at 20 degrees in peripheral vision would be interfered with (crowded) by another character anywhere within 10 degrees of the letter. For a target letter only 5 degrees from the center of the fovea, the crowding zone would extend only 2.5 degrees from the target. In other words, the spatial extent of crowding (the size of the crowding zone) gets smaller for targets closer to foveal fixation.

Denis Pelli (2004) and colleagues proposed an explanation for the crowding phenomenon. According to their explanation, the neural representation of the critical features of a target letter (such as the vertical and horizontal strokes of the letter E) is commingled with the neural representations of the features of the flanking targets if the flankers are within the crowding zone. The commingling or overlapping of the features would produce a jumbled neural representation making recognition of the target letter difficult or impossible. The lack of proper separation of the neural representation of features of the target letter from the flankers in peripheral vision might be related to the reduced allocation of visual cortex for processing peripheral vision. The crowding phenomenon is thought to pose a major impediment to pattern recognition in peripheral vision.

Macular degeneration in youth and old age

The majority of people with low vision have visual-field loss, that is, blind spots (scotomas) somewhere in the visual field. If there is field loss in the macular region, it is said to be *central-field loss* or *central-vision loss*. The most common form of macular disease is *macular degeneration*.

There are several forms of macular degeneration that occur early in life, sometimes collectively termed juvenile macular degeneration (JMD). They include Stargardt disease, Best disease, and X-linked retinoschisis. Stargardt disease is the most common of these. It is an inherited disorder, usually with an autosomal recessive inheritance pattern, related to a mutation in the ABCA4 gene. Visual impairment emerges in childhood or adolescence and may progress into adulthood resulting in acuity reduction to 20/200 or less. In addition to the loss of central vision, people with Stargardt disease may experience sensitivity to bright light and some loss of color vision.

The onset of Stargardt disease early in life and its relatively slow progression may facilitate adaptation to this form of low vision. Children with supportive parents and appropriate special education services often perform well at school, at college, and beyond.

In Chapter 6, I'll discuss the reading difficulties encountered by people with central-field loss. In a study conducted in my laboratory (Legge et al., 1992), we found that participants with JMD (mostly Stargardt disease) read magnified print substantially faster than acuity-matched participants with AMD. It is unclear whether the better reading performance of those with JMD is due to differences in the retinal condition or the greater lifetime experience of people with early onset of macular degeneration.

AMD is the leading cause of low vision in developed countries. In the United States, nearly half of all low vision is due to AMD. The prevalence of AMD rises sharply with increasing age above 65 years and is much higher among white Americans than black Americans.

An early sign of AMD is the appearance of small whitish deposits in the macula called drusen (a German word, with the singular form "druse"), illustrated in Figure 5.1B. Drusen are composed of aggregated debris (fatty proteins) and formed between the choroid and RPE. Small drusen can be seen in healthy eyes, but when they become medium or large in size, they are signs of macular degeneration. According to one scale, "small" is less than 63 microns, "medium" from 63 to 125 microns, and "large" greater than 125 microns. Hundred microns is equal to one tenth of a millimeter.

There are two major forms of AMD—dry and wet (Figures 5.1C and 5.1D)—with the dry form accounting for about 90% of the cases. In dry AMD, the medium or large drusen are associated with damage to the adjacent RPE cells and loss of function in the corresponding retinal photoreceptors (rods and cones). In advanced forms of dry AMD, also called geographic atrophy (GA), there is patchy loss of vision (small scotomas) in the macula. If the patchy loss does not include the fovea, acuity may remain high.

In wet AMD, also termed choroidal neovascularization (CNV), new, unwanted blood vessels form in the choroid. These new vessels (neovascularization) may penetrate through the bounding membrane of the choroid (Bruch's membrane) and infiltrate into the RPE. The vessels may hemorrhage, releasing blood, and cause scarring that damages photoreceptors throughout the macular portion of the retina. The growth of the unwanted blood vessels is promoted by the release of vascular endothelial growth factor (VEGF). This is a protein which is produced by the body, usually helpful in promoting the growth of blood vessels in early development or in restoring blood flow after injury. However, an excess secretion of VEGF in the retina is damaging.

Historically, wet AMD was considered to be more threatening to vision than dry AMD. But, helpful treatment has now been developed for wet AMD. The treatment involves injections into the eye of agents that inhibit the growth of the unwanted blood vessels, termed anti-VEGF drugs. Typically, multiple injections are required over many months. The treatment may slow, halt, or even reverse the decline in acuity typical of untreated wet AMD. Anti-VEGF treatment has become standard for wet AMD, and also has applications in the treatment of other retinal diseases including diabetic retinopathy and retinal vein occlusion. Box 5.1 has more details about anti-VEGF therapy for wet AMD.

Box 5.1 Anti-VEGF treatment for wet AMD

Anti-VEGF drugs injected into the eye to treat wet AMD include Avastin (generic bevacizumab), Lucentis (generic ranibizumab), and Eylea (generic aflibercept).

The development of effective therapy for wet AMD has an interesting history, described by Kim & D'Amore (2012). Since the mid-20th century, ophthalmologists speculated that areas of retinal damage due to diabetic retinopathy and macular degeneration responded to a lack of oxygen by producing an unidentified chemical signal, termed factor X, that promoted the development of unwanted blood vessels (termed neovascularization). Parallel work in cancer research was showing that tumor growth also spawned the growth of new blood vessels. In the 1990s, factor X was identified as a protein generated by cells when they were short of oxygen and named VEGF. Could anti-VEGF drugs be developed to inhibit disease-related neovascularization? Drug companies initiated research on therapies culminating in the development of the anti-VEGF drug Avastin. Following clinical trials, the U.S. FDA approved Avastin for the treatment of colon cancer in 2004. Meanwhile, ophthalmologists began evaluating the efficacy of Avastin and the chemically related drug Lucentis as a treatment for wet AMD.

In 2006, Philip Rosenfeld from the Bascom Palmer Eye Institute at the University of Miami and his colleagues reported on a clinical trial of the efficacy of Lucentis in treating wet AMD. Their study described data from 716 patients with wet AMD at 96 sites in the United States; the patients were divided into three groups—two groups with different dosages of Lucentis and a control group with ineffective "sham" treatment. The patients were treated monthly for two years with injections into the vitreous chamber of the eye. The primary outcome variable was visual acuity, measured with the ETDRS chart. As expected, the control group with sham treatment showed a progressive decline in acuity over the two years, losing an average of two lines of acuity (0.2 logMAR) after one year and three lines of acuity (0.3 logMAR) after two years. The two Lucentis treatment groups showed an average improvement of a little over one line in acuity after one year and remained at this level after two years. Comparing the Lucentis groups and the control group after two years, there was an average change in acuity of four lines, one line better for the treatment groups and three lines decline for the control group. While the Lucentis treatment groups showed only a small improvement in acuity, the most important finding was that the anti-VEGF treatment appeared to slow or halt the progression of acuity loss in wet AMD.

Until recently, there has been no treatment for dry AMD. Research has focused on the hypothesis that AMD is related to an inflammatory response associated with drusen. In 2023, the U.S. Food and Drug Administration (FDA) approved two drugs to treat GA, the advanced form of dry AMD. These drugs, injected into the eye, appear to slow down the rate of growth of patches of retinal degeneration in GA, but improvements in visual functioning are yet to be demonstrated.

There has been research on the benefits of nutritional supplements for slowing the progression of macular degeneration. Evidence from the Age-Related Eye Disease Study (AREDS) conducted by the National Eye Institute has shown that people with dry AMD at an intermediate stage of the disease and who are at high risk for developing advanced-stage AMD can lower the risk by about 25% by taking a specific formulation of antioxidant vitamins. An updated formula, called The AREDS2, includes vitamins C and E, zinc, cupric oxide, lutein, and zeaxanthin and is incorporated into commercially available vitamin pills. For people with no AMD or early AMD, the AREDS2 supplements do not seem to provide any benefit.

Age is the strongest risk factor for macular degeneration, but cigarette smoking is the most preventable risk factor. According to a 2006 report by Khan et al., people who smoked a pack a day for 40 years tripled their risk of AMD. The same study showed that secondhand smoking is also a risk factor for AMD.

There is some evidence that exercise may reduce the risk of AMD. In 2017, a study led by Myra McGuinness from the Center for Eye Research Australia reported on a review of nine studies. The review indicated an association between exercise and a reduced risk of early onset AMD and reduced risk of more advanced AMD. The association may not be causal but may be due to overall lifestyle factors such as a healthy diet.

There is also a genetic predisposition to AMD, with more than 30 genes implicated in AMD. Gene variants on chromosomes 1 and 10 are especially important in elevating the risk for AMD.

Impact of macular degeneration on vision

AMD is often bilateral, affecting both eyes but not necessarily with the same time of onset or progression. Someone with central-field loss in both eyes from advanced AMD will have low vision. What are the visual characteristics of macular degeneration?

Metamorphopsia

In the letter quoted at the beginning of this chapter, Molly wrote about the visual symptoms that first prompted her to visit her doctor, leading to the diagnosis of macular degeneration: "The first indication was a sudden distortion of the right side of people's faces with the distortion hindering my reading, especially of numbers." And then later, "the upright wooden window frames opposite now appear to bend and sway out." Molly was describing an early visual sign of macular degeneration, the appearance of spatial distortions noticeable in central vision called *metamorphopsia.* These distortions may arise from irregularities in the images formed on the retina in the early stages of macular degeneration. Think, for example, of distortions to a printed photo if the page is warped or slightly crumpled.

In 1947, the Swiss ophthalmologist Marc Amsler (1891–1968) described a set of grid patterns composed of lines to test for metamorphopsia. An Amsler grid is shown in Figure 5.3A. The idea was that people at risk for macular degeneration would hang a copy of the Amsler grid on a wall at home. They would frequently (daily or weekly) fixate on the dot at the center of the chart and determine whether the grid retained its regular form. If they noticed any distortions in the grid, possibly as indicated in Figure 5.3B, they were instructed to immediately visit their eye doctor. In the mid-20th century, not much could be done to treat macular degeneration. Subsequently, therapies began to emerge, with the most successful so far being the anti-VEGF

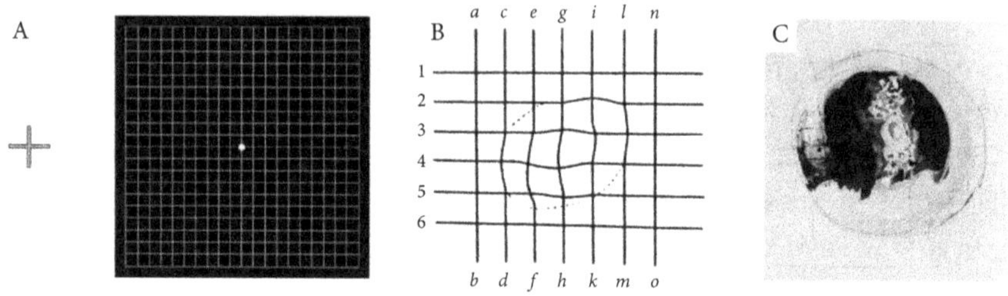

Figure 5.3 Metamorphopsia. A. Picture of an Amsler grid. If a person at risk notices distortion of the pattern of horizontal and vertical lines, it may be a warning sign of macular disease. B. Sample distorted grid pattern depicting a possible form of metamorphopsia in macular disease, prepared by Richard Förster in 1862. C. Drawing by the Norwegian artist Edvard Munch, depicting his own experience with a blind spot and distorted retinal image due to a hemorrhage in the eye. B and C are reproduced from Figures 11 and 9A, respectively, in Marmor (2000). A brief history of macular grids: From Thomas Reid to Edvard Munch and Marc Amsler. *Survey of Ophthalmology*, *44*(4), 343–353.

treatments for wet AMD. With possible treatments at hand, there is good reason to detect macular degeneration early.

In an article published in 2000, Michael Marmor described some of the historical precursors of the Amsler grid. The distorted grid pattern in Figure 5.3B, produced by the German ophthalmologist Richard Förster in 1862, was possibly the first depiction of metamorphopsia in the medical literature. Marmor also described the personal sketches of the Norwegian artist Edvard Munch (1863–1944), famous for his painting "The Scream." Munch suffered a hemorrhage in his eye in his 60s. He drew sketches to represent the progression of his abnormal vision through the affected eye. Figure 5.3C shows an example of his sketch of a macular blind spot superimposed on a hand-drawn grid. Apparently, the effects of the hemorrhage eventually dissipated, so the blind spot was not permanent.

How good is the Amsler grid at detecting metamorphopsia and hence macular degeneration? Analyses by Michael Crossland and Gary Rubin (2007) at the Institute for Ophthalmology in London and by Emily Wiecek (2015a, b) and colleagues at the Schepens Eye Research Institute in Boston have shown that self-reported metamorphopsia and distortions on the Amsler grid are not very sensitive or specific in detecting early macular degeneration. Wiecek and colleagues reported that 70 of 74 participants with several forms of macular disease saw some distortions in a carefully controlled computerized version of the Amsler grid. But, unlike Molly, most of these participants did not report seeing distortions in their daily lives.

If metamorphopsia is demonstrably present in early macular degeneration, why don't people notice distortions of scenes more often? If the problem is present in one eye and not in the other, the abnormality in the eye with the disease may be masked by good vision in the healthy eye. In other cases where small blind spots (scotomas) are present, the perceptual filling in, similar to the filling in at the normal blind spot, may hamper awareness of a gap in a scene. So, while metamorphopsia is commonly present in early macular degeneration, it is not a reliable early warning sign. Nevertheless, for people at risk, checking vision using the Amsler grid at home is still thought to be beneficial.

Reduced acuity and contrast sensitivity

Scotoma size is often represented by the number of degrees of central vision blotted out. For example, a scotoma covering 10 degrees of central vision, if perfectly circular and centered on the fovea, would extend 5 degrees into peripheral vision in all directions. We would expect acuity and contrast sensitivity to be no better than the corresponding values in the normal eye at 5 degrees in peripheral vision. Table 5.1 shows the comparison of acuities in normal peripheral vision and the corresponding acuities of patients with central scotomas of varying sizes. The values for normal, healthy peripheral vision are computed from the formula provided in Chapter 4. The acuities for patients with central-field loss were reported by Eleanor Faye in her 1976 book and referred to central scotomas extending to the indicated retinal location. For example, for patients with a central scotoma extending to 5 degrees, Faye found acuities to be 20/60.

Table 5.1 Acuity in normal peripheral vision and in central-field loss

Distance in peripheral vision (°)	Healthy peripheral vision	Patients with central-field loss (Faye, 1976)	Scotoma coverage
2.5	20/36	20/40	Fovea
5	20/53	20/60	Much of macula
10	20/86	20/100	All of central vision
20	20/150	20/200	Extending into peripheral vision
30	20/220	20/400	Extending farther into peripheral vision

Table 5.1 shows fairly good agreement between the estimated acuities in healthy peripheral vision and the corresponding central-field loss acuities. The patient acuities are slightly poorer. This difference could be due to several factors—clinical vs. laboratory precision of measurements or greater variability in the results for the patients. It may also be the case that the retina outside the boundary of a patient's central scotoma is not as healthy as the corresponding retinal location in normal healthy eyes.

Eleanor Faye (1923–2020), director of Low Vision Services at the Lighthouse in New York City, was one of the first ophthalmologists to devote her practice to low vision. She was a pioneer in raising the profile of low vision in ophthalmology.

It's clear that as scotomas get larger, acuity declines, and there will be a corresponding need for greater magnification.

People with central-field loss from macular degeneration benefit from magnifying devices. Hand-held optical magnifiers or stand magnifiers that sit on a page of text may be effective for people with moderate acuity reduction. E-readers with built-in print-size adjustment are helpful for many people with macular degeneration. Portable electronic magnifiers and desktop closed-circuit television (CCTV) magnifiers have become very popular, especially for people with more severe acuity reduction. As described in Molly's letter at the beginning of this chapter, there can be ergonomic challenges in navigating an optical or electronic magnifier along lines of hard-copy text. Head-mounted displays have been developed as high-tech electronic magnifiers for low vision including macular degeneration. They allow hands-free scanning of text but have not yet achieved wide acceptance for reasons reviewed by Andrew Miller (2023) and colleagues. For computer access, screen magnification software is widely available and is very helpful.

What about contrast sensitivity? Many research studies have shown that contrast sensitivity also declines in normal peripheral vision. This means that there is less tolerance to poor text contrast in peripheral vision than in central vision. Hans Strasburger (2011) and colleagues have documented the interactions between character contrast, size, and location in peripheral vision. Their findings would lead us to expect that for people with central-field loss, there would be a correlation between reduced acuity and reduced contrast sensitivity. A study by Ying-Zi Xiong and colleagues, published in 2020, verified this prediction. They compared acuity measured with the ETDRS chart and contrast sensitivity measured with the Pelli–Robson chart for 232 people with AMD (eyes tested separately for many, bringing the total to 353 eyes). Their analysis showed a correlation between the reduction in acuity and the reduction in contrast sensitivity. For example, on average, a 70-year-old person with AMD and mild acuity reduction to 20/60 would reach the tenth contrast step on the Pelli–Robson chart (Figure 3.3) with a corresponding Pelli–Robson score of 1.34. A person with more advanced AMD and acuity of 20/200 would only read down to the seventh contrast step on the Pelli–Robson chart having a score of 0.9. Recall that adults with healthy, normal vision will typically reach the fourteenth contrast step on the chart. In short, people with AMD typically have reduced contrast sensitivity, meaning that they require better contrast to see things.

Microperimetry and the preferred retinal locus

It is challenging to measure the visual fields of people with central-field loss. The kinetic and static forms of perimetry, discussed in Chapter 4, for measuring peripheral-field loss, rely on steady eye fixation by the patient. If the patient doesn't reliably image the fixation target on the fovea, we lose the correspondence between the visual-field location of the test target and the stimulated location on the retina. For example, if we can assume foveal fixation and if a test target is presented on a display screen five degrees above the fixation target, we have a good idea of the location on the retina stimulated. But, if we are uncertain that the patient is imaging the fixation target on the fovea, we can't be sure where a particular test target lands on the retina.

People with central-field loss cannot see targets imaged on the fovea. When asked to fixate on a target, some people will try to image the target on the fovea despite the lack of vision there. Others consistently image the fixation target on a specific retinal location outside the boundary of the scotoma that retains vision. This location on the retina is termed the *preferred retinal locus* (PRL).

High-tech instruments have been developed for measuring the central visual field and for determining the retinal location of the PRL. These instruments do not rely on foveal fixation. These include the Nidek and MAIA (Macular Analyzer Integrity Assessment) microperimeters.

During a test with one of these instruments, the subject faces a display screen. A camera captures a video image of the retina (using invisible infrared illumination). Computer software analyzes the image in real time and identifies retinal landmarks, so that the device can track eye movements and present stimuli at known locations on the retina in relation to these landmarks. The examiner is provided with a screen image of the patient's retina while the patient attempts to look at a fixation target such as a small circle or a cross. The examiner can see the retinal location of a stimulus in relation to anatomical landmarks such as retinal blood vessels or the optic disc. The instrument can be used to monitor directly where stimuli are placed on the retina, so it has great advantages for field mapping and other applications. The term *microperimetry* refers to measurements of retinal sensitivity at a grid of points covering a limited region of the visual field including the macula. During the test, the patient is asked to respond when they see briefly flashed spots of light. From the patient's perspective, testing is similar to the visual-field testing with the Humphrey Field Analyzer, described in Chapter 4.

Figure 5.4 shows two retinal photographs from a Nidek MP1 used in my lab. The photo on the left is from the eye of a person with a normal, healthy macula, and the photo on the right is from the eye of a person with wet macular degeneration. The colored squares with numbers are light-sensitivity measures (in dB units) from the MP1 microperimetry test; higher values and green colors mean greater light sensitivity. For the eye with macular degeneration, the open red squares within the scotoma region mean that even the brightest perimetry targets could not be seen. The blue dots show the retinal locations of a fixation cross during a test of fixation stability. In the test, the patient is asked to steadily fixate on a small cross on the display screen for 30 seconds. The blue dots indicate the location of the image of the cross on the retina recorded 25 times per second.

For the person with a normal macula (left panel in the figure), the blue dots form a tight cluster at the fovea, meaning that fixation is steady with very little movement of the eyes during the test; foveal fixation is good. For the person

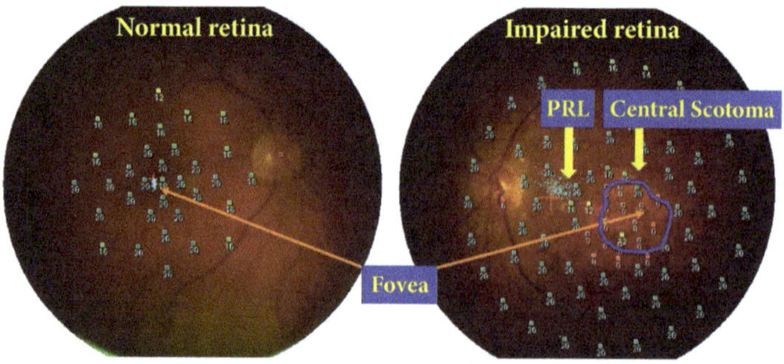

Figure 5.4 Photos of the macula of eyes of two people taken with a Nidek MP1 microperimeter. Left: Normal macula. Right: Macula with wet AMD. The color coding and numbers represent the light sensitivities of tested locations of the macula. The clusters of blue dots represent the retinal location of a fixation target during a test of fixation stability.

with macular degeneration (right panel in the figure), the blue dots cluster outside the scotoma near its left side at the PRL. The scatter of the blue dots for the person with macular degeneration is much greater than for the person with normal vision, meaning that during the fixation test, gaze direction is less stable. Less steady fixation is characteristic of most people with central-field loss. We'll return to the impact of this instability in Chapter 6 when we discuss reading.

Because of the importance of the PRL for people with central-field loss and its potential implications for rehabilitation, researchers have studied the properties of the PRL in detail. Box 5.2 briefly reviews some of the findings.

Box 5.2 Properties of the PRL in macular degeneration

Location

Many people with central-field loss spontaneously adopt a PRL, although they may not be consciously aware of doing so. Donald Fletcher and Ronald Schuchard (1997) reported that in a study of 824 patients with central scotomas, 84% of the tested eyes had a PRL, and of these, 86% of the PRLs were close to the edge of the scotoma. What determines the choice of location on the retina of the PRL? Sing-Hang Cheung and I (2005) reviewed literature on the properties of the PRL. We found that there is a high prevalence for adopting a PRL leftward in the visual field from the central scotoma. We pointed out that this would seem to be maladaptive for reading, since imaging a word in the PRL would mean that text to its right would be obscured by the scotoma. Likely, factors other than facility with reading caused the selection of PRL location.

Acuity

The fovea is the retinal location with the highest acuity in the normal eye. It would be reasonable to think that if foveal vision is lost, people would choose the retinal location with the highest remaining acuity for their PRL. However, research has shown that this is not the case. In a 2018 report, Jean-Baptiste Bernard and Susana Chung, at the University of California, Berkeley, used a scanning-laser ophthalmoscope (SLO) to position acuity targets at several points around the scotoma boundaries of subjects with central-field loss. They found that their subjects did not use the retinal regions with the highest acuity for their PRL.

An SLO is an instrument that uses a laser to "paint" a raster image, similar to a TV image, on the retina. Optics is used so that reflected light from the retina can be used to create an image of the retina on a TV monitor for viewing by the examiner. If the laser uses infrared (IR) light, it is not visible to the patient. But, if the laser uses visible light (usually long-wavelength red light), it can be seen by the patient as a red field of light.

The raster can be modulated to produce test stimuli, such as acuity letters, at known locations on the retina.

"Pseudofovea"

The PRL is sometimes termed a "pseudofovea" because it takes on some of the functionality of the normal fovea. Does the PRL become more fovea-like in its perceptual processing? As we discussed earlier in this chapter and as illustrated in Figure 5.2, the crowding effect is more pronounced in peripheral vision. Crowding would seem to adversely affect target recognition at the PRL. In 2013, Susana Chung showed that the spatial extent of crowding is reduced at the PRL location in the peripheral vision of people with macular degeneration. It seems that with long-term use of a PRL, the visual pathways adapt to reduce the impact of crowding.

Training

Does training on particular visual tasks enhance visual performance with a PRL in macular degeneration? Susana Chung (2011) showed that a form of perceptual training resulted in a 53% improvement in reading speed for magnified print by people with macular degeneration. A subsequent study by Luminita Tarita-Nistor (2014) and colleagues at the Toronto Western Research Institute demonstrated a similar training-related improvement in reading speed and also a small improvement in acuity (equivalent to one line on the ETDRS chart).

Adaptation of eye movements

The adoption of a PRL for fixation outside the fovea is an impressive form of adaptation. Instead of reflexively moving the eyes to try to fixate objects of interest on the unseeing fovea, people with central-field loss move their eyes to fixate targets of interest on their PRL. The PRL becomes a new retinal reference point for eye movements and for attending to objects of interest.

Since the PRL is offset from the anatomical fovea, a person will need to shift their gaze to look at objects of interest such as a friend's face. This can be accomplished by a head turn or by rotating the eyes. In either case, it may seem as if the person with the PRL is looking in a different direction. This can be socially awkward if the friend is unaware of the cause of the unusual gaze behavior. The social awkwardness associated with the use of PRL in casual meetings can be embarrassing if the person with macular degeneration fails to recognize the acquaintance. The acquaintance may wonder, "why doesn't she look at me, and why doesn't she acknowledge knowing me and say hello?"

A judge with central-field loss told me about her strategy for dealing with this problem in addressing witnesses and attorneys in court. She wanted them to feel comfortable. She practiced by having her court clerk stand next to a witness. She learned how far from the witness her clerk needed to be so that when she looked at the clerk with her PRL, it appeared as if she was actually looking at the witness. She was learning to compensate for the offset of her PRL in order to put others at ease.

The size and shape of scotomas are often different in the two eyes, with one eye having better vision than the other. Microperimeters are designed to identify PRL locations monocularly, that is, one eye at a time. Frequently, PRLs in the two eyes are found to be at noncorresponding retinal locations; for instance, to the left of a scotoma in one eye and to the right of a scotoma in the other eye. In a 2023 review article entitled *What Is a Preferred Retinal Locus?* Luminita Tarita-Nistor and colleagues have made a strong case that most everyday viewing is binocular and that PRLs in central-field loss should be viewed as a binocular adaptation. They present evidence indicating that during binocular viewing, the PRL in the better eye often dictates a shift in the PRL of the poorer eye to a corresponding retinal location. In some cases, this might mean that during binocular fixation, the target may actually be imaged within the scotoma in the poorer eye.

In normal vision, eye movements are used to bring targets of interest into the fovea; we say that the fovea is the reference for eye movements. In the presence of central-field loss, the reference for eye movements moves to the PRL, that is, to a location on the retina outside the central scotoma. In a 2021 article, Preeti Verghese and colleagues reviewed current understanding of the time course for adapting eye movements to a PRL. The development of a PRL, as measured with a fixation test by a microperimeter, appears to take several months after the onset of central-field loss. It may take substantially longer, perhaps years, for saccadic eye movements (like those in reading or visual search) to fully adapt. Pursuit eye movements are used to track moving objects such as a person or a vehicle. Verghese et al. reported that visual pursuit may lag behind moving targets in cases of central-field loss. Imagine, for example, trying to track the flight of a ball, a moving car, or a bicycle. You are trying to keep your PRL locked on the moving target, but your eyes are falling behind. Not only is the target harder to see as it gets away from your PRL, but the target might also disappear entirely into your scotoma. People with central-field loss often complain of suddenly losing sight of targets. In short, while adapting eye movements to use a PRL in the presence of central-field loss is a remarkable form of visual adaptation, eye-movement control remains a challenge.

Blind spots and hallucinations—things seen and not seen

Pictorial representations of central-field loss frequently show a picture with a missing area at the center sometimes depicted as a black spot. This is not an accurate representation of the experience of most people with central-field loss. In 2012, Donald Fletcher and colleagues reported on a survey of 153 consecutive AMD patients who visited the low-vision clinic at the California Pacific Medical Center in San Francisco. The patients had their central fields measured. They were asked whether they saw blind spots or defects in their vision and whether they noticed objects disappearing from view. Central scotomas were present in both eyes of 88% of the patients, with absolute scotomas in at least one eye of 66%. Fifty-six percent of the patients with binocular scotomas were completely unaware of their blind spots, with scotoma sizes covering up to 30 degrees of central vision. Of course, these patients knew that they had a vision problem, but it didn't manifest as awareness of a gap or hole in their visual field. Two patients reported fleeting perception of their blind spots; one reported seeing a dark spot on the ceiling when first waking up in the morning. Forty-four percent of the patients with binocular central scotomas reported that things sometimes disappeared, especially letters or numbers when reading. One lady reported that a cockroach disappeared in her vision when she tried to step on it.

It seems surprising that someone with a large blind spot in their central vision wouldn't perceive a large gap in everyday scenes. But, recall the observations in the previous chapter—people with normal vision are not perceptually aware of the blind region behind them or the natural blind spot in their peripheral field; glaucoma patients are also typically not perceptually aware of their peripheral-field loss. It seems that the absence of vision, whether a part of normal visual experience or due to eye disease, is not represented in the brain as a gap or blank portion of the visual field.

While blind spots in the visual field may not be perceived, there are instances in which people with low vision experience visual hallucinations. These hallucinations are fairly common in people with central-field loss, but they can also occur in people with other forms of low vision. The condition of experiencing visual hallucinations, without hallucinations in other sensory systems and without any associated mental disorder, is called Charles Bonnet Syndrome. This condition was first identified by the Swiss naturalist Charles Bonnet in 1760 when he reported the visual hallucinations of his grandfather. A vivid description of Charles Bonnet hallucinations was given in a 2013 *New*

York Times article by Maxine Kumin entitled "*Seeing Things*."[1] Kumin had wet macular degeneration. She first began to notice unusual imagery in her peripheral vision when she was a car passenger: "... trees by the side of the road morphed into towering brick walls suggestive of a maximum-security prison, sometimes intricately patterned with what looked like droplets of colored sugar." Then, later, while reading a story at home, she noticed that "the lines of print were invaded. Bold patterns in vivid colors, striped, polka-dotted, some outlined in black like a Rouault painting, took over." In other instances, she saw the shapes of faceless hooded people, which then faded from view. Kumin's article also contains a vivid description of her experience receiving monthly anti-VEGF injections to treat her wet AMD.

Someone who experiences Charles Bonnet hallucinations for the first time may find them disturbing, fearing that they are symptoms of a psychiatric disorder. But, it is well-established that visual hallucinations can occur in individuals with low vision in the absence of psychiatric or other neurological disorders. The hallucinations are sometimes categorized as simple or complex. The simple hallucinations are described as geometrical shapes or branching patterns. The complex hallucinations may contain people, faces, animals, birds, flowers, or other readily identifiable objects. Usually, the images are not menacing. Having low vision myself, I have experienced simple visual hallucinations. Sometimes after a demanding outdoor run on a bright sunny day, when entering the dimmer interior of my house, I have "seen" colorful spirals or radial patterns shimmering in waves. If I had a poetic turn of mind, I would probably describe them as exotic flower blooms or as a fireworks display.

The cause of Charles Bonnet Syndrome is not well-understood and is not considered to be prognostic of additional vision problems. In a review article published in 2016, Linda Pang reviewed several possible theories for the syndrome. One general idea is that reduced visual input from eye disease may sometimes result in enhanced excitability of neurons along the deprived visual pathway, causing hallucinatory imagery. The phenomenon may be similar to the phantom limbs experienced by some people with amputated limbs.

There is no medical or drug therapy for Charles Bonnet Syndrome. In the case of Maxine Kumin, her hallucinations faded over time. This is true for many others. The bottom line is that this strange syndrome, sometimes accompanying low vision, is not a matter of major concern.

[1] https://www.nytimes.com/2013/02/03/opinion/sunday/seeing-things.html.

Experiencing central-field loss

While we can describe how objective measures of acuity, contrast sensitivity, and the visual field are affected by macular degeneration and other disorders of the macula, it is difficult to accurately simulate the experience of living with central-field loss. Box 5.3 briefly discusses why simulating central-field loss is so challenging.

Box 5.3 Why it's difficult to simulate central-field loss

The most straightforward way to represent central-field loss is to gray out or otherwise obscure the center of a picture such as in Figure 5.5B. Marmor and Marmor (2010) produced more sophisticated pictorial simulations by introducing progressive blur outside of the simulated scotoma to represent declining acuity in peripheral vision. Going a step beyond static pictures, there are cellphone apps that allow users to actively inspect their surroundings using the cellphone camera, producing images on the screen with the central portion of the image modified to simulate vision with macular degeneration.

These techniques convey the major point that valuable information is missing for the person with central-field loss. But, these simulations yield a picture with a big gap in the center. As we saw earlier in this chapter, most people with central scotomas are not perceptually aware of a large gap in their visual fields. Furthermore, in a real setting, a person with a central scotoma that covers a target of interest, such as the two boys in Figure 5.5, can shift their gaze so that the faces of the boys are no longer obscured. Just as in normal vision, people with central scotomas deploy eye movements in inspecting scenes. To more accurately simulate central-field loss, we would need to track the gaze of a person with normal vision and continuously update the images they see with a simulated central scotoma. Several studies have used eye trackers and video displays to create simulations that allow eye movements while blanking out central vision. Most people with central-field loss also develop a PRL outside their scotoma, enhancing the effectiveness of eye movement control and possibly enhancing the perceptual capabilities of peripheral vision in the region of the PRL. In 2013, MiYoung Kwon and colleagues at the University of Southern California conducted a study to see whether normally sighted subjects could be induced to develop a PRL in the presence of a simulated central scotoma. They trained their participants with simulated central scotomas over several hours across several days in tasks requiring visual fixation and visual search. The participants began to rely on a specific region of peripheral vision outside the simulated scotoma for performing these tasks, similar to the development of a PRL in macular degeneration. Their project may have produced the best simulation yet of central-field loss for people with normal vision. But even in this case, the simulation may not take into account the long-term perceptual and eye-movement adaptations experienced by people with naturally occurring central-field loss.

Typical pictures demonstrating central-field loss show a scene with a blurred, grayed-out, or black region in the middle representing the central scotoma. A particularly well-known simulation is found on the National Eye Institute website and reproduced in Figure 5.5.

An original image (Panel A) shows two boys, each holding a ball. The modified image (Panel B) simulating macular degeneration has a large gap at the center with the faces of the boys obscured. But, as we saw earlier in this chapter, most people with central scotomas don't report a large gap in their visual fields. Deanna Taylor (2018) and colleagues at the City University of London interviewed 29 people with dry AMD and asked them to describe the appearance of scenes in their daily lives. The investigators' goal was to obtain first-person descriptions of perceptual experience with AMD. They divided their participants into three groups based on retinal exams—early, intermediate, and severe (GA) forms of dry AMD. They analyzed transcripts of the interviews. They identified 31 language descriptors used by their participants and categorized them into a few major types. The three most-common descriptor categories were: (1) blur; (2) missing parts; and (3) distortions. Here are sample descriptions from participants in the three AMD groups:

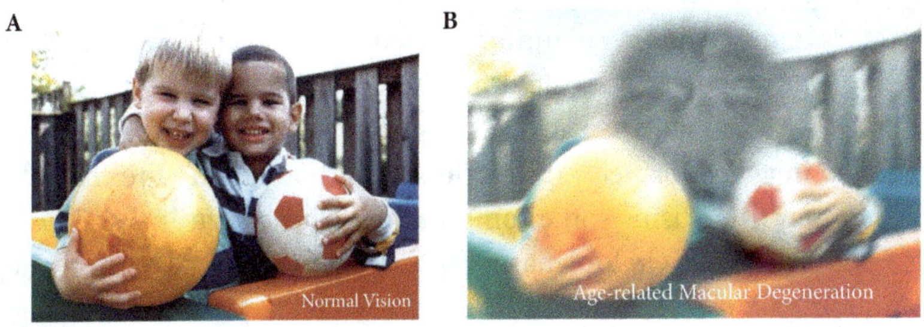

Figure 5.5 A. Original image showing two boys, each holding a ball. B. Image modified to represent central-field loss. The faces of the two boys are obscured. Reproduced from the National Eye Institute website.
https://medialibrary.nei.nih.gov/search?keywords=&category=Eye%20Disease%20Simulations

- Early AMD: "*I don't draw my curtains so I look outside, and I can see on the house opposite, **I see two chimneys instead of one**.*"
- Intermediate AMD: "*Well it's things like when I was standing on the station today, when you're looking at a long platform, it **can look (like) a wavy line**.*"
- Severe AMD: "*It's like if I'm looking at a scene, something on television or even out in the road, it's—there's **part of it missing**. There's **part of it missing** there. I can't see the whole picture anymore.*"

The frequent reference to blur and missing parts in the Taylor et al. study is reminiscent of the account given to me by a lady who described her first awareness of her macular degeneration. Here is my paraphrasing of her description: "My apartment overlooks the parking lot. I looked out to see where our car was parked. But, when I looked at each car, it was a blur, and I couldn't tell which one was ours." Taylor and colleagues also showed their participants the picture of the two boys (Figure 5.5), both the original image and the version modified to simulate central-vision loss. They asked in a neutral way how similar was the modified image compared with their vision. Only two of the participants agreed that the modified picture was a good representation of their visual experience. Apparently, most of the people in this study, all with dry AMD, did not perceive a sizable gap in their visual fields. The authors acknowledged, however, that the picture with the large gap in the center might be representative of the visual experience of people with more extensive central-field loss.

People with central-field loss often mention being frustrated in recognizing friends and family. Loss of central vision means that face recognition must rely on peripheral vision which has reduced acuity and contrast sensitivity. In Chapters 2 and 3, I pointed out that reduced acuity and contrast sensitivity have an adverse impact on face recognition, so we would also expect that these factors hamper face recognition for people with central-field loss. Two additional factors may add to the difficulty. First, as I mentioned earlier in this chapter, a person with central-field loss must alter their gaze direction so that the face image is formed on functioning retina outside the central scotoma. They may do so using some combination of head turn and eye position. A person with central-field loss may feel socially uncomfortable turning their head to look at someone because it appears as if they are not making eye contact. Second, the crowding phenomenon might have an impact on face recognition. All faces have the same basic features—eyes, nose, eyebrows, and mouth. Distinguishing one face from another may use subtle distinctions in the shape and position of these features, as well as overall head shape and hairline.

Evidence discussed earlier in this chapter indicates that crowding of adjacent facial features could hamper face recognition, similar to the crowding of letters in words that may hamper reading. Andrew Logan (2020) and colleagues at Glasgow Caledonian University in Scotland investigated this possibility. They tested 20 subjects with dry AMD, 20 subjects with wet AMD, and a group of 20 age-matched normally sighted controls. They used computer-generated faces as test stimuli. They morphed the faces to produce subtle differences based on either internal face features (position and shapes of the mouth, nose, eyes, and eyebrows) or external features (head shape and hairline). Subjects were shown sets of four faces, three of them the same face and one different, and were asked to indicate the odd face. Not surprisingly, both AMD groups were less sensitive to small changes in both external and internal face features compared with the controls. But the researchers found that both AMD groups were more disadvantaged in identifying the odd face when there were differences in the internal face features compared with differences in external features. The researchers proposed that the greater difficulty with using internal features for face recognition in AMD was due to visual crowding in peripheral vision.

In a 2000 report, Linda Weaver Moore from Xavier University in Cincinnati, Ohio, described a qualitative study of participants with severe visual impairment from macular degeneration. She recorded interviews of eight women who ranged in age from 63 to 85 years. All were living at home—four with their husbands, two with family members, and two on their own. Despite acknowledging the difficulties associated with vision impairment, all of the women maintained a positive attitude. Like Molly, quoted at the beginning of this chapter, most of the women expressed appreciation for having good sight for most of their lives. They had all come to terms with the reality of vision impairment. Moore described the humorous analogy used by one of the ladies to characterize the permanent nature of her condition: "When you lose your center vision, it's just like your virginity; once it's gone, it's gone." All of the women regretted the loss of independence, especially driving. They described valued activities that were difficult or no longer possible such as sewing, reading the newspaper or putting on makeup. But, they also described adaptations such as the use of audio books, paratransit, and new cooking strategies. The women worried about social interaction and when or if to tell acquaintances about their impaired vision. Some reported fear of further vision declines or that impaired vision might be a forerunner of mental decline.

We have had many participants with macular degeneration visit my laboratory. Our research focuses on the ability of these patients to read or perform other daily activities using their remaining peripheral vision. We emphasize the value of remaining vision despite the loss of central vision; the cup is at least half full not half empty. Our AMD visitors participate in research out of interest and to contribute to knowledge that may benefit others in the future through improved rehabilitation methods or assistive technology. Some of the AMD participants have come to my classes to speak to my normally sighted students. One energetic retired nun told us about her depression following the onset of vision loss from AMD. She soon realized that several older nuns in her order shared her disability. She became a peer counselor. She felt rejuvenated, and she gained a new sense of purpose by helping other sisters. After participating in our lab research, she said how excited she was to learn about the details of her central scotoma and how she had developed a PRL. She asked for a printout of her field map from our MP1 microperimeter. She took it home to show her friends.

The three major dimensions of low vision

In Chapters 2–5, we've considered the three major ways of describing low vision—reduced acuity, reduced contrast sensitivity, and visual-field loss. We divided the discussion of field loss into peripheral loss (Chapter 4) and central-field loss in the current chapter. Acuity is the best-known measure of low vision. Many people know their acuity as a Snellen fraction, such as 20/100 (6/30) or 20/400 (6/120). Knowledge of acuity can help in guiding the prescription of optical or electronic magnifiers for reading and distance vision. Most people with low vision also know that poor contrast is a major impediment in their daily lives, but few people have had a test of contrast sensitivity. Clinics that specialize in low-vision rehabilitation are increasingly administering the Pelli–Robson or Mars tests to their clients. Rehabilitation strategies focusing on enhancing the contrast of objects in the home—plates on the table, measuring cups on the kitchen counter, furniture in the living room—are of great importance. Visual-field loss is difficult to measure and understand but is of great importance to the majority of people with low vision.

In Part II of this book, I'll discuss the impact of the different forms of low vision on two major activities of daily living—reading and mobility.

PART II

THE IMPACT OF LOW VISION ON DAILY LIFE

6
Reading with Low Vision

Is the Glass Half Empty or Half Full?

Reading difficulty is the primary reason for people to seek help from low-vision clinics. In this chapter, I will discuss how the three major dimensions of low vision help us to understand reading difficulty. Reduced acuity is related to print size and the requirement for magnification. Reduced contrast sensitivity is related to the need for high-contrast text and good lighting. Visual-field loss, especially central-field loss, is related to the number of text characters visible at each glance, a number termed the *visual span.* I will also discuss fonts for low vision and the need for an adequate display size.

• • • • •

Why is print reading important?

Do you remember learning to read? I learned to read twice. The first time was when I was at home for a year at the age of six, recovering from the severe illness that resulted in my low vision. A home teacher came once or twice a week. Because my impaired vision was too low to read regular print, she drew large letters with a black marker on white cardboard. I must have loved learning to read. I remember looking through my parents' daily newspaper to find the headlines, holding the paper close to my face so I could read the big print.

A year later, at the age of seven, I was enrolled in a school for the blind. I learned to read for the second time, this time with my fingers. I learned to read Braille. The first-grade teacher showed me flashcards with raised dot patterns to feel, first letters and then words. Soon, I was reading sentences and then children's books in Braille.

Throughout my life, I've been both a print reader of highly magnified print and a Braille reader. I rely on Braille for my lecture notes in class. I consult my notes by touch while maintaining eye contact with the students. I rely

Low Vision. Gordon E. Legge, Oxford University Press. © Oxford University Press (2026).
DOI: 10.1093/9780198946960.003.0007

on print reading for technical material such as math equations and graphics. I also use audio for reading—screen reader software on my computer and audio books.

A few years ago, while I was waiting for a doctor's appointment, I was reading a braille magazine. A neighbor who happened to be in the waiting room tapped me on the shoulder. "Isn't it amazing how you can read that with your fingers? It's incredible!" We chatted briefly. I acknowledged my Braille-reading skill and then remarked that it is equally amazing how the eyes can interpret tiny black patterns on a page as meaningful language. Reading, whether by the eyes or fingers, is an astounding human capacity and of enormous value in our culture.

Print reading is a challenge for almost everyone with low vision. For this reason, low vision is sometimes defined as difficulty reading newspaper text at a typical viewing distance of 40 cm (16 inches). While a definition of low vision based on reading hard-copy newspapers is becoming dated, the basic point remains; print accessibility is a challenge for almost everyone with low vision.

Traditional hard-copy reading has not been inclusive of people who are blind or have low vision. Since Gutenberg's invention of the printing press in the 15th century, people with low vision have been disadvantaged in text communication—with major impact on education, employment, recreation, and activities of daily life. In 1962, Marshall McLuhan, in his famous essay *The Gutenberg Galaxy*, referred to the invention of movable type as bringing about the "tyranny of the visual."

After Gutenberg's invention, the availability of hard-copy printed materials expanded and literacy increased. Success in society became dependent on the ability to read, requiring good visual acuity. The "tyranny of the visual" persisted for centuries and has excluded many people with impaired vision from the literate mainstream.

Happily, in the words of Bob Dylan, "the times they are a-changin." The accelerating transition to the use of digital documents brings about new opportunities for people with visual impairment. Digital documents on computers and mobile devices permit customization of print size, spacing, font style, color of both text and background, and page layout to optimize reading displays for people with low vision. In many cases, digital text can also be rendered in audio or Braille formats.

I have faced the challenge of text accessibility throughout my life. I currently rely on three sensory channels for reading—vision of highly magnified text on my computer screen or closed-circuit television (CCTV) magnifier (Figure 6.1), listening to computer-generated text-to-speech or audio books,

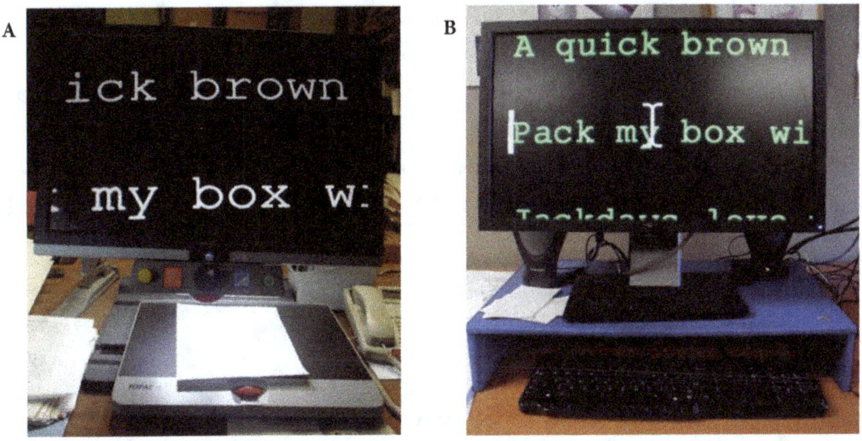

Figure 6.1 A. Magnified text on a closed-circuit TV (CCTV) magnifier. B. Magnified text on a computer screen using the screen-magnification software ZoomText.

and tactile input from Braille. I am writing and editing this chapter with the help of the screen reader program JAWS (Job Access With Speech) that reads my text aloud. I am also looking at very large print on my computer screen. The widening availability of digital text has vastly increased text accessibility for me and many others with low vision.

Results of an online survey of digital reading by people with low vision, led by Yueh-Hsun (Walter) Wu (2020) in my laboratory, showed that vision is the primary mode of access to text. Seventy-five percent of our survey participants did more than half of their reading visually, while some also made use of listening and Braille. Even many people with moderate-to-severe acuity reduction consider vision to be their primary method for accessing text. With high magnification, some people with acuities as low as 20/2000 can read. It is important to recognize that low vision, even very low vision, is compatible with useful visual reading, provided that adequate magnification is feasible. In our survey, we also found that people with low vision rely more heavily on digital reading than hard-copy reading for work, education, news, pleasure, and spot reading (short items such as recipes and medical labels).

In my professional life as a professor with a research interest in low vision, I've frequently been consulted by people struggling with reading. Older faculty colleagues have sometimes approached me for advice about accessing text. They have age-related macular degeneration (AMD) or some other age-related form of vision impairment that threatens their reading. They are anxious and discouraged. Since reading is pivotal to life as a professor, the loss of access to text seems catastrophic. I usually give them my "glass half full, glass half empty" talk. Yes, reading is going to be more challenging with low vision. But, there are several options for addressing this challenge. I tell them about devices that offer optical or electronic magnification for reading and the possibility of audio access to books, smartphones, and computers. I refer them to suitable resources. In other words, the glass is at least half-full! Reading can remain a key part of both their professional and personal lives.

Print size and magnification

Before beginning this section, you may want to have a look at Box 6.1. It reviews the important concept of angular print size and defines typical units for measuring both angular and physical print size.

Box 6.1 Print size preliminaries

To understand the impact of print size in normal and low vision, we briefly review two topics—the concept of *angular print size* and the units for measuring both angular print size and physical print size.

The legibility of text depends on the physical size of the printed letters and the reader's viewing distance. Angular print size takes these two factors into account and is well-approximated by the ratio of physical print size to viewing distance. A typical viewing distance for normally sighted readers is 40 cm (16 inches). This distance is sometimes used in calculations of angular print size as a default. Often, the angular print size of a font's lowercase "x" is used to represent the font's angular print size. As we discussed in Chapter 2, visual angles can be expressed in several units including radians, degrees, or minutes of arc. For example, if the x-height on a page is 1.0 cm and the viewing distance is 40 cm, the angular print size in radians is approximately 1/40 = 0.025 radians, which converts to 1.43 degrees or 86 minutes of arc. Recall that there are 57.3 degrees in one radian and 60 minutes of arc in one degree.

Representing print size in terms of visual angles makes sense because angular size determines retinal-image size.

Software programs and type designers represent print size in terms of the physical size of print on the page or screen without taking viewing distance into account. The units of physical print size are often points (1 point equals 1/72 of an inch). The sizes of letters in a given font typically vary in height and width; for instance, capital letters (such as "H" or "L") and letters with ascenders and descenders (such as "b" and "p") have greater vertical extent than other lowercase letters such as "x" or "c." The overall measure of print size in a font is *body size*.

Historically, body size was the physical height of the metal "sorts" that carried the faces of the letters used in printing. Body size is now defined as the distance from the ascender line to the descender line plus a small additional space or gap, which serves to separate ascenders and descenders of adjacent lines. It is an overall measure of the size of print in a font, such as 12-point Times Roman. Most letters in the font, especially the lowercase letters that comprise most narrative text, have a smaller vertical extent. The height of a lowercase "x" is often thought to be more representative of a font's print size than body size when studying reading vision. In Times Roman, the x-height is only 45% of the body size. For example, in 12-point Times Roman, the x-height is only 5.4 points (equal to 0.075 inches or 1.9 mm). Figure 6.2 shows examples of 9-point and 90-point Times Roman print with the corresponding x-heights of 4 points and 40 points.

Acuity letters represent the smallest angular print size that a person can read on an acuity chart. But, imagine trying to read a book when the letters are at your acuity limit and just barely legible. Reading will be effortful and slow. Numerous studies have shown that print size must be substantially larger than acuity letters for fluent reading. The angular print size required for someone to achieve their maximum reading speed is termed their *critical print size* (CPS).

For people with normal vision, studies have shown that the CPS is approximately 0.2 degrees (x-height), which is roughly two-and-a-half times larger than acuity letters. The range of print sizes yielding maximum reading speed for normally sighted readers extends from the CPS value of 0.2 degrees to 2 degrees, a factor of 10. This is the range of print sizes for fluent reading with normal vision. Figure 6.2 shows samples of text in 9-point and 90-point Times Roman. If read from a distance of 40 cm (16 inches), the corresponding x-heights are 0.2 degrees and 2.0 degrees, representing the lower and upper bounds of the fluent range. For print sizes outside of this range (either larger or smaller), reading speed slows down.

Charles Bigelow at the School of Print Media at the Rochester Institute of Technology and I published a review examining the hypothesis that the distribution of print sizes in both contemporary and historical sources of text falls within the fluent range for normally sighted readers (Legge & Bigelow, 2011). We conjectured that type designers and typographers are aware, at least implicitly, of the print-size constraints on reading imposed by the human visual system. We compiled data on print sizes in contemporary hard-copy sources including 360 U.S. newspapers, 200 hardcover novels, and 100 paperback novels. The average print sizes were close to but slightly

This sentence is printed with 9-pt Times Roman and an x-height of approximately 4-pt, while the following large print is 90-pt Times Roman with an x-height of 40-pt.

90-pt Times

x-height 40

Figure 6.2 Illustration of text printed in 9-point Times Roman with an x-height of 4 points (1.4 mm) and 90-point Times Roman with an x-height of 40 points (14 mm).

larger than the 0.2 degree estimate of CPS for a reading distance of 40 cm. Presumably, economic factors and user convenience impose pressures to minimize print size and keep texts compact but with the constraint that the print be larger than the CPS for normally sighted readers. We also gathered historical data on print sizes for books and type foundry specimens from the 16th and 18th centuries. We focused on texts using serifed Roman types because of their continuous use to the present. These historical sources also used print sizes close to but slightly larger than the CPS value of 0.2 degrees. An interesting exception was the production of Protestant bibles in the 16th century with tiny print, much smaller than the CPS of 0.2 degrees. These bibles must have been difficult to read. They may have been produced as inexpensive, portable, and clandestine religious texts during the religious confrontations of the period of the Counter-Reformation in Europe. These small-print bibles from the 16th century pale in miniaturization to the 2003 Guinness Book of World Records for the smallest book. Pawan Sinha at MIT and colleagues printed the New Testament of the King James Bible on a 5-mm square silicon chip. They used very-large-scale integration technology used in the production of microchips. Ten lines of the print would fit in the width of a human hair, and the tiny, inscribed letters would need to be magnified 600 times to be read by the naked human eye.

Many studies have also shown that people with low vision require print to be substantially larger than their individual acuity letters for them to achieve their maximum reading speed. CPS values for low vision can be three or more times larger than their acuity letters and correspond to angular print sizes not available in most everyday text.

The primary method for facilitating low-vision reading is magnification, which refers to increasing the angular print size for the reader.

Because angular print size is determined by the ratio of physical print size to viewing distance, magnification can be accomplished either by enlarging the physical print size or by reducing the viewing distance, or some combination of the two. Print in hard-copy text cannot be changed in physical size without reprinting the text. Most hard-copy text is composed of print whose physical size is too small to read with low vision at a comfortable viewing distance. A few publications are available in large print formats. In 1999, Aries Arditi, then at the Lighthouse Guild in New York, recommended that large print materials should be at least 16 to 18 points. Even when large print is an option, there are practical limitations on the sizes of pages and books. For this reason, large print rarely exceeds 20 points. For people with moderate or severe low vision, 20-point print provides insufficient magnification.

When the print on the page is too small for a reader, the simplest method of magnification is to reduce the viewing distance, that is, bring the text closer to the eyes. Reducing the viewing distance proportionately increases the angular print size. For instance, viewing the newspaper from 20 cm rather than 40 cm (a factor of 2) is equivalent to magnifying the print size by a factor of 2.

Reducing viewing distance requires the reader to focus at the nearer distance. Young people who can focus over a wide range, or people who are myopic (shortsighted), may be able to focus at short viewing distances of 10 or 20 cm. But, most people require a lens to focus on print at very short viewing distances. Lenses used for this purpose are optical magnifiers.

By the way, most older adults with normal vision usually require reading glasses or bifocals to focus on text at a comfortable reading distance of 40 cm (16 inches). This is because after about 50 years of age, people develop presbyopia (the reduced ability to focus). Although reading glasses for presbyopia are not called magnifiers, they do serve the purpose of aiding focus at a desired reading distance.

Optical magnifiers are especially valuable for accessing hard-copy text. They come in three general types—hand-held, spectacle-mounted, or stand magnifiers that rest on the page. There are three challenges associated with the use of optical magnifiers. First, the enlargement of the letters in a portion of a page by a magnifier limits the field of view. Typically, the higher the magnification (the larger the angular size of the letters), the fewer the letters visible in the magnified view. Several studies in my laboratory and elsewhere have examined how reading speed is affected by the number of simultaneously visible letters in a magnifier's field of view, termed the magnifier's *window size*. For text that drifts automatically through the field of view, like the scrolling news headlines in New York's Times Square, maximum reading speed can be achieved with a window of as few as five characters. When a low-vision reader needs to move a magnifier manually through text, a window of at least eight characters is required to achieve maximum reading speed. As magnification increases, it becomes more difficult to meet these window-size requirements.

The second challenge is the motor skill required to move the magnifier across the lines of text. This process is sometimes termed *page navigation* and imposes demands on eye or head movements and manual dexterity (Beckmann & Legge, 1996).

The third challenge is lighting. The higher the magnification, the closer the magnifier needs to be to the page. Placing the magnifier close to the page can block illumination from a lamp or overhead lights. Some optical magnifiers have built-in light bulbs to provide adequate illumination of the text.

Optical magnifiers are effective reading aids for people with mild forms of low vision. For people with acuities worse than about 20/100 (6/30), requiring magnification of 6X or more, optical magnifiers become challenging to use effectively for the three reasons just discussed.

A major step in alleviating the problems associated with high-power optical magnifiers came in the late 1960s with the invention of CCTV magnifiers by Samuel M. Genensky (1969) (1927–2009) and colleagues at the Rand Corporation in California. Sam was inspired by his own lifetime experience with low vision (Genensky, 2001). At birth, drops of silver nitrate solution were put in Sam's eyes as a standard procedure in Massachusetts at the time to protect against the transmission of infection from mother to infant. But, the solution was not adequately diluted and caused burns to his eyes that resulted in permanent severe low vision (acuity of 20/1000). Despite his vision disability, Sam received his bachelor's degree in physics and PhD in applied mathematics from Brown University. He was employed as a mathematician at the Rand Corporation. Throughout his early life, he contrived creative optical solutions for accessing hard-copy print. In the late 1960s, he and his colleagues at Rand built the first prototype CCTV magnifier. An article in *Reader's Digest* in 1971 brought this invention to the public's attention. The article was entitled "Sam Genensky's Marvelous Seeing Machine." I was one of the early adopters, acquiring a CCTV magnifier during my days as a PhD student in the mid-1970s. I continue to use CCTV magnifiers at home and at work to the present day (Figure 6.1A).

On the only occasion when I met Sam Genensky, he gave me a valuable tip. Like me, Sam sometimes used high-power binoculars for distance viewing. Also like me, Sam relied on vision in his better eye. Instead of holding the weight of heavy binoculars up to his two eyes, Sam recommended taking the binoculars apart, yielding two separate monoculars, each easier and lighter to handle for monocular viewing by the better eye.

Figure 6.1A shows the display of text on my CCTV magnifier. The device includes a video camera, pointed downward, imaging a page of text lying on a movable X-Y table. The camera zoom is adjustable, allowing for high magnification, up to 64 times or more (the ratio of character size on the screen to character size on the hard-copy page). The user can view different portions of the page by moving the table left/right or forward/back beneath the camera. I have adjusted the magnification so that the x-height on the screen is 3.3 cm (1.3 inches), about 19 times larger than the characters on the page (Courier 10 point). I view the screen from a distance of 33 cm (13 inches), with the result that the angular character size is almost 6 degrees. I also prefer bright letters on a dark background rather than the conventional dark letters on a white background. Some people with low vision have higher acuity and read better with reversed-contrast text. CCTV magnifiers are designed to include options for reversing contrast.

The original CCTV magnifiers were desktop devices. Subsequently, portable electronic magnifiers have become available. These are handheld devices with a built-in liquid-crystal display (LCD) screen, a range of zoom, and the capability for contrast reversal. The user moves the magnifier across a page containing text. There are now many portable electronic magnifiers on the market. The American Foundation for the Blind maintains a list of CCTVs/video magnifiers.[1]

Another leap forward toward reading accessibility for low vision was the advent of computer software for screen magnification of digital text. Figure 6.1B shows text magnified by the software program ZoomText on my computer display. Like the CCTV magnifiers, screen magnification software is designed with a wide range of zoom and the capacity for contrast reversal. The user can navigate lines of text that don't all fit on the screen by moving the mouse or by taking advantage of the program's auto scrolling capability.

CCTV magnifiers and computers allow zooming of text size so that both reduced viewing distance and physical print size can be adjusted to provide magnification. In a study conducted in my laboratory at the University of Minnesota, led by Christina Granquist (2018), we found that most people with low vision combine print zoom and shorter viewing distance to enhance text visibility on computer screens. On the whole, people rely more on zoom than shorter viewing distance for magnification. Box 6.2 gives a numerical example illustrating the greater reliance on zoom.

Box 6.2 Combining print zoom and viewing distance to magnify print on digital displays

In their 2018 article, Granquist et al. gave an example of how a person with 20/200 acuity might combine print zoom and reduced viewing distance to achieve adequate magnification for reading text on a digital display. Since the person's acuity letters are 10 times larger than the acuity letters of a normally sighted person with 20/20 acuity, we would predict that the angular size of print for comfortable reading should be at least 10 times larger for this person with low vision. Put another way, the ratio of print size to viewing distance should be at least 10 times larger.

Based on the data from their survey of digital reading by people with low vision, Granquist et al. estimated that a typical reader with 20/200 acuity would zoom letter size on the screen to six times the size of normally sighted readers and would reduce

[1] https://www.afb.org/blindness-and-low-vision/using-technology/assistive-technology-products/video-magnifiers.

viewing distance by a factor of 2.8 times (for instance, from 50 cm to about 18 cm). The combined effect of these two operations would be to increase the size to distance ratio by a factor of 16.8. In other words, the combined effect of print zoom and shorter viewing distance is equivalent to magnification of angular print size by 16.8 times. This is a little more than the tenfold difference in acuity. Often, people with low vision seem to require print magnification for reading that exceeds a simple prediction based on acuity.

Granquist et al. also found that low-vision readers usually rely more on print zoom than shorter viewing distance to achieve their required magnification. Why do they bother with changing print size? Why don't they leave the print size unchanged and get very close to the text, that is, adopt a very short viewing distance? In our example, the person could achieve the required size/distance ratio by reducing the viewing distance by a factor of 16.8 compared with the normal viewing distance, for instance from 50 to 3 cm. Disadvantages of this strategy would include ergonomic challenges in getting close to and maintaining such a short viewing distance from screens (especially laptops with hinged screens behind the keyboard). Moreover, most people would not be able to focus on the text at such a short distance. A high-power optical magnifier could, in principle, be used for focusing at very short viewing distances. In practice, however, most people with low vision prefer to use a combination of print zoom and viewing distance to achieve magnification of print on digital displays rather than using strong, optical magnifiers to read small print at a very short viewing distance.

Modern digital technology has given birth to three additional categories of reading aids for low vision—magnifier apps on smartphones and tablets, text-to-speech apps on smartphones and tablets, and head-mounted displays (HMDs). Magnification on smart devices is built-in as a zoom feature, helpful for low-vision reading. There are also third-party apps that facilitate the use of a phone or tablet as an electronic magnifier.

Most smart devices have built-in screen readers that convert digital text to computer speech—VoiceOver on Apple and TalkBack on Android. These screen readers have made smart devices accessible and are widely used by blind and low-vision users. There are also smartphone apps that use optical character recognition software to convert camera shots of hard-copy text to computer speech.

HMDs, used for gaming and other mainstream applications, have been adapted for low-vision magnification and can be used for reading. They have the advantage of allowing hands-free use but typically rely on head scanning to track across lines of text.

Hilde van der Aa from Amsterdam University in the Netherlands and the Lighthouse Guild in New York City led a team that evaluated four

HMDs designed for low vision (van der Aa et al., 2024). The four devices were eSight4, Eyedaptic EYE3, Eyedaptic EYE4, and IrisVision Inspire. The researchers tested 15 subjects with heterogeneous forms of low vision. They compared performance with and without the HMDs on three types of daily activities—reading, visual search, and hand–eye coordination. There were six reading tasks: "Reading a page from a book, scanning a printed recipe to find the amount of flour needed, reading a street sign at 6 meters, identifying a banknote, finding a web address displayed on a tablet computer, and reading a digital thermostat at 1 meter." In separate weekly sessions, subjects were given about 40 minutes of training with each HMD before testing. The subjects were also surveyed on their satisfaction with the HMD devices.

As expected, given the zooming features of the devices, the subjects had improved acuity on the letter chart through the HMDs. Many of the subjects were unable to complete the reading tasks unaided. The HMDs allowed more of them to succeed on completing four of the reading tasks—reading a page of text, a recipe, a street sign, or a banknote. Nevertheless, the authors summarize their findings: "Results suggest that whereas clinical test performance improved with head-mounted displays, real-world daily activity performance remained mostly unchanged or declined from baseline, contributing to overall dissatisfaction with the devices." Some other reports have been more positive about HMD magnifiers. It is also possible that the subjects in the van der Aa study might have performed better and changed their opinions after more extensive use of the devices at home. As I mentioned in Chapter 5, Andrew Miller (2023) and colleagues have reviewed reasons why HMDs have not yet received wide acceptance as low-vision aids. The reasons include high cost, ergonomic challenges, and embarrassing appearance when wearing an HMD in public.

Display size

The CCTV and computer displays shown in Figure 6.1 illustrate a major challenge for reading magnified text on electronic displays. As the print size gets larger, the number of visible characters on a line gets smaller, and the number of visible lines on the screen also gets smaller. One way of approaching this challenge is to use a bigger display. Many people with low vision invest in large computer displays. But, of course, people with low vision may also want to use devices with smaller displays such as laptops, tablets, or cell phones.

My computer display, shown in Figure 6.1B, has about 14 characters per line (including spaces) at my preferred magnification. It's evident from the photo that I can see only a portion of the line of text. I need to use the mouse to scroll horizontally to see the rest of the line of text. This requirement for manual scrolling, sometimes termed page navigation, imposes a burden on reading for me and for others who use magnified computer text.

One way around this line-length problem would be to format the text onto shorter lines that entirely fit on my screen. E-readers or web pages can be designed to reformat magnified text in this way. Because I use high magnification, I would need text to be formatted into lines with only about 14 characters each. This solution raises two new questions: How few characters per line can be tolerated while sustaining good reading speed and how am I going to cope if I want to read on a much smaller display such as my cell phone?

There is an important practical tradeoff between print size and display size. For a display of a given size, the larger the print, the fewer the characters that can be displayed on a line of text. And, for print of a given size, the smaller the display, the fewer the characters that can be displayed at one time. This tradeoff is illustrated in Figure 6.3. The figure illustrates the rendering of text in three print sizes on three displays of different sizes—laptop, tablet, and phone. Panel A shows that text composed of a given number of characters per line (about 10 character spaces per line) can be presented at a larger size (higher magnification) on a laptop than on a tablet or phone. Panel B shows that more text of a given print size can fit on a line using a laptop than using a phone; in the example, there are about 35 characters per line on the laptop but only 10 characters of the same size per line on the phone.

How many character spaces per line are required to maintain good reading performance? In a study conducted in my laboratory led by Nilsu Atilgan and Ying-Zi Xiong (2020), we measured reading speed for a range of print sizes in three display formats—laptop, tablet, and cell phone. The goal was to determine how the joint requirements for print size and display size would affect reading performance. We measured reading speed in words per minute for normally sighted subjects and low-vision subjects. In the experiment, our subjects read one-minute excerpts from Grimms' Fairy Tales for eight print sizes and the three display formats. The number of words read was recorded and scored as reading speed in words per minute.

We discovered that low-vision readers require at least nine characters per line to approach their maximum reading speed and normally sighted readers require at least 13 characters per line. The smaller requirement in low vision may be due to two factors—a smaller visual span for reading (see later in this chapter for more on the visual span) and overall slower reading. This means that for effective reading, a person with low vision would need a display that meets two constraints: the display must accommodate at least nine characters per line and the characters must exceed the reader's CPS. In our study, some of our subjects with lower acuity could not meet the dual

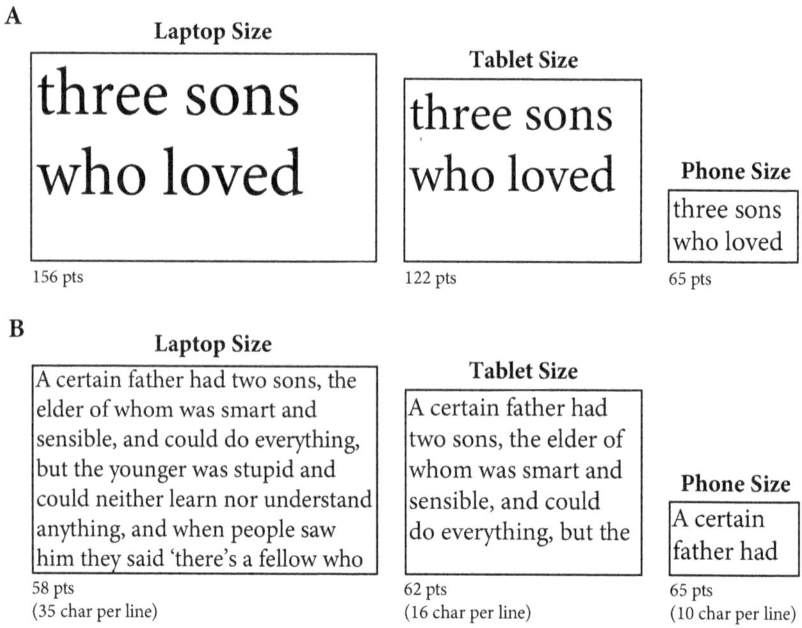

Figure 6.3 Illustration of the trade-off between print size and display size. Panel A shows text with an equal number of character spaces per line for three types of displays—laptop, tablet, and mobile phone. The ten-character spaces per line have much higher magnification on the laptop than on the phone. Panel B shows text with a similar print size on the three displays. In this case, single lines contain many more characters on the laptop (about 35) than on the phone (about 10). In this figure, the sizes of laptop, tablet, and phone have been scaled down to fit the page layout. (Adapted from Atilgan, et al. (2020). Reconciling print-size and display-size constraints on reading. *Proceedings of the National Academy of Sciences*, *117*(48), 30276–30284, Fig. 2.)

constraints for effective reading on the smaller displays (phone and tablet); they could not simultaneously achieve sufficiently large characters and more than nine characters per line.

We created a web-based app in conjunction with this research, intended to allow clinicians, rehab specialists, and/or people with low vision themselves to estimate the display sizes and print sizes they will need for fluent reading. The app is called MyReadingDisplay.[2] The user enters acuity, preferred viewing distance, and preferred font (if any) and the app calculates the minimum display size required to meet the dual constraints of print size and display size.

[2] https://myreadingdisplay.umn.edu/.

Measuring reading performance

If we want to assess the impact of text properties on reading, we need a method for measuring visual reading ability. Recent articles by Gary Rubin (2013) and Wolfgang Radner (2017) have reviewed clinical tests for assessing visual aspects of reading in both normal and low vision. Several of the tests are based on measuring reading speed in words per minute. Miles Tinker at the University of Minnesota introduced reading speed long ago as a measure of reading performance. A review of his many contributions to understanding the effects of typographic variables on normally sighted reading is given in his 1963 book *Legibility of Print.*

Reading speed is straightforward to measure, is sensitive to changes in both the properties of the text and the reader's eye condition, and is functionally significant for readers.

Figure 6.4 illustrates an eye chart for measuring reading speed at different print sizes, called the MNREAD reading acuity chart. It was developed in my laboratory at the University of Minnesota in the early 1990s. Its name derives from the postal code for Minnesota (MN) and from its use in measuring reading. The MNREAD chart incorporates several of the design principles described in Chapter 2 for the ETDRS acuity chart, including the same geometric progression of print sizes (in 0.1 log unit steps corresponding to a reduction of x-height to 80% of the previous line), uniform layout across print sizes, and the use of the logMAR scale for measuring print size. Unlike conventional eye charts, MNREAD is composed of short sentences rather than strings of unrelated letters. All of the sentences are formatted into three lines and have exactly 60 characters (including spaces). The vocabulary and sentence construction were chosen so that the test can be used with children eight years of age and older. The MNREAD chart is printed on two sides and is composed of 19 sentences. At a 40 cm (16 inches) viewing distance, print sizes range from Snellen ratios of 20/400 to 20/6.3. This wide range accommodates most people with both normal and low vision. The 20/6.3 letters are more than three times smaller than 20/20 letters, tinier text than anyone can read. If low-vision testing requires letters larger than 20/400, shorter viewing distances can be used (20 cm or even 10 cm), yielding corresponding increases in angular print size to 20/800 or 20/1600.

In the test, subjects are instructed to read the sentences aloud as quickly and accurately as possible. The examiner records the time taken for each sentence and the number of missed words or words read in error (if any).

These measurements are converted to reading speed in words per minute and plotted as a function of print size. Figure 6.5 shows sample data for one

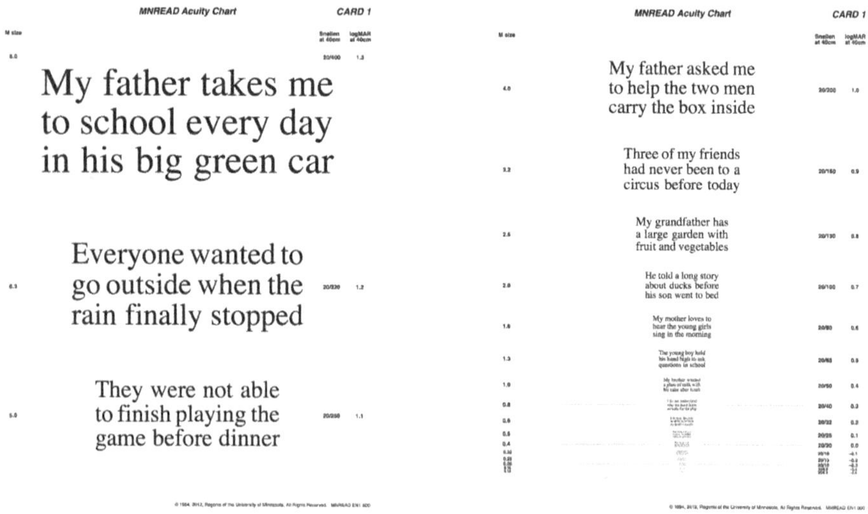
MNREAD Acuity Chart
CARD 1
My father takes me
to school every day
in his big green car
Everyone wanted to
go outside when the
rain finally stopped
They were not able
to finish playing the
game before dinner
MNREAD Acuity Chart
CARD 1
My father asked me
to help the two men
carry the box inside
Three of my friends
had never been to a
circus before today
My grandfather has
a large garden with
fruit and vegetables
He told a long story
about ducks before
his son went to bed
My mother loves to
hear the young girls
sing in the morning

Figure 6.4 The MNREAD chart. It includes 19 test sentences, ranging in print size from 20/6.3 (−0.5 logMAR) to 20/400 (1.3 logMAR), which are printed on two sides of a card measuring 11 by 14 inches.

normally sighted subject and one low-vision subject with AMD. Reading speed in words per minute (wpm) is plotted on the vertical scale. Angular print size is shown on the lower horizontal scale in both Snellen notation and logMAR units. The corresponding font size in points is shown on the upper horizontal scale. Please refer to Box 6.1 for a reminder about the distinction between font size and angular print size. The correspondence between numerical values of angular print size and font size in Figure 6.5 is specific to the reading distance of 40 cm used in the test and to the Times Roman font used on the MNREAD chart. The data points show the reading speeds of the two subjects at the indicated print sizes. The curves have a typical shape. Moving from small to large print, reading speed rises rapidly and then becomes stable at large print sizes.

The plots show three salient features of reading performance. *Reading acuity* is the smallest print size at which the subject can read at all, shown by the open arrows at the left end of each curve. The reading acuity obtained from MNREAD is usually close in value to letter acuity obtained from a chart such as ETDRS. The CPS occurs at the bend in the curve, shown by the filled arrows, and indicates the smallest print size for which the person can achieve their maximum reading speed. As you would expect, the reading acuity and CPS values for the AMD subject are larger than those for the normally sighted subject. The CPS, which is usually substantially larger than acuity letters, can guide magnifier prescription in low vision. In the figure, the CPS for the AMD subject is about 0.8 logMAR, which corresponds to a font size of about 24 points. This person would not be able to read 12-point print comfortably on a computer screen or in a book without the help of magnification. Keziah Latham (2023) from Anglia Ruskin University in the United Kingdom and colleagues have shown that a low-vision reader's selection of their smallest comfortable print size is usually close to the CPS measured by the MNREAD test.

The third salient feature of the plots is *maximum reading speed.* It is shown by the vertical scale value for the flat parts of the curves (dashed lines). In the example shown, the maximum reading speed is about 300 wpm for the normally sighted subject and about 100 wpm for the AMD subject. Often, people with low vision, especially those with AMD, read more slowly than those with normal vision, even when they have sufficient magnification such that the print size exceeds their CPS. This difference in maximum reading speeds means that factors other than print size can have a deleterious effect on low-vision reading. We'll discuss these factors in the section below on *Reading with Central-Field Loss.*

The MNREAD test has three major applications in low vision. First, it can be used in the prescription of magnifiers by indicating the goal print

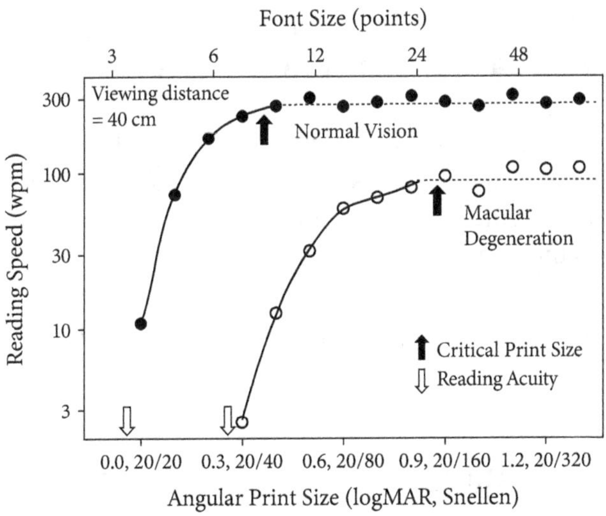

Figure 6.5 Sample MNREAD test data for one normally sighted subject (upper curve) and one subject with age-related macular degeneration (lower curve). Reading speed is shown on the vertical scale. Angular print size is shown on the lower horizontal scale and font size on the upper horizontal scale.

size for reading. Second, knowing an individual's maximum reading speed can be helpful in rehabilitation strategies. In an influential 1993 article by Stephen Whittaker from the Pennsylvania College of Optometry and Jan Lovie-Kitchin from the Queensland University of Technology in Australia, the authors identified three functionally distinct levels of reading speed. They referred to 40 wpm as "spot reading," effective for short but important tasks such as reading price tags, medicine labels, phone numbers, and addresses. This speed would likely be too tedious and effortful for reading long texts such as a novel. They identified 160 wpm as the boundary for "high fluent" reading, effective for lengthy passages. In between, they identified 80 wpm as "fluent reading," effective for short narrative texts such as messages, short articles, or recipes. A low-vision person whose maximum reading speed is 40 wpm would find vision important and useful for spot reading tasks but might prefer audio reading for novels or other lengthy texts.

A third application of MNREAD is in clinical trials of eye treatments or interventions. Researchers may want to know if their treatment improves reading. An assessment of reading before and after treatment can demonstrate whether the treatment results in improvement in reading acuity, CPS, and/or reading speed. It is possible, for example, that the treatment might not improve reading acuity or CPS but might enhance maximum reading speed.

Impact of text variables on low-vision reading

The impact of many text variables on low-vision reading has been studied. I reviewed many of these studies in my 2007 book, and there have been many more studies since. According to an online publication by the American Council of the Blind (2011), the most important text variables are print size, contrast, spacing, and font style. All of these are modifiable by digital devices. We've already talked about print size. Let's take a look at the other variables.

Contrast and lighting

In Chapter 3, I described the importance of contrast for low vision and how contrast sensitivity is measured. Most people with low vision have reduced contrast sensitivity as well as reduced acuity. In the context of reading, contrast refers to the difference in light intensity between letters and their background. Figure 3.2 in Chapter 3 illustrates examples of diminishing contrast of text and also the distinction between two text polarities—regular text with black letters on a white background and contrast-reversed text with white letters on a black background.

For normally sighted subjects, contrast polarity has very little effect on reading speed and only a weak effect on reading acuity. But, some people with low vision read faster and more comfortably with bright letters on a black background. I'm one of them as you've seen with the photos of my reading displays in Figure 6.1.

The advantage of reversed contrast in low vision is sometimes related to abnormal light scatter in the eye, which reduces the contrast of text images on the retina. In advanced cataract, cloudiness of the crystalline lens in the eye can produce abnormal light scatter. The benefit due to reversed-contrast text occurs because a white background with black text produces more light scatter in the eye than a dark page with white print. In my case, the abnormal light scatter comes from my cloudy cornea rather than from my crystalline lens. Some forms of retinal disease are also associated with improved reading with reversed-contrast text. In particular, a substantial proportion of people with retinitis pigmentosa (RP) benefit from reversed-contrast text. The reason for the benefit for RP readers is not yet understood. Most CCTV magnifiers and other electronic displays for low-vision reading include options for reversed contrast. The capacity for contrast reversal is an advantage of electronic magnification over optical magnification for low vision.

Normally sighted readers can tolerate substantial loss of text contrast. In several studies conducted in my laboratory, we showed that normally sighted readers can sustain their maximum reading speed down to a critical contrast of 5%–10% (Legge et al., 1987, 1990). Readers may complain about low-contrast print and it may be fatiguing on the eyes, but at least for short passages, they can maintain fast reading.

People with low vision typically have poorer contrast sensitivity, meaning that they have less tolerance for low-contrast text. For those with a severe loss in contrast sensitivity like me, reading speed decreases with any reduction from maximum text contrast. In 2010, Michael Crossland, at Moorfields Eye Hospital in London, and colleagues reported that the maximum contrasts on the Amazon Kindle and Sony e-Reader were both about 63%. Although these contrast levels are satisfactory for people with normal vision, they would be problematic for some low-vision readers. For this reason, digital devices with the highest contrast displays are especially valuable for individuals with low vision.

Common sense tells us that good lighting is important for reading. The Illuminating Engineering Society of North America (IESNA) recommended about 400 lux illumination for reading by normally sighted readers. This is the level that would typically be found in a well-lit office. Light levels may need to be higher for older people because they tend to have smaller pupils and also more light absorption by the optics of the eye. The average 60-year-old eye may have only about one third of the light reaching the retina compared with the average 20-year-old eye (Weale, 1963).

How bright should lighting be for reading with low vision? Studies of this question have focused primarily on people with macular degeneration. There is consensus that some improvement in reading acuity and CPS can be achieved with moderate enhancement of lighting. For example, in separate studies by Alexandra Bowers (2001), then at Glasgow Caledonian University in Scotland, and William Seiple (2018) at the Lighthouse Guild in New York, a substantial increase in page lighting from typical home levels resulted in a factor of 2 improvement in reading acuity and CPS, that is, the AMD study participants could read smaller print under the higher light levels. The benefits for maximum reading speed under brighter lighting were weaker. The Seiple study found almost no improvement in maximum reading speed due to bright lighting, while the Bowers study found an improvement of about 35% in reading speed from dim home lighting (50 lux illumination) to typical eye-clinic lighting (600 lux). Bowers and colleagues recommended brighter lighting for AMD reading (2,000 lux). A task lamp positioned 8–10 inches from a page on the desk might illuminate the page at 2,000 lux. Brighter light beyond this level would not likely be helpful for reading and might become uncomfortable.

Both the Bowers and Seiple studies were conducted with hard-copy reading. How bright are computer displays relative to the findings of these two studies? When a white page of hard-copy print is illuminated with 2,000 lux illumination, the reflected light reaching the reader's eye has a luminance of approximately 500 cd/m^2. Modern LCD computer monitors and some E-readers, such as iPads, can achieve screen luminance levels close to 500 cd/m^2.

Text on a modern computer display will often be brighter than hard-copy text viewed in typical home or office lighting. Try this simple experiment. View a page of text on your monitor, and then, print it in hard copy. Hold the printed version next to the monitor with typical home or office lighting. You will usually find that the on-screen version is brighter than the hard-copy text. Given that people with AMD and some other forms of low vision may read better with enhanced lighting, digital reading on computers or bright E-readers may often have advantages over hard-copy reading.

Bright ambient lighting can sometimes have adverse effects on digital reading. The contrast of text on a computer display can be washed out by light from windows, direct sunlight, or other bright lights. The brighter the display, the less the contrast will be diluted by these glare sources. I am particularly susceptible to glare. In my campus office, there are bright windows covering the wall near my desk. I use Venetian blinds to control lighting from the windows nearest to my desktop computer to keep down glare.

Bright light is not always desirable for reading. People with photophobia from conditions such as migraine or traumatic brain injury may choose subdued lighting for reading. People with achromatopsia will typically prefer low illumination for reading as well as magnified print.

To briefly summarize, people with low vision usually have a greater requirement for high-contrast text compared with normally sighted readers. Low-vision reading will often benefit from a brighter display and from care in controlling excessive light from external glare sources.

What about the color of the source of illumination for reading? James Wolffsohn (2012) from Aston University in England and colleagues tested the reading performance of a group of 107 people with low vision, most of whom had AMD. The subjects read with optical magnifiers fitted with LED bulbs, matched for illumination level, but varying in color temperature. Color temperature refers to the wavelength spectrum of the light and varied from 6,000 Kelvin (similar to natural daylight) to 2,700 Kelvin, which was redder and "warmer" in appearance. Across the low-vision group as a whole, there were no significant effects of color temperature on reading speed, CPS, or reading acuity. The researchers also asked their subjects for their preferences for the different types of illumination. The researchers found that their subjects had slightly faster reading speeds (9%) for their preferred form of lighting. Given these individual differences, it may be helpful for people with low vision to try different types of light sources for reading.

In my 2007 book on reading with normal and low vision, I reviewed earlier findings on the impact of text and background color on reading. The conclusion, which still stands, is that the luminance contrast of the text is the most important for low-vision reading, whether displayed as bright letters on a dark background or dark letters on a bright background. Color has weaker and more idiosyncratic effects on reading. To reiterate the recommendations from Chapter 3, if color is employed in text, use colors from the middle of the visible spectrum (green or yellow) or white for the bright areas and either black or colors from the ends of the visible spectrum (blue or red) for the dark areas of text.

Fonts and spacing

There have been many recommendations for the most suitable fonts for low vision, and several efforts have been made to design fonts specifically for low vision. Undoubtedly, individuals have preferences, but evidence is lacking for special design features benefiting general low-vision use.

A common belief is that sans serif fonts, such as Arial and Verdana, are more legible than serif fonts for low vision. But, a study by Luminita Tarita-Nistor (2013) and colleagues at the Toronto Western Hospital did not support this belief. They compared AMD reading with four fonts—Times Roman (serif), Arial (sans serif), Courier (serif), and Andale (sans serif). They found that reading acuity was best with Courier, and there were no differences between the four fonts in maximum reading speed.

Another common belief is that bold print is desirable for low vision. But, Susana Chung (2018) and J. B. Bernard at the University of California at Berkeley varied stroke thickness in the Courier font and measured reading performance for a group of subjects with AMD. They found no evidence for improved reading performance for stroke widths bolder than the standard Courier stroke thickness.

APHont and Tiresias are fonts that have been designed exclusively for low-vision readers, but there is no strong evidence showing advantages of these special fonts over mainstream fonts. A review by Russell-Minda et al. (2007) concluded that there is little empirical evidence for an optimally legible font for low vision.

More recently, two fonts have been designed specifically for readers with macular degeneration, Eido and Maxular Rx. Sample sentences in these fonts are shown in Figure 6.6 along with the mainstream fonts Times Roman, Courier, and Helvetica. It is possible that people with central-field loss from macular degeneration might benefit from fonts designed for reading in peripheral vision. For example, the modification of letter spacing or shape might help alleviate the crowding effect we discussed in Chapter 5. Maxular Rx was designed to have extra spacing between letters, to have a large x-height (in relation to overall font size), to be bold, and to eliminate sharp angles. Eido was designed to simplify letter shapes while at the same time emphasizing distinctiveness between letters, both properties designed to reduce crowding.

In a study conducted in my laboratory at the University of Minnesota, led by Ying-Zi Xiong (2018), we measured reading performance across a range of print sizes for groups of subjects with macular degeneration and normal vision. Subjects were tested with the two new fonts—Eido and Maxular

Rx—and also the mainstream fonts Times Roman, Helvetica, and Courier. Our findings showed that Maxular Rx could be read with the smallest print size by both the normally sighted subjects and those with macular degeneration; in other words, reading acuity was best with Maxular Rx. But, for print larger than the CPS, the subjects with macular degeneration read fastest with Times Roman. Overall, there was a tradeoff based on spacing between letters for people with macular degeneration. Fonts with greater spacing (Maxular Rx, Courier) were legible to a smaller print size, but Times Roman with narrower spacing could be read faster when the print exceeded the reader's CPS. The between-letter spacing in a font may be a property that has an impact on low-vision reading. When small print is needed, as in medicine labels, fonts such as Maxular Rx or Courier may be advantageous for low vision. When print size is not a limiting factor, fonts with tighter spacing, such as Times Roman, may be more effective.

What about the spacing between lines? Studies of reading with macular degeneration have shown little or no benefit from extra spacing between lines (Chung et al., 2008; Calabrèse et al., 2010). But, another study showed that combining double-line spacing and double between-word spacing was helpful for subjects with macular degeneration (Blackmore-Wright et al., 2013).

Overall, fonts designed to have wider between-letter spacing may be helpful in reading print near the reader's acuity limit. Extra-wide spacing between lines and words may be helpful for some readers with low vision.

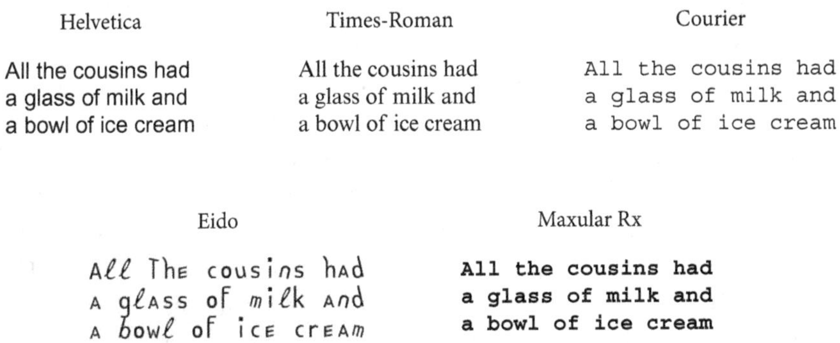

Figure 6.6 An MNREAD sentence is rendered with each of the five fonts used in the study by Xiong et al. (2018). Eido and Maxular Rx were designed specifically for macular degeneration. Times Roman, Helvetica, and Courier are mainstream fonts. Print size for the five fonts is matched in x-height.

Reading with central-field loss

People who lose central vision usually have major difficulty with reading, a situation faced by people with advanced AMD.

Why is central-field loss so detrimental to reading? People with central blind spots must use their peripheral vision for reading. We know that peripheral vision has poorer acuity, so we would expect magnification to help—and it does. But, even with adequate magnification, many people with central-field loss cannot achieve the same reading fluency as normally sighted readers. For example, in Figure 6.5, the MNREAD test data show that the AMD subject (lower curve) has a maximum reading speed of about 100 words per minute, well below the value of about 300 words per minute for the normally sighted subject. Even when the print size is larger than the AMD subject's CPS, they read slowly. This means that something other than print magnification is limiting their reading speed. The concept of *visual span* helps to explain the problem.

Figure 6.7 introduces the concept of visual span and explains why reading with a central scotoma is difficult. The left panel of the figure is a diagram showing what information is available in a single-eye fixation by a normally sighted person. There is only a small region at the center of the visual field in which text letters can be accurately recognized. For people with normal vision, this region is only about 9 or 10 letters wide. We say that the normal visual span for reading is about 10 letters. Outside this region, the crowding effect makes the letters too indistinct to be recognized reliably. When a person with normal vision reads, their eyes jump from word to word along a line of text. These eye movements are called reading saccades. The reader proceeds through the text with a series of eye fixations, separated by saccades, recognizing a cluster of letters on each fixation.

The right panel of the figure simulates a reading fixation with a central blind spot. The 2-D geometry of the normal visual span becomes ring-shaped. It is no longer possible to recognize all the letters on a horizontal line of text passing through the center of the normal visual span. Recall from Chapter 5 that most people with central-field loss eventually adopt a preferred retinal locus (PRL) for fixation outside the central blind spot. The PRL is usually near the edge of the blind spot, but we still don't know what factors determine whether the PRL is left, right, above, or below the blind spot. Young people with early onset forms of macular disease, such as Stargardt disease, tend to adopt a PRL below the scotoma in the visual field. This is generally regarded as best for reading. But, many older people with AMD adopt a PRL to the left or right of the scotoma. This is generally thought to

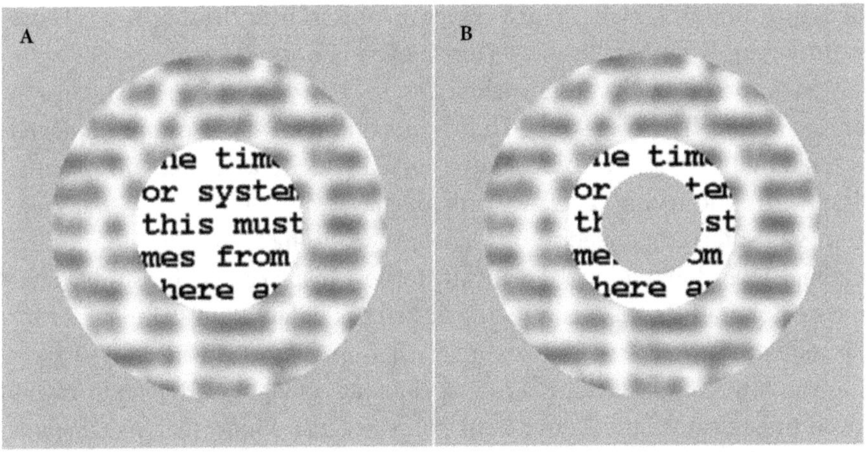

Figure 6.7 A diagram illustrating the concept of visual span. Panel A illustrates that in normal vision, there is only a small region of the visual field in which letters can be recognized accurately without moving the eyes. A reader can identify about 10 letters on a line of text passing through the center of this region, "this_must." This reader's visual span is said to be 10 characters wide. Panel B shows that the region of reliable letter recognition becomes ring-shaped in the presence of a central scotoma and that the maximum number of visible letters on a line of text is reduced. The reader with a central scotoma has a smaller visual span.

be maladaptive for reading because text characters on the line being read will disappear into the scotoma, and because only a small cluster of letters would be recognizable to the left or right of the scotoma. Whatever the choice of PRL, we would expect the number of recognizable letters on each fixation to be reduced. For example, in Figure 6.7B, a lower PRL would see the six letters "here a" and a PRL to the right of the blind spot would only see the two letters "st." In other words, the person with central-field loss will have a smaller visual span for reading. Think of it as a smaller window for seeing chunks of text on each eye fixation.

In my lab, we have developed two methods for estimating the size of the visual span for reading (Legge et al., 2001). One method was based on the time it takes to read words of different lengths. The second method involved a series of trials in which a test subject tried to identify strings of three letters (trigrams) presented briefly at varying distances to the left and right of fixation. We used trigrams rather than single letters in order to include the effects of letter crowding between adjacent letters in text. Using these methods, we found that the visual span for normally sighted readers is about 9 or 10 letters under good viewing conditions, but it gets smaller for letters near the acuity limit or for letters with very low contrast near the threshold. These are situations when reading slows down even in normal vision.

Because people with central-field loss must rely on their peripheral vision for reading, we have also studied how well peripheral vision can be deployed for reading by people with normal vision. If you are a person with normal vision, imagine trying to read words displayed in your lower visual field. In a 1998 study conducted in our lab, led by Susana Chung, we found that reading slows down quite dramatically for text displaced farther and farther into peripheral vision, even when print size is enlarged to compensate for the reduction in acuity. For example, when text was displaced 20 degrees into the lower visual field, reading speed was only about one sixth of the speed in central vision. In our 2001 study, we also found that visual spans for normally sighted readers get smaller in peripheral vision. These findings led us to hypothesize that a reduction in the size of the visual span is a factor contributing to the reading difficulty of people with central-field loss.

We tested this hypothesis in a study led by Allen Cheong (2008). She measured reading speeds and visual spans for a group of 13 subjects with AMD and a group of age-matched normally sighted controls. The normally sighted group had a mean visual span of 8.7 letters. The AMD group, with a range of disease severity, had a mean visual span of 5.2 letters. One AMD subject had a visual span of only 2.7 letters. It would not be surprising to find that a person who could recognize only two or three letters on each fixation would read much more slowly than a normally sighted person who recognizes eight or nine letters on each fixation. Allen found, however, that shrinkage of the visual span by itself was not sufficient to explain the slower reading of her AMD subjects. The data indicated that the time course for recognizing letters was also longer in AMD subjects than in the normally sighted controls. Statistical analysis indicated that both the reduced size of the visual span and the longer time required for letter recognition jointly contributed to slower reading. A 2004 study by Michael Crossland and colleagues has shown that people with central-field loss who rely on a PRL for fixation have less stable fixation; the eyes drift more when attempting to fixate on a letter or other targets. It may well be the case that the longer time required for letter and word recognition is related to less steady fixation.

In short, the reading difficulties of people with central-field loss, even when they have adequate magnification, may be due to a combination of a reduced number of letters visible on each fixation (reduced visual span) and increased time required for recognizing those letters.

Summary of how text properties and vision status affect reading

We now know much more about how different characteristics of low vision impact reading and how to optimize text for visual reading. For people with low vision, the migration of text from hard copy to digital formats offers great promise for the customization of text properties and enhancing accessibility. While visual reading may often be a challenge, be assured that for many people with low vision, the glass is at least half full.

To summarize the impact of text variables on low-vision reading:

- Print size and display size matter. Magnification is usually necessary for text characters to exceed the reader's CPS. The display of text needs to accommodate a critical number of characters on each line.
- High-contrast text is often essential.
- Contrast reversal (bright letters on a dark background) is helpful for some people with low vision.
- Bright displays can be helpful, especially for reading print near the acuity limit.
- There may be individual differences in font preferences, but specific fonts don't have clear advantages for low vision. Fonts that emphasize letter spacing may be helpful when people read near their acuity limit.

We can also summarize the impact on reading of the three major dimensions of low vision:

- Reduced acuity has a major impact on the print size and display size requirements for reading.
- People with low contrast sensitivity require high-contrast text. People who experience light scatter in the optics of the eye, such as people with advanced cataract, experience glare effects and will often benefit from reversed-contrast text. Some people with RP and some other forms of retinal disease also read better with reversed-contrast text.
- People with central-field loss from AMD and other maculopathies must rely on peripheral vision to read. They will require print magnification. Even with sufficient magnification, they may still read slowly because of a combination of reduced visual span, longer time to recognize letters, and less stable eye fixations in reading.

7

Mobility and Low Vision

Getting Around on Foot

Mobility is a major challenge for many people with low vision. Mobility refers to getting around on foot, by car, or by public transportation. It includes mobility within the home, the neighborhood, the community, and the world. In this chapter, we will consider several perspectives on pedestrian mobility with low vision. What visual and nonvisual cues are used by people with low vision in getting around? What is the influence of variations in lighting? How can architects and designers enhance the visual accessibility of buildings for people with low vision? In the next chapter, we'll turn to driving with low vision.

• • • • •

Independent mobility is an important prerequisite for full participation in modern society. It figures in employment, education, commerce, social interaction, and recreation. The ability to remain mobile with vision impairment, whether low vision or blindness, is so important that a specialized form of vision rehabilitation has been developed to address it, termed orientation and mobility (O&M). Beginning in the 1960s, several university programs began graduating specialists who could train visually impaired pedestrians in mobility skills. The goals of the O&M training are to enable the visually impaired person to travel safely and effectively through the environment while maintaining awareness of their current location, heading, and the presence of relevant nearby people, vehicles, or objects. An additional component of effective mobility is to travel with confidence and without fear.

The impact of low vision on mobility depends on the type and severity of vision impairment. Figure 7.1 shows an indoor hallway scene. The top two panels compare a clear view with a view simulating reduced acuity. With low acuity, the near table is recognizable, the mid-distance table is detectable as a blob but not recognizable, and the far tables are essentially invisible. The two lower panels compare a wide-field view of a hallway with a view through a narrow field severely restricted to 7.5 degrees. While central vision is intact

Low Vision. Gordon E. Legge, Oxford University Press. © Oxford University Press (2026).
DOI: 10.1093/9780198946960.003.0008

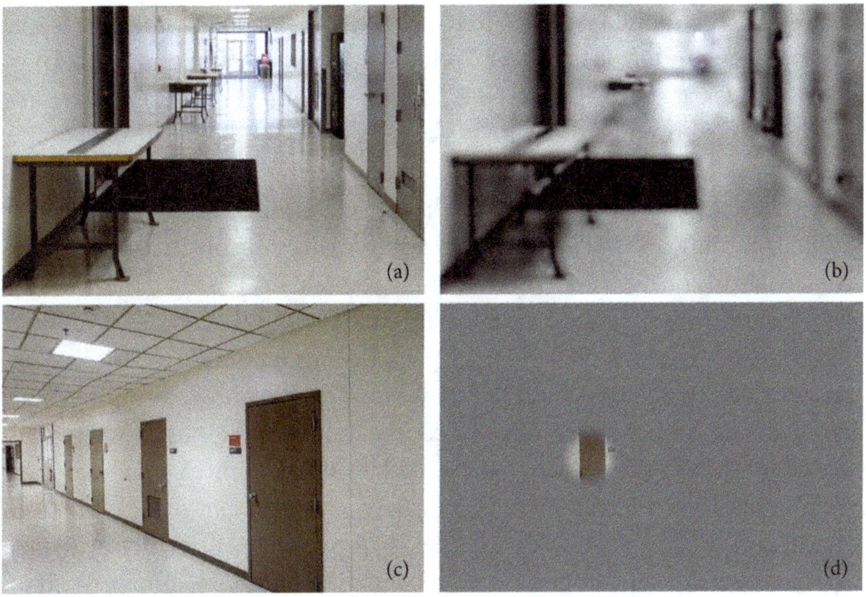

Figure 7.1 Hallway scenes illustrating the impact of impaired vision. The top pair of panels compares clear vision with a simulation of reduced acuity (20/250) and reduced contrast sensitivity (1.0 Pelli-Robson measure). The bottom pair of panels compares a wide field of view with simulation of severe field restriction (7.5 degrees diameter). Adapted from Creem-Regehr et al. (2021). How can basic research on spatial cognition enhance the visual accessibility of architecture for people with low vision? *Cognitive Research: Principles and Implications*, 6(1), 3.

in the view with the narrow field, adjacent doors on the right are out of sight. Later in this chapter, we'll look at the impact of reduced acuity, reduced contrast sensitivity, and field loss on mobility in more detail.

There are three major components of pedestrian mobility—obstacle avoidance, environmental awareness, and wayfinding. *Obstacle avoidance* is the ability to take the next step safely without bumping into things or tripping. Many people who are visually impaired deal effectively with obstacle avoidance using a white cane, guide dog, or their own low vision. *Environmental awareness* refers to the accurate perception of the distance, direction, and identity of objects in the immediate environment. Sometimes, low vision is sufficient to avoid obstacles but insufficient for identifying nearby objects (is it a trash bin or a mailbox?) or for estimating the distance to objects. *Wayfinding* refers to the ability to learn layouts and plan and follow routes from place to place while keeping track of one's current position and heading. Low vision can impede wayfinding when visual landmarks are not visible or directional signage is not legible.

Safety during mobility is a primary concern for people with low vision. Most people with low vision have accidentally encountered obstacles. They have had to learn strategies to avoid bumping into things including tripping hazards on the ground such as toys, stools, benches, and pets; objects to the side such as door jambs, tables, chairs, or people; and head-level items such as tree branches, awnings, or chandeliers. I had a nasty fall in my campus building, coming around a corner and tripping over the outstretched legs of a student sitting on the floor. My coffee mug went flying. I incurred a fractured arm. I'm now more cautious in rounding corners.

Mobility hazards also include uncertain footing, especially steps, slippery surfaces (ice, wet showers, and highly waxed floors), as well as uneven surfaces such as gravel or irregularly placed flagstones. I enjoy outdoor activities including hikes in the woods, but I usually avoid terrain in which visually guided foot placement is necessary for safety.

In older age, when low vision is the most prevalent, difficulty in seeing steps or obstacles on the ground or recognizing uneven footing can combine with reduced balance to increase the risk of falling. Of course, falls in old age can be dangerous and even life-threatening. Fear of falling itself is a major issue for seniors with low vision and an impediment to mobility. There has been extensive research into the greater risk factors for falling with low vision, especially among seniors. In Box 7.1, I review some of the research findings.

Box 7.1 Research on falls by older adults with low vision

Falls are dangerous for everyone but particularly for older adults. More than 25% of people over the age of 65 fall at least once each year, and falls are the leading type of injury causing death in seniors. A U.S. study of falls by people aged 65 years and older, culminating in Emergency Department visits, indicated that 79.2% of the falls occurred in the home, with the most-common locations being the bedroom, bathroom, and stairs (Moreland et al., 2021). A team led by Kathleen Colón-Emeric (2024) at Duke University in North Carolina reviewed many studies identifying risk factors for falling and interventions to prevent falls. The review indicated that exercise programs focused on leg strengthening and better balance can reduce the risk of falling in older people.

Are the risks of falling higher for people with eye disease? A team led by Jung Yin Tsang (2023) at the University of Manchester reviewed primary-care health records of patients in England, collected from 2007 to 2020. The team examined data from groups of patients with three of the most common types of eye disease—410,476 with cataract, 75,622 with AMD, and 90,177 with glaucoma—each group compared with age- and sex-matched control groups with about five times as many individuals. The three eye-disease groups all exhibited higher rates of falls (25%–38% higher) and also fractures (18%–31% higher) than their comparison groups.

Joanne Wood (2011) from Queensland University of Technology in Brisbane Australia and colleagues studied falls and other injuries in a group of 76 people with AMD with a mean age of 77. The participants with AMD received a thorough eye exam at the beginning of the study and then reported monthly for a year on falling incidents and injuries of other types. More than half the group reported at least one fall during the year, and 74% of the group reported either a fall or other injuries during the year. The leading causes of falling were tripping and loss of balance, and the leading types of other injuries were lacerations and collisions with obstacles. Reduced contrast sensitivity was the vision measure with the strongest association with falls and other injuries.

A study by Jin (2024) and colleagues reported on results from the United States National Health and Aging Trends Study (NHATS), which included measures of visual acuity and contrast sensitivity, as well as number of falls. The sample included 2,951 older adults (Medicare recipients aged 71 years and older), of which 27.6% were classified as having vision impairment. The group with vision impairment had 25% more falls per year than the group with normal vision. The authors found that reduced contrast sensitivity, but not reduced acuity, was associated with a higher prevalence of falls. Overall, the evidence indicates that reduced contrast sensitivity is a major visual risk factor for falls. This makes intuitive sense since failing to see steps or curbs or tripping over objects under foot is often related to the low contrast of hazards rather than their small size.

The review cited above by Colón-Emeric and colleagues indicated that exercise programs reduce the risk of falls for seniors. Would exercise programs also be beneficial for seniors with low vision? John Campbell (2005) and colleagues at Otago University in Dunedin, New Zealand, conducted a randomized controlled study to address this issue. Seniors, aged 75 years and older, with visual acuity of 20/80 (6/24) or worse were randomly assigned to four intervention conditions—home-safety assessment and modifications delivered by an occupational therapist, an exercise program delivered at home by a physical therapist, a program with both home modifications and exercise, and a control group with social visits only. There were between 97 and 100 participants per group. The home modifications included attending to loose floor coverings, enhancing the contrast of step edges, installing grab bars and stair rails, improving lighting, and reducing glare. The exercise program involved at least three sessions a week for 30 minutes of leg strengthening and balance training that increased in difficulty and outdoor walking at least twice a week. The control group with social visits received two one-hour home visits by research staff. The group with home-safety modifications had fewer falls during the yearlong trial (an average of 0.65 falls per person) than the group with the exercise program (1.30 falls per person). The exercise group did not differ significantly from the group receiving only social visits. These results indicate that the home modifications were effective in reducing falls and that the exercise program did not provide significant benefit. Curiously, the combined program (home modifications plus exercise) was not as effective as the home modifications alone. One issue with the exercise program was that most of the participants did not adhere fully to the demands of the program throughout the year of the trial. More recently, a team led by Jian-Yu E (2020) at Johns Hopkins University reviewed several studies evaluating interventions to reduce falls in seniors with low vision and found only weak evidence for the benefits of both exercise programs and home modifications in reducing the prevalence of falls.

Despite equivocal evidence, it seems likely to me that home modifications, guided by an experienced occupational therapist, will reduce the risk of falling for seniors with low vision. Similarly, the strong evidence for the benefits of exercise for reducing the risk of falls in normally sighted seniors should also apply to seniors with low vision if they adhere to appropriately designed programs.

How do we study the impact of environmental factors such as lighting or a person's vision condition on mobility? Researchers have adopted several strategies. One approach is to use survey questions to ask people with low vision to rate their level of difficulty in navigating in dim illumination or other challenging mobility conditions. A second approach is to ask subjects to walk through an obstacle course with harmless objects such as foam pillars or cardboard boxes and count the number of contacts (bumps) the subject makes with an obstacle; the more the contacts, the greater the impact of the variable under study such as reduced lighting. A third approach is to compare a subject's walking speed in an open area with their walking speed when they need to avoid obstacles. People with low vision may slow down to avoid obstacles. Yet another approach is to measure the ability of a person to detect and recognize obstacles from specific distances. In my lab, we have done several studies in which subjects with both normal and low vision were asked to identify the presence of a step or ramp ahead at varying distances and under various lighting and contrast conditions (Bochsler et al., 2013; Legge et al., 2010). Of special importance, researchers have evaluated the ability of blind and low-vision subjects to judge when it is safe to cross a street in the presence of traffic. For example, Shirin Hassan (2012) at Indiana University asked groups of subjects—normally sighted, low vision, and blind—to rate the safety of crossing streets when there were cars approaching from different distances. She found that the judgments of the group with low vision were as accurate as those of the normally sighted group, but the judgments of the blind group, who relied on sound, were less accurate.

Nonvisual cues in mobility

What sorts of cues are useful in mobility, especially for obstacle avoidance? People who are blind must use nonvisual cues, and people with low vision may sometimes rely on nonvisual cues. Touch can be used to explore the environment by probing ahead with one's hand or a cane. Features felt under foot can be informative such as tactile textures at the edges of subway or bus platforms, the tactile domes signaling the edge of a street crossing, the grass–cement boundary on a residential sidewalk, a boundary between a carpeted and non-carpeted floor, and the incline of a ramp. These tactile cues under foot are often supplemented by color contrast, providing additional help for people with low vision. I've noticed that the tactile domes at street crossings are colored bright red or yellow in some cities, which is helpful for me. In my hometown of Minneapolis, the domes are often brown and less salient for me as warning markers at street crossings. Railings can provide both physical support and a cue to the presence of steps or ramps. Follow the railing and when it bends down, you are at the top of the stairs. Usually, when the railing ends, you are at the bottom of the stairs. I have occasionally encountered staircase railings that end before the last step or two, posing a significant hazard to nonvisual mobility.

Environmental sounds are also important for mobility. Traffic sounds can be used to avoid crossing at the wrong time or to define a path parallel to traffic flow. Sounds made by other people can also be important; hearing a person talking, sneezing, or walking can be a nonvisual cue to their proximity. Stable sound sources are also helpful as acoustic landmarks in mobility such as the sound made by an outdoor water fountain or the hum of an indoor vending machine. Accessible pedestrian signals use auditory tones or spoken messages to guide people to a street crossing, inform them when it is safe to cross, and sometimes provide an auditory target for staying on course while crossing the street. Perceiving the directions of sound sources is important in mobility and relies on differences in the time or intensity of sounds reaching the two ears. For this reason, good hearing is helpful in mobility for people with impaired vision. People who have both vision impairment and hearing impairment (termed dual-sensory loss) encounter additional challenges in mobility.

Many obstacles in the environment don't emit sounds, such as walls, benches, posts, trash cans, tree trunks, and branches. It is possible to probe silent obstacles with echolocation. Bats and dolphins generate sounds and learn about objects in their environments from the echoes bouncing back from the objects. Humans can make use of echoes to acquire information about the environment. Imagine, for example, stepping into an empty room with your eyes closed and clapping. You will probably be able to tell whether you are in a small, echoic space like a bathroom or a larger, more muffled space like a bedroom. You may have had the experience of navigating in a dark room and sensing the presence of a nearby wall without seeing it. Studies of blind and blindfolded subjects in the 1940s revealed that they could sense the presence of a nearby wall without vision. This ability was termed *facial vision* because it seemed to be associated with feeling of pressure on the face. Subsequent research by Daniel Ashmead and Robert Wall (2002) at Vanderbilt University has shown that "facial vision" can be understood as an acoustic cue, produced by a change in the low-frequency spectrum of sounds near a large surface such as a wall.

The use of a white cane can take advantage of echolocation. The tapping of the metal tip of the cane on the ground produces a useful signal for generating echoes. People can also generate sounds with finger snaps, claps, or tongue clicks to produce echoes. Some blind individuals become experts in using echolocation to probe the environment for objects and obstacles. Daniel Kish is a prominent advocate for the value of echolocation in blind mobility. Kish lost his vision to retinal blastoma, a cancer of the eye, at the age of 13 months. Subsequently, he taught himself to use tongue clicks for echolocation to explore the presence of objects around him. In 2000, he founded a nonprofit organization called World Access for the Blind to teach blind children how to use echolocation to enhance their mobility. Have a look at his TED talk.[1] As a child, I had a blind friend who would use echolocation to play tag. We would sometimes play in a field with trees. My friend would run, pausing every few seconds to clap. From the tree echoes, he kept his bearings and perhaps sensed the positions of other kids in the game.

Santani Teng (2012) and colleagues at the University of California at Berkeley showed that expert blind echolocators can make rather precise judgments about the directions of objects ahead. These researchers also showed that acuity for echolocation was correlated with the age of onset of blindness—the earlier the onset of blindness, the better the echolocation. Teng et al. also showed that normally sighted individuals could be trained to improve their echolocation ability. It is likely that some people with low vision make use of echolocation as well.

Effective mobility also relies on maintaining a desired heading, that is, staying on course. Imagine you are crossing the street at a four-way intersection. You want to follow a straight line without veering into the traffic lanes. People with good vision easily cross by sighting landmarks on the far corner.

[1] https://www.ted.com/talks/daniel_kish_how_i_use_sonar_to_navigate_the_world?language=en.

White lines on a crosswalk can provide visual guidance for people with low vision who have trouble sighting a visual target across the street. When visual or auditory landmarks are not accessible, people with impaired vision may need to rely on vestibular and kinesthetic body-centered cues to follow a straight line without veering. The vestibular system plays an important role in maintaining balance and good posture and in signaling head movement. The vestibular system is composed of sensory organs in the inner ear—the semicircular canals and the otoliths. The semicircular canals code for three dimensions of head rotation and the otoliths code for linear accelerations. In principle, changes in speed or direction during mobility—walking, driving, or while being pushed in a wheelchair—can be sensed by the vestibular system. Kinesthetic signals come from muscle receptors about limb motion, especially legs and ankles, and provide body-centered information about walking direction.

How accurately can people maintain a straight line while walking without visual or auditory landmarks? There are stories about people with good vision lost in a snow blizzard or in the forest and who found that they had walked in a circle while trying to find their way home. Why did they veer away from a straight line? One unproven theory held that such veering was related to slight differences in leg length. Researchers interested in orientation and mobility skills have investigated the accuracy with which people can walk a straight line nonvisually. In a study in my lab at the University of Minnesota, led by Chris Kallie (2007), we conducted extensive measurements with small groups of blind subjects and blindfolded normally sighted subjects. They repeatedly attempted to walk a straight line for a distance of 30 feet (9.14 meters) in a large empty classroom. They wore earmuffs to block auditory cues. How much veering would we observe? Would the blind subjects veer more or less than the blindfolded sighted subjects? Performance was quite good. Across approximately 40 trials completed by each subject, average veering errors for individuals ranged from 1.47 feet (0.45 m) to 5.7 feet (1.74 m) after walking 30 feet. We thought blind subjects might perform better than blindfolded sighted subjects because of more everyday experience walking without sight. On the other hand, sighted subjects might do better owing to their prior visual experience in calibrating body-centered signals with straight-line walking. In the end, we found no significant difference between the two groups. Based on data from some follow-up experiments, we developed a model to explain the veering behavior we observed. We attributed veering to three sources: initial misalignment with the straight-ahead direction, systematic bias in stepping direction (rightward or leftward) by some subjects, and small variable errors in direction introduced on each step. We described this latter source of error as "undetectable motor noise," that is, errors on each step so small as to be undetectable from body-centered cues. We estimated that these step-by-step errors averaged about 1.3 degrees in direction. After many steps, the cumulative effect of these step-by-step errors would result in significant veering away from a straight line. David Guth (2008), an orientation and mobility researcher at Western Michigan University, has shown that a training procedure can be helpful in reducing veering by some blind pedestrians. The training involved the use of acoustic feedback to alert subjects when they deviated systematically from the straight ahead. Ultimately, however, the Kallie et al. findings indicate that small errors, accumulating step-by-step, will result in errors in straight-line walking if there are no external cues for error correction.

Distance cues useful in low vision

One of the most important functions of vision is to provide information about the identity and layout of objects in the nearby environment. Judging distances to visible objects is called *depth perception*. People with normal vision effortlessly survey their environments and move among nearby objects, whether furniture in a room, toys on a playground, or rocks and trees in a meadow. How might low vision affect depth perception? Vision scientists have devoted a great deal of effort to classifying visual-depth cues and to measuring the accuracy of human depth perception. Relatively little research has been done on low-vision depth perception. For people with moderate or severe visual impairment, access to some depth cues is limited or lost.

Visual depth cues can be classified into three broad categories—binocular cues that make use of two eyes, motion cues due to an observer's motion through the environment, and pictorial cues that are present in pictures or in a stationary view of a scene.

Binocular cues

A major advantage of having two eyes is stereoscopic depth perception, the ability to infer depth based on the slightly different views of objects seen by the two eyes. Stereopsis is most useful for nearby activities involving depth such as threading a needle, pouring liquid into a glass, or grasping an object. Effective stereopsis requires proper alignment of the two eyes and equivalent vision status in the two eyes. Misalignment of the eyes or unequal vision in the left and right eyes is a risk factor for deficient stereopsis. Many people with low vision have one eye that is much better than the other eye. A study led by Ying-Zi Xiong (2021) at the University of Minnesota reported data showing that many people with macular degeneration, glaucoma, retinitis pigmentosa (RP), and cataracts have substantial differences in acuity and contrast sensitivity in their two eyes. A 2021 review of binocular status in low vision, led by Janelle Tong at the University of New South Wales in Australia, pointed out that such interocular differences often result in misalignment of the two eyes, termed convergence dysfunction. Several studies, reviewed by Tong and colleagues, have shown that many individuals with macular degeneration, glaucoma, and RP have reduced or no access to depth information from stereopsis. Since depth judgments from stereo vision are the most accurate for near distances, deficient stereopsis is likely to have a greater impact on reaching and grasping and less impact on mobility. But, stereopsis may be helpful in noticing curbs or other single steps. Failing to see a step can lead to falling, which can have serious health consequences, such as hip fractures. Tong et al. reviewed several studies of the association between falls and deficits in stereo vision. They concluded that the association is not definitive and is hard to disentangle from deficits in other vision measures such as acuity. In summary, in many cases of moderate or severe low vision, stereoscopic depth perception is likely to be compromised, but the impact on mobility may be slight.

Motion cues

Motion parallax is an alternative method for acquiring depth information and may be useful to people with low vision who lack stereo vision. Instead of viewing a scene with two eyes from slightly different viewpoints as in stereo, motion parallax involves moving the head and/or body left or right to view a scene from two vantage points. Even if vision is functional in only one eye, this type of motion provides information about distance. You can demonstrate motion parallax with a simple experiment. Close one eye. Align your two index fingers with several inches of separation between them along the line of sight of your open eye. Now, if you move your head left or right while maintaining your gaze straight ahead, your nearer finger will move farther into your peripheral vision than the more distant finger. Your head motion changes the angle of view of the nearer object more than the more distant object. The differential offsets of the two objects in your visual field provide information about their relative depth. Motion parallax has two major advantages for low vision. First, motion parallax only requires one functioning eye. Second, the observer determines the separation between the two vantage points by choosing the extent of head motion, whereas stereopsis relies on the fixed separation of the two eyes in the head. I have no stereo depth perception, but I have often used motion parallax. If I'm not sure about the distance of an object, I'll sometimes move my head to the left or right or even take a sidestep and observe how much the object of interest shifts in my field of view. If there is no noticeable shift, I know that the object is very far away. In brief, motion parallax is a depth cue potentially useful for people with low vision, but it is not known if it is widely used.

Pictorial cues

Pictorial depth cues are used by artists in painting to portray depth. They are also available in static views of real scenes and require just one eye. Textbooks on art or perception list many pictorial cues, some more important than others and some likely to be more accessible than others in low vision. Perspective is the best-known pictorial cue. As we discussed in detail in Chapter 2, the same object, viewed at a greater distance, subtends a proportionately smaller visual angle. Diminishing size in a picture or in a visual image may convey information about distance. A famous example is linear perspective in which parallel lines appear to converge in the distance. Railroad tracks are often used as an example. Of more immediate relevance to most people with low vision, the parallel edges of a long, straight sidewalk will converge in the distance, whether in a perspective drawing or in a real-world retinal image. For linear perspective to be useful for someone with low vision, the contrast of the converging edges would need to be above the person's contrast threshold and acuity would need to be sufficient to see the diminishing separation of the edges in the visual image.

Familiar size is another important pictorial depth cue. If you know the approximate physical size of an object, such as a person or a soda can, then its angular size in a visual image can be informative about its distance. If the image of the person is tiny, you know they are far away. The use of this cue requires knowing the identity of the object. In some cases of low vision, acuity may not be sufficient to recognize the object. Yes, I see something out there, but I don't know what it is. If you have no idea what the object is, familiar size will not be helpful in estimating distance. Sometimes guesswork can be helpful and sometimes lead to mistakes. I see a vertical elongated form across the street on the sidewalk. Is it my neighbor? I call out "Hello Jack." There's no response. Then, I figure out that it's not Jack, but his tall trash bin at the curb. Yes, I have occasionally found myself addressing inanimate objects.

A distance cue that is robust with low acuity and does not require identification of an object is illustrated in Figure 7.2. The two photos show a frisbee lying on a patio near a brick wall. The camera's view is straight ahead in both images, but the camera is nearer to the wall in the right image. In the nearer view, the frisbee is located lower in the picture than in the more distant image on the left. A person with low acuity might not be able to identify the frisbee but could estimate its distance based on its vertical location in the visual field. This cue is called "height in the picture plane" or "angle of declination." It refers to the inverse relationship between the distance to an object on the ground and the angular distance in the visual field between the line of sight ahead and the object.

For those who are interested, here is the calculation underlying this distance cue. For a person with standing eye height H (height of the eye above the ground) looking straight ahead (parallel to the flat ground surface) and an object on the ground that makes angle A in the lower visual field, the distance D to the object is H divided by the tangent of A: D = H/tanA. For example, suppose eye height H is 5 feet (about average for adult women), if the angle

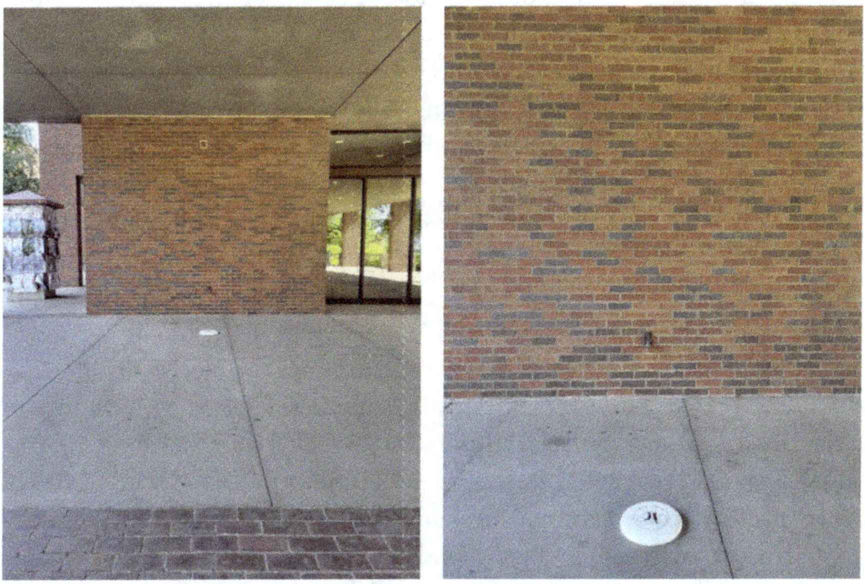

Figure 7.2 An illustration of angle of declination as a distance cue.

A is 2 degrees, then the distance D is 5/tan (2) = 5/.035 = 143 feet. But, if the object appears 30 degrees below the line of sight, the distance is D = 5/tan (30) = 5/0.58 = 8.6 feet.

While our visual system and brain do not make explicit numerical calculations, our experience allows us to make implicit judgments about the distances of objects on the ground plane based on the angular offset between the straight-ahead line of sight and objects in the lower visual field. An alternative strategy for judging the distance to an object on the ground might be for a person to tilt their head or eyes down to fixate on the target and to estimate the distance from the extent of their head tilt.

Can people actually use this cue? Margaret Tarampi (2010) and colleagues at the University of Utah tested distance perception with normally sighted college students. The subjects viewed a black box on the floor of a large room at distances ranging from 1.5 to 6 meters. On some trials, they viewed the target with their normal vision, and on other trials, they viewed the target through blurring goggles that reduced acuity severely to about 20/700 (with a visual field of about 70 degrees in diameter). After viewing the target on each trial, the subject was blindfolded and attempted to walk to the location of the target. An experimenter removed the box so there would be no collision. The accuracy of walking to the target blindfolded was used as an estimate of distance perception with and without artificial acuity reduction. The subjects were equally accurate in blind walking to the target location whether they had viewed the target with normal vision or severe blur. The investigators interpreted the results to mean that their subjects used angle of declination as a distance cue and that this cue is robust against severe acuity reduction. They also suggested that the visibility of the floor–wall boundary in the room may have helped as a reference for estimating angle of declination and hence distance to the target boxes.

In the photo on the right in Figure 7.2, the visible boundary between the wall and the patio floor is located lower in the picture than in the photo on the left, indicating a viewpoint closer to the wall. An experiment in my lab has implicated the floor–wall boundary as a useful cue for judging room size (Legge et al., 2016). We had groups of subjects with normal vision and low vision visit six rooms in our campus building. The rooms varied in size from 8 by 15 feet to 24 by 27 feet. From the doorway, the subjects were asked to view the space and estimate the length and width of the rooms. Our low-vision subjects had a wide range of conditions ranging from someone with a very narrow field and an acuity of 20/32 to someone with acuity close to 20/2000. How effectively would people with low vision be able to estimate room size? We were surprised to discover that there was no significant difference in accuracy between the room-size estimates of the normally sighted and low-vision subjects. Our results showed that even very low vision can be effective in interpreting room size. We think that the angle of declination of the floor–wall boundary provided the cue that enabled our low-vision subjects to make good room-size estimates. If so, accessible design for low vision should include good contrast between floors and walls.

Another study in my lab, led by Andrew Freedman (2019), further supported the salience of the floor–wall boundary for indoor mobility with low vision. We used head-mounted eye-tracking equipment to assess the gaze direction of a group of subjects with low vision while they walked around an indoor course and attempted to identify objects to the left and right of the travel path. We found that the low-vision subjects spent more time looking at floor–wall boundaries in the room than normally sighted controls.

To summarize, of the many distance cues available in normal vision, some are more resistant to low vision than others. Motion parallax may be available for estimating distance when stereopsis is not available. Perspective and familiar size are likely to be helpful in low vision but of declining value with poorer acuity and contrast sensitivity. Angle of declination, also known as height in the picture plane, is a depth cue that may be particularly resistant to acuity loss.

Impact of lighting

Three aspects of lighting affect mobility—overall light level, directional lighting, and glare.

Overall light level

Overall lighting is represented by phrases such as "it's a very bright day," "I'm dazzled by this intense lighting," "this is a dim room; please turn up the lights," "I can't see anything in this dimly lit restaurant," or "I can't find my way in the dark at night." There are three broad domains of overall lighting, determined by the responsiveness of photoreceptor cells (rods and cones) in the retina. *Photopic* (daylight) lighting refers to conditions when lighting is sufficient to stimulate the cone photoreceptors in the retina and too bright for the rod photoreceptors. Photopic lighting is typically available outdoors in daylight (sun or clouds) and in indoors with overhead illumination. *Scotopic* (nighttime) lighting refers to conditions when only the rods are responsive, as on a moonless night or in a dark building without the lights on. *Mesopic* (twilight) vision is a range of lighting levels in which both rods and cones are responsive. Examples include lighting half an hour after sunset or lighting at night in a residential area with streetlights. Box 7.2 briefly describes numerical values for light levels corresponding to these three domains of vision.

Box 7.2 Light measurement

Numerical levels of illumination can be assessed with a light meter that measures the light flux falling on a surface in the space, such as the floor or tabletop. The metric units of illumination are lux (lx). Another common unit of illumination is the foot-candle (ft-c). To convert illuminance in foot-candles to lux, multiply by 10.76. The lowest light level for photopic vision is in the range of 20–50 lux.

The response of the photoreceptors in the eye will depend on the luminance of a surface viewed by the eye. The metric unit for luminance is candelas per meter squared, written cd/m^2. The surface luminance seen by the eye depends on both the light flux falling on that surface measured in lux and the reflectance of the surface. A surface's reflectance can range from a maximum of 1.0 (all light is reflected from the surface) to a minimum of 0 (the surface absorbs all light falling on it). A high-reflectance surface, such as a piece of white paper, will have a much higher luminance when viewed by the eye than a low-reflectance surface, such as black felt, for the same level of illumination. The formula for converting illuminance I in lux to luminance L in cd/m^2 for a surface with reflectance R is:

$$L = IR/\pi$$

The lower bound for photopic vision is a luminance of approximately 5 cd/m^2. This level of luminance could arise from surface illumination of about 50 lux falling on a dark surface with reflectance of about 0.3 or from 20 lux illumination on a surface with high reflectance of about 0.8 such as white paper.

Mesopic vision ranges from about 0.001 to 5 cd/m^2 and scotopic vision for light levels below 0.001 cd/m^2.

For details on numerical measurements of light and color, consult Wyszecki and Stiles (1982).

The impact of overall light level on low-vision mobility depends on the eye condition. As we saw in Chapter 3, people with achromatopsia, who lack cone photoreceptors, find photopic lighting to be dazzling and uncomfortable. They need to use dark glasses and other strategies for mobility.

At the other extreme, RP is a disorder in which rods lose their function before the cones. The result is that people with RP have deficits in night vision; they are severely affected in their mobility under scotopic and even mesopic lighting.

Thomas Kuyk (1996, 1998) and colleagues at the Veterans Affairs Medical Center and the University of Alabama at Birmingham (UAB) conducted a major study of factors, including lighting, affecting low-vision mobility. They tested 88 veterans, mostly males averaging mid-60s in age, with varying types and degrees of vision impairment. The subjects were tested on three types of mobility routes: (1) a well-controlled indoor obstacle course, 3–5 feet in width bounded by walls, doors, cabinets, and benches, with foam cylinders on the floor and suspended from the ceiling acting as obstacles to be avoided; (2) a 500-feet path through hallways on two floors of a medical center with serendipitous obstacles such as chairs along the walls, a copy machine, house-cleaning carts, and pedestrians; and (3) an outdoor route covering three-and-half blocks in a mixed residential and small business area, with street crossings, and obstacles such as posts, broken pavement and curbs, tree branches and shrubs, and other pedestrians. The researchers recorded the time taken to complete the routes and the number of contacts with obstacles or other "incidents" such as stumbles or long pauses. To evaluate the impact of lighting, they measured mobility under photopic and mesopic conditions. The photopic condition utilized typical indoor lighting for the lab and hallway routes and daylight (usually sunny, but sometimes cloudy) conditions for the outdoor routes. To test mobility under mesopic lighting, the subjects wore wrap-around dark glasses that reduced illumination to mesopic levels, similar to dim restaurant lighting or early evening travel outdoors.

Throughout testing, an O&M specialist accompanied the subjects to score performance and to ensure safety. The mobility performance of the subjects on the lab obstacle course was similar to and correlated with performance on the real-world hallway and outdoor routes, confirming the validity of the lab testing. In all three settings, the subjects took more time to complete the routes with mesopic lighting, ranging from 35% longer for the outdoor routes to 47% longer for the lab obstacle course. Clearly, the low-vision subjects slowed down in mesopic lighting. Perhaps, more importantly, the number of contacts with obstacles or other mobility incidents increased substantially in mesopic lighting, by 110% in the lab obstacle course, 121% in the hallway route, and 291% in the outdoor routes. The big difference between the percentage increase in indoor and outdoor mobility incidents is hard to interpret but may be due to the greater environmental variability in the outdoor routes.

Under mesopic lighting, the low-vision subjects in this study walked more slowly and were at greater risk of bumping into things. There are two caveats to consider in evaluating this study. First, the study did not include an age-matched control group of subjects with normal vision. My intuition is that normal controls might have walked a little more slowly through the three types of routes under mesopic conditions but would still have avoided contacting most or all of the obstacles. In other words, normally sighted controls would likely have experienced fewer disadvantages in mobility in the mesopic lighting condition. A second caveat is that the low-vision subjects in the study were not permitted to use aids such as a white cane or dog guide under the mesopic lighting conditions. At least, some of them would likely use such aids in their everyday mobility, especially in low lighting.

Some other studies have shown that within the photopic (daylight) range, low-vision subjects don't necessarily require unusually bright lighting. For example, in a study in my laboratory led by Quan Lei (2024), we tested the ability of a group of 13 low-vision subjects with a variety of eye conditions to identify ramps or steps ahead on a walkway. The subjects also provided ratings of confidence in their judgments. We varied photopic luminance of the stimuli over a 100:1 range of typical indoor lighting. Although we found no significant difference across light levels in the ability to recognize steps and ramps ahead, subjects' confidence ratings decreased in dimmer lighting; they were less sure of what they saw.

Dim lighting (mesopic or scotopic levels) reduces visual acuity and contrast sensitivity for everyone. Normally sighted older adults experience greater difficulty in dim lighting than young adults due to a reduced range of pupil dilation and reduced transmission of light through the optics of the eye. According to an estimate by Weale (1963), the average 60-year-old eye admits about one-third the amount of light to the retina of the average 20-year-old eye. It is not surprising that older people often complain of difficulty in low illumination. People with low vision due to retinal disorders that affect the rod photoreceptors experience even greater difficulties in dim lighting. We have already mentioned the severe problems encountered at night by people with RP. People with macular degeneration also report difficulties with night vision.

Cynthia Owsley (2006) and colleagues at UAB developed a Low Luminance Questionnaire (LLQ) to assess the impact of dim lighting on daily activities of people with low vision. To develop the questionnaire, the researchers collected input from 80 participants in focus groups. The groups consisted primarily of people with age-related macular degeneration (AMD), ranging from early to advanced conditions, and also age-matched individuals with normal vision. Participants were asked about problems or concerns they had about activities in dim lighting or at night. The responses of the participants were analyzed to identify important themes. Problems with driving elicited the most comments, followed by psychosocial concerns, general vision limitations, adapting to changes in lighting, and difficulties with mobility and reading. The researchers created 32 questions to probe the themes derived from the focus group data. The questions were framed so that answers could range from high scores representing no difficulty with the activity to low scores indicating that the person was unable to do the activity. Examples of the 32 questions on the LLQ include the following:

- Do you have difficulty reading menus in dimly lit restaurants?
- Because of your vision, are you bothered that you have difficulty moving around in a darkened theater?
- While driving at night, do headlights from oncoming cars cause you difficulty?
- Do you feel bad or depressed about your ability to see at night or under poor lighting conditions?

The newly designed LLQ was administered to 125 subjects. Scores were lower for AMD subjects than for subjects with normal vision, with lower scores being associated with more severe macular disease. Although the LLQ was originally designed for macular degeneration, it can also be used to assess the impact of low lighting on people with other causes of low vision.

Sudden changes in lighting from bright to dim require the eyes to dark adapt and can pose an additional challenge for everyone. Think about going into a darkened theater or finding your way to bed after turning off the hall or bedroom light. Studies have shown that the time required for dark adaptation is substantially longer in older adults than in young adults. Research findings from Cynthia Owsley and colleagues at UAB, as reviewed in a 2011 article by Owsley, indicate that this extended period of dark adaptation is related to slower regeneration of the light-absorbing pigment (rhodopsin) in the rod photoreceptors in the retina. The time to achieve full dark adaptation can be several minutes longer for older people than for young adults.

Consistent with findings from the LLQ described above, people with AMD report extra difficulties in sudden transitions from bright to dim lighting requiring dark adaptation. A study led by M. Scott Alexander at Simon Fraser University in British Columbia, described in two articles in 2014 (2014a, 2014b), sought to document the impact of a change in lighting on mobility by comparing subjects with advanced AMD and age-matched controls. The investigators tested their subjects in three lighting conditions—photopic lighting similar to a well-lit office (600 lux), mesopic lighting equivalent to moonlight (about 0.7 lux), and after a sudden transition from the photopic to mesopic lighting (lights suddenly dimmed from 600 lux to about 0.7 lux). In the mobility test, subjects walked along a wooden sidewalk in the lab for several meters. A precision foot placement task required the subjects to step on the center of several irregularly spaced, low-contrast patches (20 cm by 15 cm in size) on the sidewalk. In the photopic lighting condition, the AMD and control subjects were about equally accurate in their foot placements. The controls continued to step accurately in the dim lighting and sudden transition conditions. But, the AMD subjects made greater foot-placement errors in the mesopic-lighting condition and even greater errors in foot placement in the sudden transition of lighting. The researchers also compared the performance of AMD subjects and controls in negotiating a step up or down (curb) on the sidewalk in the three lighting conditions. Here again, the AMD subjects exhibited greater deficits than the controls under the mesopic and sudden transition conditions. The Alexander study illustrates mobility deficits experienced by people with macular degeneration in low illumination and dark adaptation. Difficulties in accurate foot placement in uneven terrain or in negotiating steps in dim illumination are significant risk factors for falls and injuries.

Why might people with macular degeneration exhibit severe deficits under low illumination? We often think of the macula as a region dominated by the cone photoreceptors and specialized for high-acuity daylight vision. Shouldn't macular disease primarily affect daylight vision while leaving night vision intact? Although the fovea at the center of the macula is exclusively populated by cones, the macula as a whole contains many rods. Surprising to many, the rods outnumber the cones by about nine to one in the macula of young normally sighted adults, including a rod-dominated area surrounding the fovea (Curcio et al., 2000). It is now understood that macular degeneration, even in its early stages, involves the loss of rod photoreceptors in the macular region. It is likely that the loss of rod function in people with AMD has an adverse effect on mobility in dim light and in dark adaptation.

Lighting arrangement

The placement of lights in a space can also have an impact on low-vision mobility. While it is often assumed that diffuse overhead lighting is best for low vision, the strategic placement of directional lights can be used to highlight salient environmental features such as steps or hazards. Figure 7.3 illustrates the impact of the arrangement of lighting. In the three panels, we are looking up two steps into a windowless warehouse from a workroom below it. Overhead lights are on in the warehouse. The warehouse has a desk and a chair, but let's focus on the visibility of the steps. In the left panel, there is overhead lighting in the workroom behind us. This light illuminates both the treads and risers of the steps. Contrast of the steps is low, and visibility is poor. In the middle panel, the lights behind have been switched off and the lights above the steps have been turned on. This arrangement of lighting produces good contrast between the brighter treads and dimmer risers. In the right panel, daylight from the window on the left has been added to the artificial lighting of the scene. Step contrast is reduced compared with the middle panel. This is a case in which window daylighting actually reduces the visibility of the steps.

Glare

Bright lights, whether directional or diffuse, can sometimes cause visual discomfort, a situation termed discomfort glare or photophobia. Localized light sources, such as the sun, a spotlight, or a bright lamp, can produce two types of glare and adversely affect mobility. Veiling glare is a reduction of target contrast due to the addition of light from a bright nearby source. For example, bright light from a window, falling on a step ahead, might reduce the contrast

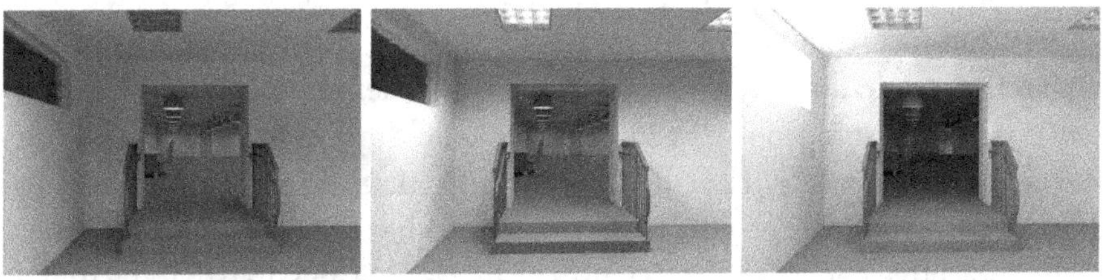

Figure 7.3 The three images show how variations in lighting arrangement can affect the visibility of steps.

between the step riser and the tread, making the step hard to see for someone with low contrast sensitivity. See, for example, the right panel in Figure 7.3. Similarly, glare light from a window, falling on a computer screen, might reduce the visibility of text on the screen.

Disability glare is a reduction of acuity or contrast sensitivity due to the presence of a bright light source somewhere in the visual field remote from the region of interest. A common example is bright sun, high in the sky, introducing glare that makes mobility along a sidewalk difficult. Light scatter in the eye due to advanced cataract can cause glare that produces the perception of halos or streaks around headlights or other bright sources and may reduce retinal-image contrast. People with advanced cataract and some forms of retinal disease—RP, macular degeneration, or diabetic retinopathy—may experience disability glare. They may try to avoid facing windows or shield their eyes from bright lights during mobility. They may wear baseball caps or side shields on their glasses to cut down on sun glare. I suffer from disability glare and use these strategies. If the sun is anywhere in my visual field, I'm in visual trouble. When I spent a visiting year in Cambridge, England, during the autumn and early winter, the sun remained close to the horizon throughout the day because of England's northern latitude. My mobility was adversely affected by the low sun angle and the short period of daylight.

Although disability glare is known to be an important mobility problem in some forms of low vision, there has been little research, with most of the empirical work on glare having been devoted to topics relevant to normal vision such as the effects of oncoming headlights in driving and refractive surgery. The best clinical tests of disability glare compare visual acuity or letter contrast sensitivity with and without an adjacent glare source (Elliott & Bullimore, 1993).

Sometimes, people with low vision who complain of glare are prescribed color-tinted lenses. The best known of these are the Corning Photochromic Filters (CPFs) and the NoIR filters from No-IR Medical. The CPFs cut out short-wavelength blue light and are said to reduce glare and protect the retina from ultraviolet or blue-light toxicity. It has been difficult for vision researchers to definitively demonstrate improvements in acuity or contrast sensitivity with tinted lenses. A 2002 review article by Frank Eperjesi and colleagues at Aston University in the UK concluded that "... a substantial amount of research has produced equivocal results and has failed to prove any consistent objective benefit of tinted lenses or filters." It is possible that the tinted lenses contribute to visual comfort even if they don't enhance performance on tests of acuity or contrast sensitivity.

Impact of deficits in acuity, contrast sensitivity, and field

There is a consensus among experts on low vision that deficits in contrast sensitivity and restriction of the visual field have more deleterious effects on mobility than reduced acuity. Why might this be the case? Suppose you have reduced acuity but good contrast sensitivity and a wide visual field. Reduced acuity means you need to be closer to a mobility hazard to see it. Mobility involves moving toward things—posts, chairs, other people, etc. If your acuity reduction is not too severe, your approach will eventually bring you close enough to the obstacle to see and avoid it. You will not see the object from as great a distance as a normally sighted person, but often, you will see obstacles in time to avoid bumping into them. Results from the Salisbury Eye Evaluation Study, a population-based study of 2,520 older adults, indicated that people were not much disabled in mobility tasks unless acuity was poorer than 20/200 (West et al., 2002).

Now, suppose you have a loss of contrast sensitivity. Even objects within your acuity range will not be visible if the obstacle has low contrast with its background. In Chapter 3 (see Figure 3.1), I described the example of my black cat Hudson. I have tripped over him when he is lying on our black slate floor, but he is easy for me to see at a greater distance when he has high contrast lying on our white bedspread.

Finally, imagine you have a narrow field of view, sometimes the case in RP or glaucoma. Even if your acuity and contrast sensitivity are quite good within your remaining narrow field, obstacles on the floor or to your left or right might fall outside your field of view. You might easily miss seeing a tripping hazard on the floor immediately ahead or a person or a post to your left or right. In a study simulating field restriction with the use of immersive virtual reality technology, Shirin Hassan (2007) and colleagues found that mobility in an obstacle course was impaired if the field of view was less than 30 degrees for low-contrast obstacles.

In the mobility study led by Thomas Kuyk, described earlier, subjects with low vision were given tests of acuity, contrast sensitivity, color discrimination, and extent of the visual field (Goldmann perimetry). The investigators wanted to know which of these visual measures were most associated with good or poor mobility performance. They also conducted a test of visual scanning. The test required a subject to find high-contrast numerals superimposed in random locations on a photograph of a street scene. How many numerals could the subject find in a ten-second interval? Kuyk and colleagues discovered that measures of visual-field extent and scanning ability were better predictors of a subject's mobility performance than measures of acuity or contrast sensitivity. Subjects with narrower visual fields made more mobility errors, while those with better scanning performance made fewer mobility errors.

Why does scanning help with mobility? Perhaps, people with narrow visual fields can compensate for their field restriction by strategic gaze shifts. Indeed, the study by Gang Luo (2008) and colleagues mentioned in Chapter 4 showed that RP subjects with very narrow fields do shift their gaze to look at portions of a scene outside their field of view. Similarly, a team led by Colas Authié (2017) in Paris showed that subjects with RP and narrow fields (10 to 25 degrees) used head and eye gaze strategies while navigating around obstacles and through open doors.

If deliberate scanning helps, then people with low vision might do better in spotting mobility hazards if they learn to employ more systematic gaze strategies while walking. Richard Ludt and Gregory Goodrich (2002) at the Western Blind Rehabilitation Center in Palo Alto, California, asked whether low-vision mobility would improve with instruction in scanning. They tested 65 older subjects, with mean age of 72.4 years, the majority with AMD. The subjects walked outdoor routes similar to those used by Kuyk and colleagues. The subjects were asked to stop and point whenever they noticed a hazard ahead. The hazards were curbs, objects on the ground, and a foam tube hanging from a tree at head height. The experimenters measured the distances at which the subjects noticed the obstacles. If the subject entirely missed seeing an obstacle, the detection distance was scored as zero. The subjects were tested before and after a training period. The training consisted of instructions to "scan the sidewalk, head to toe, for anything that's in your way" including separate instructions to look for obstacles at head level, street level, and drop-offs. Following the training, the average hazard-detection distances more than doubled. Some hazards that were entirely missed on the pretest were noticed at a distance that would enable subjects to safely avoid them. This study implies that deliberate effort in scanning the environment with eye or head movements enhances mobility safety for people with low vision.

While deliberate scanning strategies may be helpful to compensate for field loss while walking, the effort may be cognitively demanding or distracting. A friend with field loss told me that he deliberately scans the scene at critical points such as a street crossing, but he doesn't deploy scanning most of the time while walking along the sidewalk because it slows him down and demands too much of his attention.

Visual accessibility

Society can facilitate safe and effective mobility for people with low vision through environmental design.

Everyone is familiar with environmental modifications that enhance physical accessibility. Ramps are often easier than steps. There are design standards and guidelines for accessible door handles, the height and position of buttons on elevators, the width of doors and hallways, and wheelchair space for audience seating in auditoriums. By analogy, what aspects of environmental design enhance visual accessibility?

Visual accessibility of an architectural space refers to design features, which enable the use of vision to travel efficiently and safely through the space, to perceive the spatial layout of key features in the space, and to keep track of one's location and orientation within the space. The visual accessibility of a space depends on five major factors—(1) the vision status of the pedestrian (including their acuity, contrast sensitivity, and integrity of the visual field); (2) geometrical properties of the architecture (including landmarks, objects, and obstacles); (3) nature and variation of lighting (both natural and artificial); (4) surface properties (including color, texture, and gloss); and (5) contextual cues. An example of a contextual cue is a highly visible handrail indicating the presence of steps, even if the steps themselves are difficult to see.

I led an interdisciplinary research team studying visual accessibility for people with low vision. Our team included experts in vision science, cognitive science, computer science, and lighting design, with team members from the University of Minnesota, the University of Utah, and Indiana University. One major goal of our research was to identify cognitive and perceptual principles that may help architects to enhance the visual accessibility of their designs for people with low vision. These principles were reviewed by Creem-Regehr et al. (2021).

When we began work on visual accessibility, we soon discovered three reasons why enhancing visual accessibility in public spaces is a challenge. First, even in seemingly simple spaces, the five factors listed above interact in complex ways. Second, vision scientists have surprisingly little insight into the real-world visual cues determining accessibility for people with low vision. Third, the introspection of normally sighted professionals in relevant disciplines, such as architects or lighting designers or even rehabilitation specialists, is not a reliable guide for predicting problems of visual accessibility for people with low vision.

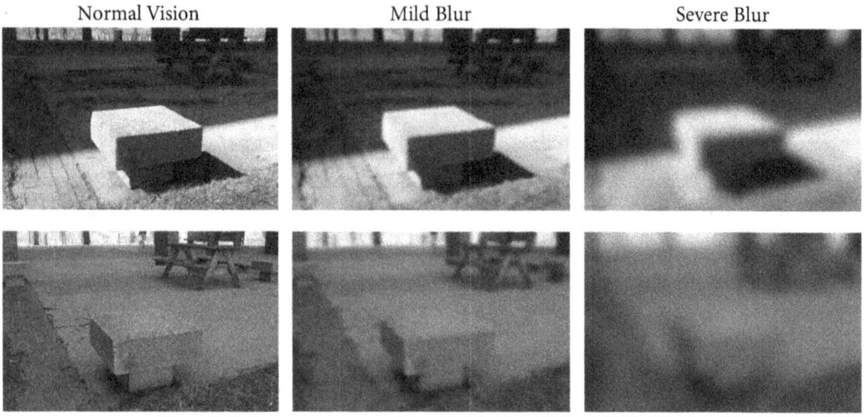

Figure 7.4 Photos of an outdoor bench in bright sunlight and overcast conditions, shown with mild and severe blur.

Hazard visibility is a major problem for low vision. Figure 7.4 illustrates an example of a potential visual hazard. The photos show an outdoor bench near my campus building, one photo taken on a bright, sunny day and the other on an overcast day. The second and third columns show the effects of mild and severe blur, simulating mild and severe acuity loss. In the sunny image, the high-contrast shadow at the front of the bench and the dark background from the building shadow provide good cues for the presence of the bench. These cues are still visible with reduced acuity as illustrated in the blurred images but rely on the presence of directional lighting from the sun. In more uniform lighting, as seen in the overcast photo, the contrast cues are diminished. The visibility of the bench is seriously compromised when acuity is reduced. I can testify personally to how painful it can be to miss seeing this bench.

Bumping into obstacles is a problem, but failing to see steps can be disastrous. Steps in an open lobby with patterned carpeting are hard to see and dangerous if missed. Similarly, cement steps in an open plaza or patio can be hard to see. Earlier in this chapter, I mentioned studies in my laboratory examining the visibility of ramps and steps. One dominant finding that will not surprise most people with low vision: A step down is usually harder to see than a step up.

Figure 7.5 shows an example of this asymmetry in the visibility of steps. An outdoor staircase has been photographed from above and from below. The mild and severely blurred versions of the photos simulate the loss of visual information associated with mild and severe acuity reduction. Even with severe blur, the steps going up are easier to see because the sunlit risers on the steps appear as high-contrast horizontal bands. The same stairs, seen from above, are invisible in severe blur.

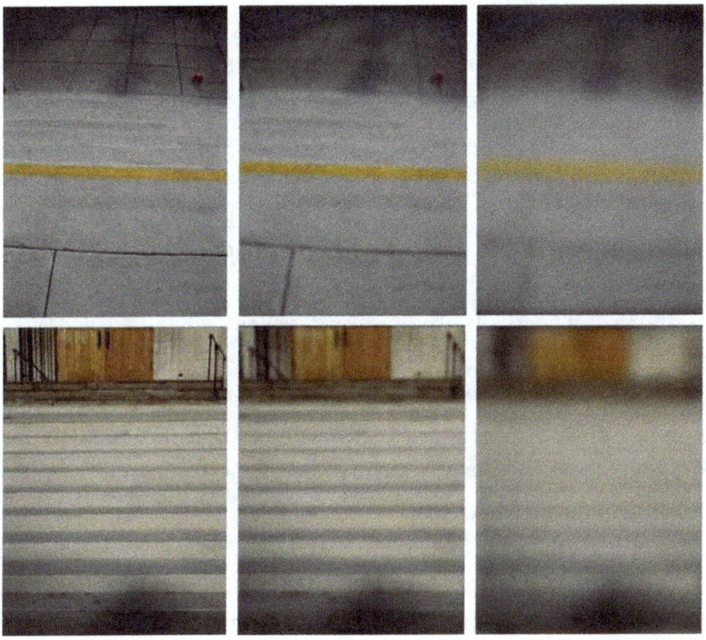

Figure 7.5 Photos of an outdoor staircase, taken from above and below, also shown with mild and severe blur.

A common strategy for enhancing the visibility of a step or flight of stairs, viewed from above, is to add a high-contrast stripe along the lip (edge) of each step. Might other marking patterns on steps be even better? Deyue Yu (2024) at The Ohio State University led a team that evaluated several additional types of markings including stripes from the back to the front of each step and diamond patterns on the steps. Across several viewing conditions, the edge stripes were the best. They also found that high-contrast baseboards on the left and right sides of the stairs enhanced judgments of the steepness of a flight of stairs.

Recommendations for enhancing visual accessibility for low vision were made in a 2015 report by the National Institute of Building Sciences (NIBS). Existing standards for visual accessibility in public spaces rely primarily on ensuring adequate light levels. A more comprehensive assessment of visual accessibility needs to take into account the vision status of the pedestrian and also the visual size and contrast of environmental features as seen by a pedestrian along a travel path. This level of analysis has typically not been practical in modern architectural design. An outcome of our research project, described by Thompson et al. (2021), is computer software for estimating the visibility of architectural hazards for people with different levels of vision impairment. The software is intended for use in conjunction with computer-aided design, when building layout and lighting can be simulated and easily modified. The user of our software (an architect or lighting designer) is asked to select a pedestrian's viewing location, a scene for evaluation, and the acuity and contrast sensitivity for a category of low vision. The software flags hazards or other features in the scene that are likely to be unseen by someone below a specified level of acuity such as 20/200. There is work to be done to validate this software and to determine its effectiveness in the hands of architects. The broader point is that there is a need for new quantitative tools for analyzing the visual accessibility of public spaces.

Wayfinding involves navigating to a building destination such as a doctor's office or the departure gate at an airport. An important aspect of successful wayfinding in public spaces is the ability to read directional signs. Imagine, for example, finding your way in an airport or medical center without being able to read the signs. The Americans with Disabilities Act (ADA) mandates the use of tactile signage for room numbers but not for directional signs for wayfinding. Tactile signs are valuable but have their limitations. They are often hard to find, even if the user expects them to be present, and many visually impaired people don't read Braille or have trouble with embossed printed characters. Most people with mild-or-moderate low vision prefer to read signs visually. In a 2017 article, Aries Arditi reviewed the current ADA standards for signage and their limitations. He pointed out that very little attention has been devoted to guidelines to enhance the accessibility of signage for people with low vision. In his article, Arditi made two proposals for public signage. First, acceptable signage should take into account the actual viewing distances and lighting conditions in which the sign is used rather than the current generic specifications of character size. This proposal would require on-site review. Second, directional signs, used for wayfinding, should be placed at a consistent height and in an approachable location so that people with low vision can get close enough to the sign for reading. I would add a third proposal: That the color of the sign itself should be chosen to contrast with its background. A white sign on a white wall is hard to see from a distance, while a black sign on a white wall is much easier to find. Good contrast is therefore important in two ways: for reading the words on the sign and for finding the sign on the wall.

In this chapter, we've been talking about mobility on foot, indoors, and outdoors. In our modern society, motor vehicles play a major role in mobility. In the next chapter, we'll consider driving with low vision.

8
Mobility and Low Vision

Let's Go for a Drive

For many people, driving is a necessity and a symbol of independence. Giving up driving can have a major impact on daily life. How do deficits in acuity, contrast sensitivity, and field restriction affect driving ability? Surprising to many, there are people with low vision who continue to drive safely. What technology is available to support their safe and effective driving? Let's look at these questions in this chapter.

• • • • •

The car is king in North America. Many people consider a car necessary for work, shopping, social interaction, recreation, and vacations. Older people often stop driving because of the onset of low vision. Younger people with low vision may never drive.

Driving in North America is a symbol of independence and personal freedom. Termination of a person's license can be psychologically devastating. It can be accompanied by social isolation and depression. I asked a friend how he felt about no longer driving. He is a man in his early 70s with the recent onset of low vision. He said, "It has had a big impact. It made me feel that my world was getting smaller. ... I really miss the freedom." Cessation of driving can be linked to health status and quality of life. Many people live farther from their families than in past generations. They may live in rural areas, senior residences, or town houses that are beyond walking distance from grocery stores, pharmacies, and places of worship.

What about alternatives to driving for getting around? Public transportation is of variable quality in urban settings and often nonexistent in suburban or rural areas. Some communities have special services such as Metro Mobility in the Twin Cities where I live. Carpooling can be an informal option. The advent of rideshare services such as Uber and Lyft has been a boon to many people who are blind or have low vision and who live in urban communities. It should be noted, however, that some people with dog guides have been denied service by rideshare drivers.

Low Vision. Gordon E. Legge, Oxford University Press. © Oxford University Press (2026).
DOI: 10.1093/9780198946960.003.0009

Are there drivers who have low vision?

Should people with low vision be allowed to drive? When I discuss this with students in my classes, opinions vary. Several questions usually arise.

If people fail the vision-screening test, should they be denied a license? Maybe not. Most of the existing vision criteria are not decisive in assessing driving ability and are not evidence-based. Instead, failure in vision screening could be a trigger for a more individualized assessment, involving an eye exam and an individual on-the-road test.

Should eye doctors report to the motor vehicle authorities on a patient whom they think should not be driving? Some U.S. states and Canadian provinces have mandatory reporting. Is this reporting a violation of a patient's privacy, or is it justified on the grounds of public safety?

What level of risk should we tolerate in allowing a particular demographic group to drive? It seems likely that reduced vision would enhance crash risk to some degree. How much risk? Compared with the safest group, would we tolerate five times the crash risk? One measure of risk is the number of crashes per million miles driven. U.S. data for 2014–2015 indicate that the safest group of drivers is aged 60–69 years, with only 2.4 crashes per million miles driven (Tefft, 2017). For 16–17-year-olds, the crash rate is almost six times higher. For 25–29-year-olds, the crash rate is more than twice that of the 60–69–year-olds. For drivers over 80 years, the crash rate is 1.8 times higher. We tolerate substantially elevated crash risks for young drivers. We don't have comparable crash risk data for drivers with low vision.

When considering whether any particular group should be allowed to drive—teenagers, octogenarians, people with low vision or other physical or cognitive disabilities—we must consider the social and economic benefit to the members of the group as well as the risk of injury to themselves or others.

How many people with low vision drive? Information to answer this question is scant. In one study, Joshua Robinson (2021) and colleagues at Vanderbilt University in Nashville, Tennessee, surveyed 335 consecutive adult low-vision patients at the Vanderbilt Eye Institute. The survey asked about driving habits and compared the responses with measures of acuity, contrast sensitivity, and field. Perhaps, surprisingly, 257 of the participants (76.7%) held an unexpired driver's license. Of them, 134 were current drivers. Of the 134 drivers, 95 met the vision requirements for a license in their state and 39 did not. Most of the participants in the Robinson study were from Tennessee, where the vision requirement for a driver's license is a monocular acuity of 20/40 or binocular acuity of 20/60. Most of the drivers had mild vision impairment. The 257 participants with valid licenses had a mean acuity of 20/52 (6/15.6). This study suggests that a substantial number of people with mild low vision continue to drive.

Visual requirements for driving

What should be the visual requirements for driving? Should people with specific levels of reduced acuity, reduced contrast sensitivity, or field loss be denied a license to drive? What is the evidence supporting existing visual requirements for a driver's license? In 2010, Cynthia Owsley and Gerald McGwin at the University of Alabama at Birmingham (UAB) reviewed the research literature on driving and visual impairment. While it stands to reason that people with severe low vision would not be safe drivers, it has been difficult to establish definitively that mild or moderate forms of vision impairment have adverse effects on driving safety.

Acuity reduction

In the U.S., many states have a requirement of best-corrected visual acuity of 20/40 or better for an unrestricted noncommercial driver's license. Nevertheless, the evidence for an association between acuity and driving safety in the range of 20/40 to 20/200 is minimal.

Concerns about discrimination against people with vision disabilities have raised questions about denying licenses to people with mild or moderate acuity reduction. Most states now allow some people with milder forms of low vision to drive, often with some restrictions. These may include daytime driving only or prohibition from highway or freeway driving. Granting a restricted license to someone with low vision may depend on their performance in a road test.

It is ironic that acuity remains the primary screening test for a driver's license, despite a lack of definitive data showing a correlation between safety and acuity. There are two likely reasons for this surprising lack of association. First, safe driving may not usually demand high acuity. Crash avoidance generally involves seeing relatively large objects such as other vehicles at a safe distance. Box 8.1 presents examples implying that someone with an acuity of 20/200 would be expected to see vehicles ahead at a safe distance. Avoiding collision with a small person, an animal, or debris on the road might put a more stringent demand on visual acuity.

Box 8.1 Seeing cars ahead on the road

A conservative rule of thumb, promoted by the American Association of Retired People (AARP), is that a driver should maintain a three-second gap behind the vehicle ahead. At a highway speed of 60 miles per hour, three seconds corresponds to 264 feet (about 80 meters). At what distance would a person with 20/200 acuity be able to see a car ahead? A typical car is about 6 feet in width. An object of this size viewed from 400 feet would subtend the same visual angle as a 20/200 acuity letter. So, in principle, a person with 20/200 vision would be able to detect a car ahead at a distance of 264 feet. In my hometown of Minneapolis, the city authorities instituted a "Twenty is Plenty" rule, a speed limit of 20 miles per hour in residential areas. At this speed, a three-second following distance would be close to 90 feet, a distance at which a person with 20/200 vision would easily see a car or truck ahead. Of course, cars on the road may often be harder to see than acuity letters on an eye chart due to the car's color, prevailing lighting, and weather conditions. Factors in addition to simple detection are also important for safety; for example, is the car ahead slowing down or braking?

Second, measurement of acuity in the eye clinic may not be representative of the visual demands of driving. Not only are the obstacles of interest—cars, bicycles, pedestrians—likely to be in motion, but the driver is also in motion. Research has shown that deficits in motion perception may contribute more to crash risk than mild acuity reduction.

Moreover, people with reduced acuity tend to self-limit their driving, often choosing to drive only in daylight or in familiar areas for reasons of safety. Some lifelong drivers with late-onset low vision may elect to stop driving altogether. My father was an experienced and good driver well into his seventies when he began experiencing vision impairment from macular degeneration. One day, he had a scare. While negotiating a construction zone, he narrowly missed hitting a flagman. He decided then and there to stop driving. Fortunately, he lived in Toronto, a large city with good public transportation. He adapted well to life without a car.

Perhaps, the most-demanding role for acuity in driving is reading signs. Sometimes, the color or shape of the sign conveys its message, removing the need to read the text. But, the characters on road signs are designed to be legible at appropriate distances by people with acuity better than 20/40. Reading the street names or numbers on signs is often important for finding your way to your destination or for learning about detours or road conditions ahead. Drivers with low vision may often have trouble reading the text on road signs because of inadequate acuity. At a conference a few years ago, I heard an eye-care professional tell this story. Her eye clinic was empty on a snowy day; many patients had canceled their appointments because of the weather. The only patient who arrived was a man with low vision who had driven 50 miles on the freeway. He had not seen the "Road Closed" signs. He commented on how light the traffic was.

The widespread availability of talking GPS software proves especially helpful to low-vision drivers as an alternative to reading signs. Not only can the software plan a route to the destination, but it can also alert the driver when a turn is required or when the speed limit changes. This is an instance in which mainstream technology has particular benefits for people with low vision.

Field loss

Many states also have a visual-field requirement for a driver's license, for the horizontal binocular field of view. This requirement is typically about 100 degrees but ranges from 60 to 150 degrees. Why is a wide field necessary for driving? Possibly to see a car approaching at an uncontrolled intersection or to spot a pedestrian entering the traffic lane from the side. At night, the effective field of view is limited primarily by the horizontal spread of the headlight pattern rather than by the driver's own visual field. According to an estimate cited by Wilkinson and McGehee (2019), the effective horizontal field of view at night from car headlights is between 35 and 45 degrees, very narrow compared with the binocular visual field of a person with normal vision.

A review of the five-year at-fault motor-vehicle crash involvement of 2,000 drivers in Alabama over 70 years of age indicated that crash risk was higher for 206 people in the group with glaucoma (Kwon et al., 2016). Among the glaucoma group, those with severe field restriction had substantially higher crash involvement. Owsley and McGwin (2010) reviewed several research studies examining the relationship between peripheral-field restriction and crash risk, much of it focusing on drivers with glaucoma. While severe binocular-field loss likely enhances risk, it is unclear whether mild forms of field loss affect driver safety.

What about drivers with a loss of central vision? In Chapter 5, we saw that people who lose their central vision from macular degeneration or other macular disorders often adopt a point of fixation in peripheral vision, usually near the edge of the blind spot (scotoma). This newly adopted point of fixation is termed the preferred retinal locus (PRL). Figure 8.1 is a schematic diagram illustrating four general cases for the location of the PRL relative to

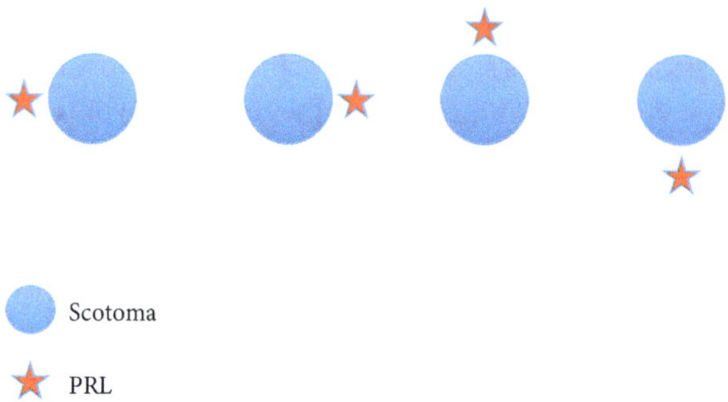

Figure 8.1 A schematic drawing of a blind spot in central vision (scotoma) with an adjacent point of fixation, termed a preferred retinal locus (PRL). Four cases are illustrated with the PRL to the left, right, above, and below the scotoma. This is a simplified representation. Central scotomas may have many shapes, and PRLs can be found near the boundary of the scotoma in any direction.

the scotoma; the PRL may be located to the left, right, above, or below the scotoma in the visual field. Imagine a driver with central-vision loss who is looking at the road ahead with their PRL. What features of the scene might be hidden by their scotoma? What hazards might be missed? When the PRL is to the left of the scotoma, objects to the right side of the road might be missed. Similarly, for a PRL to the right of the scotoma, objects on the left, potentially in the opposite lane, might be missed. What if the PRL is above the scotoma? If the driver is fixated on the road ahead, the visibility of objects in the lower field would be hindered, possibly including the road immediately in front of the car and the driver's dashboard. For a PRL below the scotoma, objects in the upper visual field might be occluded.

P. Matthew Bronstad (2013, 2015) and colleagues at the Schepens Eye Research Institute in Boston tested subjects with central-vision loss in a driving simulator. The display had a wide horizontal field exceeding 180 degrees. All the subjects were experienced drivers, although some were not currently driving. Simulator testing involved rural- and city-driving scenarios in daylight situations. The scenarios included virtual pedestrians crossing the road ahead on a collision course with the driver's car. The subjects were asked to press the horn when they saw a pedestrian. Groups of subjects were tested with the four categories of PRL in relation to the central scotoma illustrated in Figure 8.1. The investigators measured the drivers' reaction times for pressing the horn and the number of virtual pedestrians entirely missed. The experimenters also tested an age-matched control group with normal vision.

All four groups with central-vision loss had longer reaction times than the normally sighted control group. Similar to the controls, subjects with PRLs above or below the scotoma detected nearly 100% of the virtual pedestrians. The subjects with PRLs to the left or right of the central scotoma missed seeing some of the virtual pedestrians, presumably, when they were hidden by the scotoma. These results indicate that the pattern of central-vision loss, especially the location of the PRL relative to the scotoma, can have an impact on driving safety.

Do the Bronstad findings suggest that people with central-vision loss should not drive? Are they a danger to themselves and to others? A mitigating factor is the tendency for people with visual impairment to self-limit their time on the road. Dawn DeCarlo (2003) and colleagues reported that some patients with age-related macular degeneration (AMD) who visited the low-vision clinic at the UAB were still licensed drivers. Most of them had drastically restricted their driving activity. Eighty percent reported not driving at night, and most drove only about 10 miles per week.

Joanne Wood (2018) from the Queensland University of Technology in Brisbane, Australia, and colleagues reported on a study comparing driving safety ratings of a group of 33 subjects with AMD and a group of age-matched controls with normal, healthy vision. The subjects were evaluated by trained instructors during on-road driving in urban and suburban areas. The instructors provided safety ratings and counted driving errors. The AMD drivers in this study had early forms of macular degeneration; all had acuities better than 20/40 and none had central scotomas. As a group, the AMD drivers received significantly lower safety ratings than the controls and committed more driving errors, but many of the individual AMD drivers were rated as safe to drive.

Contrast sensitivity and glare

When might reduced contrast sensitivity pose a problem while driving? Possibly when spotting a white car in snow, or a snowplow in a blizzard, or a vehicle in fog, or a dark obstruction on black asphalt, or a biker or pedestrian with dark clothing at night? Few, if any, licensing authorities test for contrast sensitivity.

Similarly, glare can pose problems for drivers. Sources of glare include the sun (especially near the horizon at sunrise or sunset) in the face of the driver and oncoming headlights at night. I am unaware of any licensing authorities that administer glare tests for drivers.

Cataract can result in reduced contrast sensitivity and problems with glare. About half of the people over 75 years of age have clinically significant cataracts at some point. Undoubtedly, many older drivers have cataracts.

What is the impact on driving, and does surgery to remove cataracts reduce crash risk? Cynthia Owsley (2002) and colleagues at UAB analyzed crash statistics for three groups of drivers—those with cataract who elected to have surgery to remove the cataract, those with cataract who did not have surgery, and age-matched controls with no cataract or other eye disorders. The researchers analyzed five-year crash involvement based on publicly available police reports on auto accidents. Compared with normally sighted controls, drivers with cataracts prior to surgery drove less but had higher crash rates. The crash rate for the group who had cataract surgery was cut in half following the surgery compared with the cataract group who did not have surgery. This study was a rare demonstration of a therapeutic intervention that reduced crash risk.

Other factors

In their 2010 review of research on vision and driving, Owsley and McGwin considered several other factors potentially affecting driving safety. There is little evidence that deficits in color vision or binocularity (including stereopsis) affect driving. Problems with divided attention may account in part for increased crash rates in older drivers (Owsley et al., 1998). The use of cell phones by normally sighted drivers has emerged as a problem of divided attention. Even hands-free use of a cell phone by a driver has been shown to increase crash risk. Pedestrian mobility can also be affected by cell phone use. A blind friend of mine referred to the "temporary blindness" of a normally sighted person who was glued to their cell phone and who bumped heavily into my friend on the sidewalk.

As mentioned earlier, deficits in visual motion perception may enhance crash risk. Joanne Wood (2021) and her colleagues have shown that drivers with eye disease have slower reaction times in a test of hazard perception. These slower responses are associated with decreased sensitivity to visual motion. But to date, there are no standardized tests of motion perception for drivers.

Finally, the nature and extent of eye and head movements are relevant to vision and driving. People who have peripheral-field loss as in glaucoma or retinitis pigmentosa, or central-vision loss from macular degeneration, or hemianopia, may be able to compensate for the loss of a full visual field by strategic scanning of the eyes or head. Whether drivers with field loss learn novel scanning patterns spontaneously is unclear. Whether a training procedure would be helpful is uncertain.

Technologies to assist drivers with low vision

Mainstream technology to assist all drivers has advanced rapidly. Pushed by the U.S. federal government and the insurance industry, automakers have made several types of advanced driver assistance features standard on passenger vehicles. There is evidence that these features reduce crash risk and injuries. These features may be especially helpful for drivers with low vision. A team at four U.S. institutions, led by Rebecca Deffler (2022) at The Ohio State University, surveyed 166 current drivers, 80 with AMD and 86 with no known eye disease, about their use of and attitudes toward driver assistance technologies. The technologies in the survey were forward collision warning, forward collision avoidance, blind spot warning, lane departure warning, rearview camera, cruise control, adaptive cruise control, and GPS navigation. For the most part, the AMD group made similar use and had similar positive attitudes toward the advanced technologies as the group without eye disease. The most-commonly used technologies by both groups were GPS, cruise control, and the rearview camera. Surprisingly, the AMD group made less use of GPS and cruise control than the group with no eye disease. Perhaps, the difference was because the AMD participants drove less overall, preferred to drive in familiar areas, and tried to avoid highway driving.

Jing Xu (2022, 2023) from the Envision Research Institute in Wichita, Kansas, and the Schepens Eye Research Institute in Boston described the experiences of a low-vision driver who used the advanced auto-assist features of a Tesla Model Y car. The driver was a 53-year-old man with Stargardt disease and a recent reduction of acuity to 20/182 (6/55). He was an experienced driver. It took him three months to master the automation features of the car. His favorite features were Traffic-Aware Cruise Control, Forward Collision Avoidance, and Lane Departure Avoidance. He also made use of the car's Traffic Light and Stop Sign Control system to stop the car when he missed seeing traffic signals. Using the Navigate on the Autopilot feature, he was confident in driving on interstate highways. He described his new approach to driving as co-driving; the automation handled many routine driving tasks while he granted permission and supervised these operations. His major concern was with the lack of visual accessibility of the car's video screen. He was unable to read warning messages while driving; he could only read them after stopping when he could use a magnifier. He wanted better auditory access to the interface. Overall, the car's automation enhanced his confidence and ability to drive safely. He commented to the researchers that "having these systems is like having a second pair of eyes. The car definitely added an extra layer of

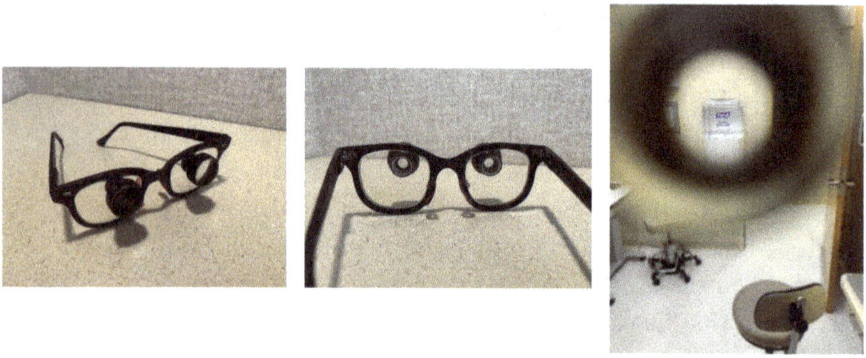

Figure 8.2 The left panel shows an overview of prescription glasses with small, bioptic telescopes on each lens. The middle panel shows a wearer's view from behind the glasses. The right panel shows an example of views through the main lens and the bioptic telescope.

safety in addition to my own vision." While this is an encouraging case study illustrating the benefits of driver-assist features for one low-vision driver, Xu and colleagues caution that it is too soon to generalize to people with other forms of low vision.

Most research on driving and low vision has focused on safety-related issues. Another important issue is the impact of low vision on following a route and finding the way to a destination. Wayfinding in unfamiliar environments often requires good acuity for reading street signs and addresses or for recognizing landmarks. Drivers with reduced acuity may minimize wayfinding problems by limiting their driving to familiar neighborhoods.

Bioptic telescopes are used by some low-vision drivers to compensate for their reduced acuity. The left panel of Figure 8.2 shows a pair of bioptic telescopes mounted on prescription glasses. The middle panel shows the bioptic telescopes as seen by a wearer putting the glasses on. The right panel shows an example of the view of the office through the main lens and the magnified view through the telescope. In more typical use, a single bioptic telescope is mounted on one lens only.

The bioptic telescope is mounted on the top of the regular prescription lens and blocks only a small portion of the field of view seen through the prescription lens. The telescope typically has a power of 2X to 4X. This level of magnification is helpful for people with mild acuity reduction. Most of the time, the low-vision driver looks through the prescription lens. But, when magnification is required to see a high-acuity target, the low-vision driver tilts their head down slightly to look through the bioptic telescope. Because the effective field of view through the telescope is reduced, the driver minimizes time looking through it, typically using it for only one or two seconds at a time. Training is required to make safe and effective use of bioptic telescopes. Training may begin with spotting static objects while standing still, then using the telescope as a passenger in a moving car, and then finally as a driver.

As of 2004, there were an estimated 4,000–5,000 drivers using bioptic telescopes in the United States (Huss & Corn, 2004). The number is now likely to be greater. Bioptic telescopes for driving are legal in more than 40 states. Richard L. Windsor (2022) and colleagues provide information about the laws governing the use of bioptic telescopes in many states via the webpage Bioptic Driving USA.[1]

The use of bioptic telescopes for driving is permitted in some countries other than the United States such as Canada and the Netherlands but not others such as the United Kingdom.

It is generally believed that bioptic telescopes are used primarily to read street signs and monitor stoplights. But, a study led by Shuhang Wang (2020) at the Schepens Eye Research Institute in Boston analyzed hours of data from 19 bioptic telescope users during on-road driving. The drivers were licensed bioptic users recruited in Massachusetts, Ohio, and Quebec. Their acuities ranged from 20/60 to 20/160 (6/18 to 6/48). There were wide variations in the use of the bioptic telescopes across the group, but overall, the drivers used their telescopes only 1.6% of the time, and about 85% of the bioptic viewing was on the road far ahead. Perhaps, they were assessing distant traffic or looking ahead to spot the next intersection. Only about 10% of the bioptic use was for reading signs and monitoring stoplights. Most of the driving occurred in familiar areas, perhaps explaining the limited use of the telescopes for sign reading. Some of the drivers may have been relying on speech-based GPS navigation software as an alternative to using the telescopes for reading signs.

Is it safe to use bioptic telescopes while driving? In a 2019 article, Mark Wilkinson and Daniel McGehee at the University of Iowa raised concerns about the demands for divided attention. Swapping attention between a bioptic view while reading a sign for one or two seconds and looking through regular glasses at the road ahead might pose an issue for safety. They advocated the use of auditory GPS guidance as a safer alternative to reliance on bioptic telescopes for reading signs. While evidence shows that bioptics are certainly used for sign reading, this is not their only function. The Wang et al. (2020) study indicated that bioptics were also used for inspecting the road ahead. Two observational studies of actual on-road driving of bioptic

[1] http://www.biopticdrivingusa.com/state-laws/.

telescope users, one led by Joanne Wood (2013) using expert evaluators in the car and one led by Mojtaba Moharrer (2020) analyzing many hours of in-the-car video recordings, failed to find any significant difference in driving safety between groups of low-vision bioptic drivers and control groups with normal vision. These studies support the case for the safe use of bioptic telescopes by drivers with low vision.

While auditory instructions from GPS navigation apps may not entirely replace the value of bioptic telescopes, it seems likely that GPS navigation software can prove especially helpful to low-vision drivers. I asked a low-vision driver (acuity 20/80) how much her visual impairment affected her driving. She said "none." She went on to say that once she had GPS to help with navigation, she felt her impaired vision had no major impact on her driving. I'm not a driver, but as a passenger, I am sometimes able to use speech-based GPS software to assist the driver. Prior to the advent of GPS, I wasn't any help at all in reading roadmaps or spotting road signs. Now, I sometimes enjoy being the navigator!

It is also noteworthy that talking GPS apps on cell phones have proven useful in pedestrian mobility for people with visual impairments. I sometimes use a talking GPS app when I'm out walking. It alerts me to the next street crossing or to things I'm passing, such as the house address or the name of a store. In short, the app conveys information to me about features of my immediate environment that lie outside my range of vision.

What about the prospect of self-driving cars (also known as autonomous vehicles or driverless cars) for use by people who are blind or who have low vision? Wouldn't it be great if those of us with vision too poor to drive could get in a self-driving car, tell it our destination, and get there safely and independently? A widely viewed YouTube video[2] produced by Google in 2012 showed a blind man in a self-driving car making his way to Taco Bell. The implication was that the future of self-driving cars would provide independent mobility for blind people. There has been some push-back. A 2018 Associated Press News article (Dearen, 2018) quoted Anil Lewis, executive director of the National Federation of the Blind's Jernigan Institute, "Although we have been held up as obvious beneficiaries of the technology in conversations and presentations, this will have just been exploitation if the systems are not accessible. ... How about instead of Taco Bell, we demonstrate a blind person independently operating an autonomous vehicle, dropping off his/her kids at school on the way to work, and maybe stopping by a Starbucks on the way?" Why this skepticism? What are some of the accessibility

[2] https://www.youtube.com/watch?v=peDy2st2XpQ.

issues for visually impaired users of driverless cars? Imagine I call a rideshare company for a pickup and a self-driving car shows up. Here are some of my concerns:

How will I identify the driverless car when it arrives among busy traffic, and will I be safe in accessing the vehicle?

How will I communicate my destination and other information to the driverless car? Will it have effective voice-recognition software, or will I be expected to use a display screen?

What kind of information will the vehicle give me during the trip about where we are and my expected time of arrival?

How will I confirm that I've arrived at the correct destination? Will I be dropped off at a safe location? Where is the building entrance when I'm dropped off?

My accessibility concerns are framed in the broader context of completing a safe and successful door-to-door trip in the absence of assistance from a human rideshare driver. Researchers with an interest in independent mobility by visually impaired travelers are beginning to address these concerns. For example, Paul Fink (2023) and colleagues at the University of Maine have developed a prototype smartphone app, called the Autonomous Vehicle Assistant (AVA) that guides a visually impaired pedestrian to a recently arrived self-driving car.

Are people with vision impairment eager to use self-driving cars? There have been a few surveys to address this question. Abigail Kuborn and Shirin Hassan (2024) at Indiana University surveyed three groups on their perceptions of self-driving cars—51 sighted subjects, 68 visually impaired (low-vision) subjects, and 65 blind subjects. Overall, more of the visually impaired subjects (blind and low vision) were positive (70% of them) than the normally sighted subjects (37% of them). Among the visually impaired, those with more severe restrictions of acuity, contrast sensitivity, or field had greater positivity. This and other surveys confirm that people with impaired vision look forward to riding in self-driving cars. But, how soon is this likely to be a common experience? More than a decade after the famous Google video of the blind man in a self-driving car, very few self-driving cars are on the road, and few visually impaired people have ridden in them. I am skeptical that I will be taking a self-driving car to the grocery store or to a doctor's appointment anytime soon, but maybe I'll be surprised.

Let's return to that big question: Should people with low vision be allowed to drive? Many experts on driving and vision rehabilitation have addressed the issues and ethics surrounding visual criteria for driving, accident risks, and discrimination against the visually impaired. My personal view is that if drivers with any form of disability, including low vision, know the rules of the road and can demonstrate safe and effective on-road performance to a qualified driving evaluator, they should be granted a license to drive. Achieving the necessary driving proficiency might require some special training or the use of assistive technology such as bioptic telescopes or GPS navigation. If the person with low vision can demonstrate driving proficiency, give them the keys to the car and wish them well on their travels!

PART III

RECOVERY OF SIGHT?

9

Childhood Low Vision

A Moving Target

The causes of impaired vision in children are different from the age-related eye diseases that afflict older adults. Advances in pediatric ophthalmology over the past few decades have had an enormous impact on the spectrum of eye disorders affecting kids, from the management of congenital cataracts to the recognition and diagnosis of cortical visual impairment (CVI). In this chapter, I'll consider some of these intriguing and inspiring developments and the impact on the visual experiences of kids with low vision.

• • • • •

Some children lose their vision in accidents. One three-year-old toddler liked to spend time with his dad. The parents, Simon-René and Monique, had a small farm, which included a vineyard. The dad was a saddler, a harness maker, with a workshop in the house. The little boy liked to play with his father's tools. One day, he accidentally poked himself in his right eye with a sharp, curved knife called a serpette. His eye became infected and then his left eye as well. He lost vision in both eyes. The little boy's name was Louis Braille. Louis became totally blind following the accident. His biographer, C. Michael Mellor, told me that he found no mention of residual vision or even light perception in Louis's correspondence. Louis attended school for two years in his village of Coupvray, France. He learned the shapes of printed letters from embossed patterns created by his father with nails hammered into wood. Then, at the age of 10, he enrolled in the residential school for the blind in Paris.

As you probably know, Louis created the Braille code for tactile reading. He completed the first version at the age of 16 in 1825. Box 9.1 provides a summary of the Braille code followed by a few comments on Braille literacy. At first, the code was rejected by normally sighted teachers of the visually impaired. They argued that tactile reading should use the same letter shapes as printed letters. After all, the sighted teachers wanted to be able to easily read the tactile letters. Many educators of the day held that any tactile code for

Low Vision. Gordon E. Legge, Oxford University Press. © Oxford University Press (2026).
DOI: 10.1093/9780198946960.003.0010

reading should "talk to the fingers in the language of the eyes." It was Louis's genius to recognize that simple configurations of dots were more legible for touch and easier to write than embossed printed letters. Louis's story is told in Mellor's compelling biography, *Louis Braille: A Touch of Genius* (2006).

Box 9.1 The Braille code and Braille literacy

Braille is not a language like English or Spanish but a code for representing the written form of a language with tactile symbols. Braille characters consist of combinations of six dots, placed in a matrix of two columns and three rows, termed a Braille "cell." The 64 possible arrangements of dots in the Braille cell (including the blank cell) comprise the 64 characters of the Braille code. Twenty-six of these characters represent the 26 letters of the English alphabet (shown in Figure 9.1). Rather than designating different Braille characters for uppercase and lowercase letters, a capitalization marker preceding a letter indicates that it is uppercase. Several additional Braille characters are used for punctuation marks. Numbers are represented in Braille by using the first 10 letters of the alphabet to represent the digits 1, 2 ... 9, 0. Numbers are distinguished from letters by a number sign character before the number.

Braille has a contracted version and an uncontracted version (shown in Figure 9.1). In uncontracted Braille, called Grade 1 Braille, there is nearly a one-to-one correspondence between printed characters and Braille characters. (An exception is the capitalization character, which does not appear in print.) Contracted Braille, called Grade 2 Braille, is the standard version used in most books, magazines, and other literary material. Unified English Braille contains 172 contractions. Examples of several types of contractions are shown in Figure 9.1. Notice that some of the 64 Braille characters, not used as letters or punctuation marks, are used as contractions, e.g., separate characters for "the," "for," and "ing." The contractions serve three purposes: to reduce the bulk of Braille, to increase reading speed, and to reduce writing time, a particular issue for those who write Braille dot by dot with a slate and stylus. The contractions reduce the length of Braille texts by about 25% (Legge et al., 1999).

Braille literacy has declined in recent years with less than 10% of legally blind students in the United States learning Braille. Students with low vision may often prefer to read visually, taking advantage of computer-based magnification or electronic magnifiers. Others may prefer to rely on audio—computer-based text-to-speech and digital audio recordings. Nevertheless, there are many advocates for the value of Braille. Modern technology makes it possible to connect Braille displays to computers and mobile phones and to emboss computer text documents in Braille. For students who are unable to rely entirely on print reading, Braille reading remains a good option. While audio access to text is valuable, advocates for Braille maintain that "listening is not literacy."

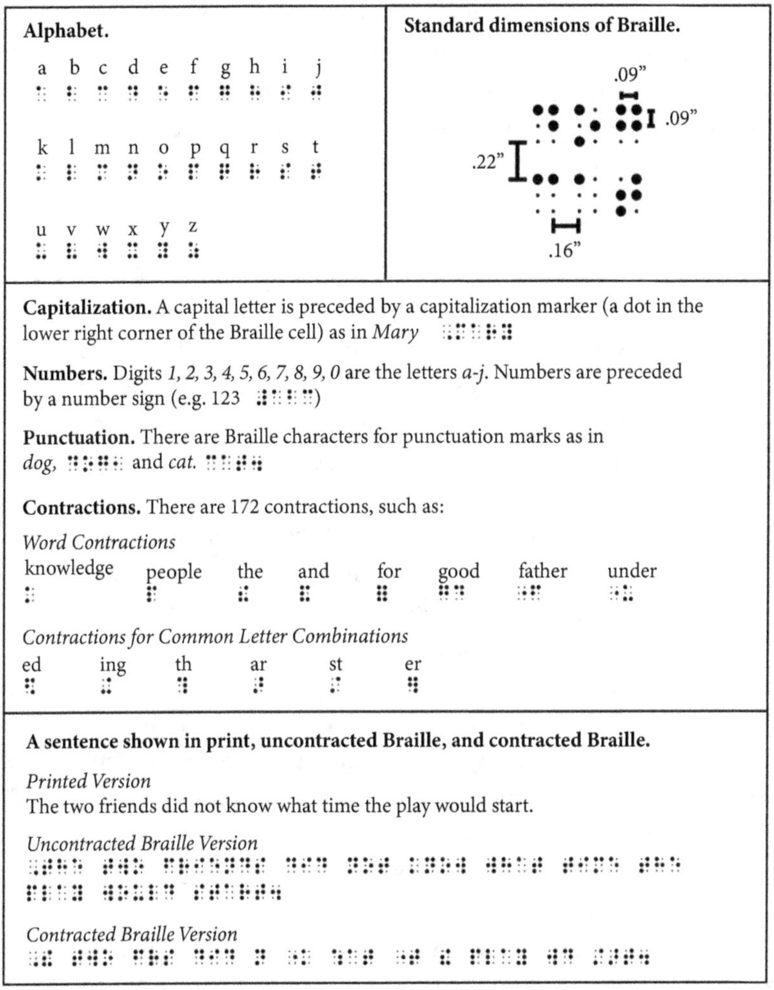

Figure 9.1 An overview of the Braille code. The six possible dot positions in each Braille cell are portrayed in outline with the actual dots shown in black. For instance, the Braille character with the top two dots of the cell represents the letter c. The top-left panel shows the Braille alphabet, and the top-right panel shows the standard dimensions of the Braille cell. The middle panel shows several features of the Braille code, including examples of the 172 contractions in Unified English Braille (UEB). The lower panel shows a printed sentence and its corresponding uncontracted and contracted Braille versions.

The Braille Challenge[1] (Braille Institute of America) is a competition meant to promote Braille literacy. Students from first grade to high school participate in activities demonstrating their skills in reading and writing Braille.

[1] https://brailleinstitute.org/braille-challenge/.

I learned Braille as a child while attending the Ontario School for the Blind. Throughout my life as a student and then as a university teacher and researcher, I've used Braille in addition to print reading and audio text to do my work. For example, when I deliver class lectures, I use Braille lecture notes, which are easier for me to access in class than printed notes or audio notes.

I had the pleasure of visiting Louis Braille's birthplace in Coupvray, just outside Paris. It is now a museum. My wife Wendy and I were the only visitors on a rainy day in August 2011. Our guide Amandine led us through the small house. She showed us many items from early 19th-century rural life in France, and several of Louis's works and inventions. Figure 9.2 is a photo of me in Simon-René's workshop where Louis's accident occurred.

I have friends of my own who lost vision in childhood accidents. Mike May lost vision at the age of three from a chemical accident and regained his vision 40 years later. His amazing story is told in Robert Kurson's book, *Crashing Through* (2007). We'll return to Mike's story in Chapter 10.

Most childhood low vision results from causes other than accidents. My own low vision is an example. I had healthy, normal vision during my early childhood. At the age of six, I survived a rare, life-threatening disease called Stevens–Johnson Syndrome (SJS), which left me with very low vision. When I was 19 years old, an unusual event gave me a new perspective on my childhood vision loss. I was seated in a row of chairs with a group of younger kids in a medical center. We were exhibits for ophthalmologists participating in continuing medical education. We were all survivors of SJS. We were there to demonstrate our eye conditions. I was the oldest in the group, and I had the most severe eye condition and lowest vision. I had survived SJS at the age of six, thanks to treatment with cortisone, a drug quite recently discovered and used to treat SJS. It was only after weeks of treatment, focusing on my survival, that the impact on my eyes was recognized. The younger kids in the workshop all had better vision than me because my case had brought attention to the risk to vision of SJS. The younger kids had received earlier and more effective eye treatment. In retrospect, I'm glad that my pioneering experience as a survivor of SJS contributed to more aggressive treatments to preserve vision for younger SJS patients.

Low vision in childhood is different from the experience of people who lose vision in adulthood. Unlike adults who may grieve the loss of their vision, children who acquire low vision early in life have little or no prior experience with normal vision. Their ability to cope with vision disability at home, in school, and in the community depends on the attitudes and actions of their parents. Some parents may fail to recognize or even deny their child's

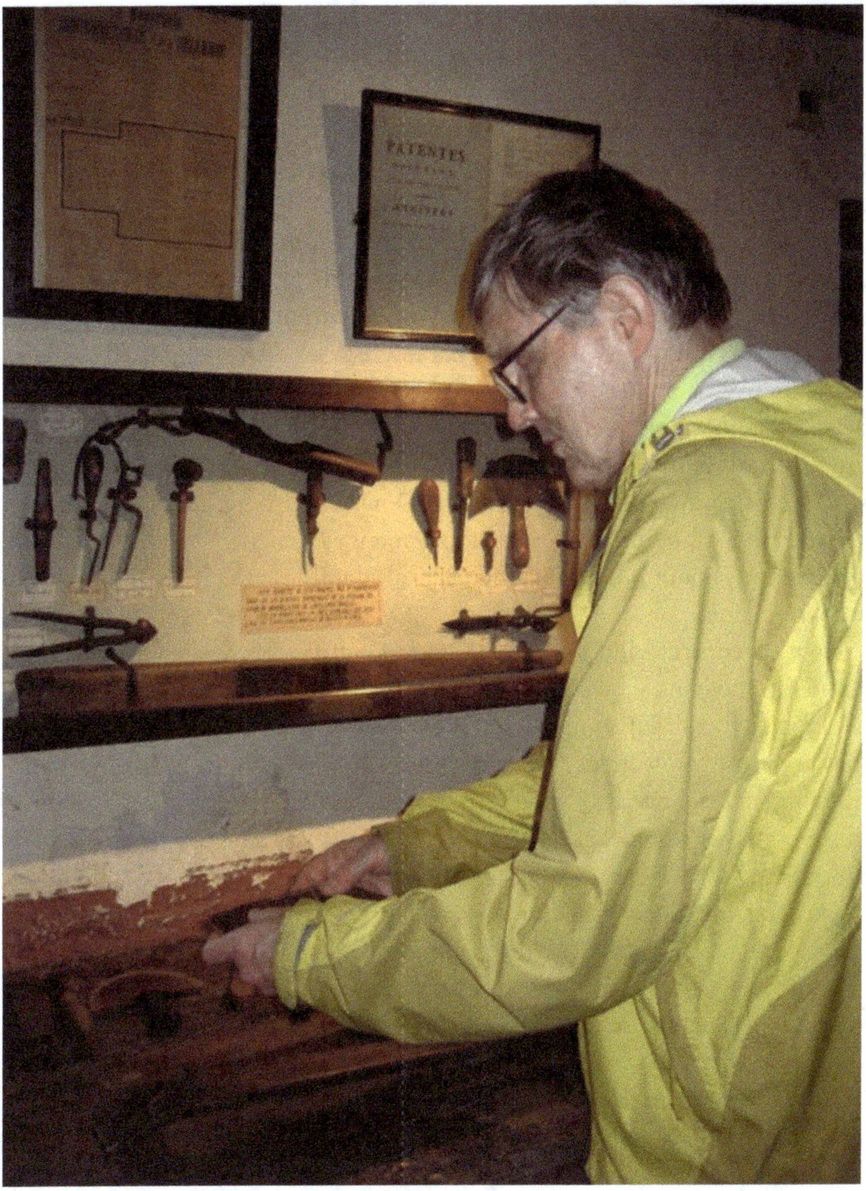

Figure 9.2 A photo at Louis Braille's birthplace in Coupvray, France (2011). The author, Gordon Legge, is inspecting the table used by Louis's father for harness making. There is a sharp tool on the table, called a serpette, like the tool that caused Louis's eye injury and resulted in his blindness.

vision impairment. A colleague told me about a friend with albinism who was unaware of having vision impairment until they went to school; the parents had not told them. Some parents may experience guilt, worrying that heredity, their lifestyle during pregnancy, or past sins was the cause of their child's disability. Most parents of kids with low vision are normally sighted themselves. They lack experience and knowledge of low vision and may not be aware of the available resources and opportunities for their children. Referrals from ophthalmologists and optometrists to rehab professionals and special educators are essential for such parents.

Andrew Solomon (2012), in his book *Far From the Tree*, distinguished between two types of childhood identities—vertical and horizontal. Vertical identities are personal traits passed down by parents to their children such as language, ethnicity, and genetic characteristics. Horizontal identities refer to distinctive characteristics not shared by a child with parents that shape life experience, often including disabilities. In his book, Solomon described the stories of families with children having 10 different types of horizontal identities including deafness, dwarfism, Down syndrome, autism, and transgender. He did not include vision impairment as a chapter, but his insightful observations about horizontal and vertical identities also apply to blindness and low vision.

How parents respond to the horizontal identities of their children can be pivotal in the child's development. Parents can be sad, disappointed, angry, in denial, or ignorant about their child's vision impairment, and sometimes, they are overly protective. They can also be supportive of the horizontal identities and special needs of their children. I was fortunate to have parents of this type. My mother learned Braille so she could write letters to me and help me with my schoolwork. My father encouraged me to play sports, taught me to play golf, and encouraged me to travel independently in our city. In short, the experience of childhood low vision depends importantly on family and community support and can be rewarding for parents and children alike. Solomon, reflecting on the trials and tribulations of the families he studied, concluded that his book's "conundrum is that most of the families described here ended up grateful for experiences they would have done anything to avoid."

Prevalence of childhood low vision

In Chapter 1, I pointed out that most low vision arises from age-related eye diseases such as glaucoma and age-related macular degeneration (AMD). The vast majority of low vision in developed countries occurs in later adulthood. But, of course, there are children with low vision as well. It is estimated by the World Health Organization that about 7% of blindness and low vision worldwide occur in childhood (Kong et al., 2012). Although the incidence of low vision in childhood is much lower than in adults, the early onset means that affected individuals will often live with impaired vision for many more years than adults who acquire low vision later in life.

The American Foundation for the Blind (AFB) has assembled estimates[2] of the number of children with impaired vision in the United States. The AFB reported that according to the 2019 American Community Survey (ACS), there were about 550,000 children (under the age of 18) with "vision difficulty." Estimates of the prevalence of vision impairment from the ACS are based on responses to the survey question, "Is this person blind or does he/she have serious difficulty seeing even when wearing glasses?" This question might enlist "yes" responses from some people who would not be included in the definitions of low vision discussed in Chapter 1. For example, some people with amblyopia who experience reduced vision in just one eye might respond yes to this question. As such, the ACS estimate of the number of young people with impaired vision cited here might be an overestimate of the number who have blindness or low vision as defined in this book.

According to the 2019 annual report of the American Printing House for the Blind (APH), there were about 55,000 children (aged 0–21 years) in the United States who were legally blind by the definitions discussed in Chapter 1. We can compare prevalence numbers from the ACS and APH with the estimates from Chan et al. (2018) reported in Chapter 1. They estimated about 5.7 million Americans over the age of 40 with impaired vision, including 1.3 million who were legally blind. Clearly, there are many fewer children with impaired vision than older adults, but the thousands of children with impaired vision represent a vitally important group.

Before we turn to specific causes of childhood low vision, let's briefly consider the development of vision in infancy in the absence of eye disorders.

Visual experience begins in the womb. Bright light and coarse pattern information can penetrate maternal tissue to reach the fetus. A team led by Vincent Reid (2017) at Lancaster University in the UK used ultrasound to monitor head turns in third trimester fetuses. They found that patterns generated by configurations of three LED lights presented to the maternal abdomen produced more fetal head turns when oriented in a face-like configuration than when oriented in an inverted face-like configuration.

Healthy human newborns have low-acuity pattern vision. In 2018, Angela Brown and colleagues at The Ohio State University reported measurements

[2] https://www.afb.org/research-and-initiatives/statistics/children-youth-vision-loss.

of the acuity and contrast sensitivity of newborn babies at the university's medical center. The investigators used square-wave grating test targets (black and white stripes varying in stripe width and contrast) and observed whether the infants moved their eyes to look at the test patterns when the patterns were moved from side to side. The ability of the baby to follow the moving targets with their eyes was an indicator that the baby could see the targets. To measure acuity or contrast sensitivity, the stripes were made narrower or lower in contrast until the baby's eyes no longer followed the movement of the stripes.

In two experiments using slightly different testing procedures, the investigators estimated newborn median acuity to be equivalent to about Snellen 20/600 (6/180). In adults, acuities this low would be categorized as severe low vision. The investigators also estimated newborn contrast thresholds to be about 0.3 (Michelson definition of contrast). This would be equivalent to being able to see only the first two or three sets of high-contrast letters on the Pelli-Robson chart (Chapter 3, Figure 3.3). These findings indicate that human newborns have very low vision at birth. Other studies have shown that infant acuity develops rapidly over the first few months of life, reaching close to 20/100 (6/30) at 12 months and nearly adult acuity by five years of age (Mayer et al., 1995).

The rapid development of pattern vision in early life requires normal visual experience. The importance of early visual experience was demonstrated in animal studies conducted by the Nobel Prize–winning researchers David Hubel and Torsten Wiesel. In the 1960s, they showed that kittens deprived of normal visual experience had irreversible deficits in cell responses in the visual cortex of the brain. Similarly, eye conditions in human infants that deprive or degrade vision early in life, such as congenital cataracts (see below), can result in failure to develop normal adult vision.

Causes of childhood low vision

There have been estimates of the prevalence of different eye disorders causing childhood vision impairment in several countries. Comparisons across studies are difficult because of variations in the years in which data were collected, differences in definitions of blindness and low vision, and healthcare disparities due to geographical and socioeconomic differences. Some countries maintain national registries that capture information about most children with impaired vision, such as the Danish National Registry of Children with Vision Impairment. Danish law requires the registration of visually impaired children, which makes them eligible for rehab services from trained vision therapists and for free access to optical and electronic aids. Line Kessel (2024) at the University of Copenhagen and colleagues have analyzed registry data on the prevalence and causes of childhood vision impairment in Denmark since 1979. They found that the prevalence of childhood vision impairment was fairly constant across this period (about 1.6 cases per 1,000 children under 18 years), but that the number of children with severe low vision and blindness has decreased. Other countries, such as the United States, have no such registry, so national estimates must be based on extrapolation from small samples.

Unlike late-onset low vision, childhood-impaired vision often results from inherited eye disorders such as albinism and several forms of inherited retinal disease. Some other forms of childhood low vision result from either premature birth (retinopathy of prematurity or deficient foveal development known as foveal hypoplasia) or birth-related neurological trauma (CVI or optic nerve atrophy). Childhood low vision can also be a secondary consequence of several diseases; in my own case, low vision was a consequence of SJS.

There is a gender difference in the prevalence of childhood-impaired vision. Unlike age-related eye diseases, which affect more women than men, studies show that more boys than girls have childhood low vision. The reasons for this gender difference are unclear. One reason may be that some inherited retinal diseases have an X-linked pattern, similar to the common forms of color blindness, which primarily affect males.

My review of the major causes of childhood-impaired vision based on studies from several developed countries indicates substantial variation but fair agreement that the leading causes are retinal diseases (including several forms of retinitis pigmentosa [RP]), optic nerve disease, albinism, CVI, and nystagmus. Of these, albinism, retinal diseases, and nystagmus predominate among those with mild or moderate forms of low vision while CVI, optic nerve disease, and retinal diseases are more common in those with severe low vision and blindness. Of course, many other diseases and conditions contribute in smaller proportions to childhood-impaired vision. Some conditions such as congenital cataract and retinopathy of prematurity, which were previously major contributors to childhood vision impairment, now account for relatively few new cases in developed countries.

In the following sections, I'll briefly describe four important causes of childhood low vision, each with their own interesting stories—albinism, congenital cataract, retinopathy of prematurity, and CVI.

Albinism and nystagmus

Albinism is a common cause of childhood low vision. The term is derived from the Latin word *albus* for white, referring to the snow-white hair of some people with the condition. Sometimes, individuals are referred to as albinos, but the National Organization for Albinism and Hypopigmentation[3] advises that many people with albinism find the term "albino" to be offensive. Similar to referencing people with many other conditions, it is more respectful to use *person-first* terminology; it is better to refer to "a person with albinism" rather than using terms such as "an albino" or "albino person."

In a 2018 autobiographical article, Cheryl Austin described how she felt stigmatized as a child by her white hair, her low vision, and the involuntary movements of her eyes (termed nystagmus):

> Children called me "albino" on the playground and, referring to my nystagmus, they asked bluntly, "Why do your eyes move like that?" Although these things were more likely said out of ignorance or curiosity rather than cruelty, their comments cut through me like knives. Rather than hold my head up high and answer their questions, I walked away and cried.

She did her best to hide her vision impairment from others. Only later as an adult did she come to terms with her low vision and become open and accepting of it: "Now, rather than view my limited vision as a disability, I now see it as something to be overcome, something in the face of which I can excel." Children with low vision in mainstream schools may often downplay or deny their vision impairment in order to fit in with their normally sighted classmates. Sometimes, they are teased or feel left out in games. Often they will have no role models with a similar vision condition. Low vision can sometimes be fairly well hidden, especially when the impairment is mild. Choosing to conceal one's condition is more difficult for those with white hair from albinism.

In some parts of the world, people with albinism are discriminated against and persecuted. In a 2018 report, Anita Franklin from Coventry University in the UK and colleagues summarized the plight of people with albinism in sub-Saharan Africa. Negative legends and folklore have led to assaults and murder. The problem was so severe that in 2008, the government of Tanzania made it a capital crime to kill people with albinism. Franklin et al. (2018)

[3] https://albinism.org/information-bulletin-what-do-you-call-me/#main.

quoted Ms. Kway-Geer, the first Member of Parliament with albinism in Tanzania:

> When I was at primary school, people used to laugh at me, tease me—some didn't even like to touch me, saying that if they touched me they would get this colour. People used to abuse me on the road when I took the buses to school. They would run after me—crowds of kids following me—shouting "zeru, zeru" (derogatory term for someone with albinism).

In 2013, the United Nations Human Rights Council called for the prevention of attacks and discrimination against people with albinism. Fortunately, in most developed countries, this form of discrimination is much less severe.

Albinism is a condition characterized by a disorder of the synthesis of the pigment melanin. Albinism has a reported prevalence of about one in 17,000 in the United States but much higher prevalence in some other countries including several African nations. According to a 2023 review by Kromberg and colleagues, prevalence data on albinism around the world are quite sparse. From the available data, they estimate a prevalence of about one in 4,000 in Africa and a lower prevalence of about one in 13,000 in Europe. The estimate of one in 17,000 in the United States comes from a 1970 publication by Witkop et al. The genetics of albinism are reviewed by Jauregui et al. (2018) and a comprehensive review of albinism is given by Summers (2009).

There are several genetic variants of albinism, including seven autosomal recessive forms of *oculo-cutaneous albinism* (OCA1–OCA7) and an X-linked form. The term "oculo-cutaneous" implies that pigmentation is absent or reduced in the skin and hair as well as the eyes. Ocular albinism (OA), a rarer condition, affects only the eyes. The genetic variants of albinism affect different molecular stages in the synthesis of melanin. Melanin refers to a group of naturally occurring pigments. It is found in plants and animals. It is responsible for the color of skin, hair, and eyes in humans. It is produced through the oxidation of the amino acid tyrosine, with the enzyme tyrosinase acting as a catalyst. A genetic mutation, resulting in the absence of tyrosinase in some humans, is responsible for OCA-1, the most pronounced form of albinism.

In the most severe form (OCA-1), there is a complete lack of melanin. The hair is white and the skin is very pale. Affected individuals are at high risk for sunburn. In the eyes, the color of the iris is gray or light blue. The lack of pigmentation in the iris results in translucency. The eyes may have a pinkish color, due to the visibility of retinal blood vessels through the translucent irises. Many people with albinism have nystagmus with onset in early infancy. Nystagmus is an involuntary oscillatory movement of the eyes. I'll comment on nystagmus in more detail later in this section. There is also a high prevalence of strabismus in albinism.

Albinism is also characterized by abnormal retinal development. There is a lack of foveal specialization termed foveal hypoplasia. The lack of foveal development means that people with albinism do not have the dense concentration of foveal cones that account for the high acuity of people with normal vision.

There is also an unusual pattern of optic nerve projections to the visual cortex. As illustrated in Figure A2 in the Appendix, the normal visual pathways transmit information from the temporal retina to the visual cortex in the hemisphere on the same side while information from the nasal retina is transmitted to the visual cortex in the opposite hemisphere. Studies of people with albinism, using visually evoked potentials (VEPs) and functional magnetic resonance imaging, have shown that optic fibers from a portion of the temporal retina also project to the opposite hemisphere. It is possible that this unusual pattern of projection might cause distortions of the visual field. But, a study by Klemen et al. (2012) of six participants with albinism failed to find a hypothetical visual-field distortion and concluded that brain plasticity compensated for the unusual pattern of optic nerve projection from retina to cortex. It therefore seems that people with albinism have intact visual fields.

What are the implications for visual perception of the unusual characteristics of albinism? The impact on vision varies across the subtypes with those having the more complete absence of melanin production (especially OCA-1) having the greatest visual deficits. The lack of development of a normal fovea means that affected individuals have reduced acuity. Those with OCA-1 may have an acuity of 20/200 (6/60) or less. Other forms of albinism may result in milder acuity reduction. Translucency of the iris allows light to leak through the iris and diffusely scatter across the retina. Affected individuals are susceptible to glare and experience photophobia. Like people with achromatopsia, described in Chapter 3, people with albinism often employ strategies to cut down on bright light and glare, such as wearing dark glasses or a billed cap.

Nystagmus, involuntary rhythmic eye movements, accompanies several congenital forms of vision impairment including albinism, congenital cataracts, achromatopsia, and optic nerve hypoplasia. These congenital forms are termed "infantile nystagmus" because of their early onset. Infantile nystagmus can also occur in the absence of any known visual abnormality, sometimes associated with a gene mutation, and is then termed "idiopathic" or "congenital motor" nystagmus. We might expect that if the eyes are continually in motion, the world might seem unstable to someone with nystagmus. But, those with congenital forms of nystagmus, whether idiopathic or associated with a known disorder such as albinism, do not perceive their visual worlds to be unsteady. Remarkably, the brain adapts to the motion and delivers a stable percept. In some forms of acquired nystagmus due to neurological disease, excessive alcohol consumption, or other causes, people may report visual scenes to be unstable. When this perceptual instability occurs, it is termed *oscillopsia*.

McLean et al. (2012) interviewed 21 people with nystagmus at the University of Leicester in the UK to understand the impact of the disorder on their daily lives. Some of them described limitations associated with reduced acuity, such as the inability to drive. Most of them were self-conscious about the appearance of their eyes and the lack of understanding by others of their condition. These concerns are reflected in the quote from Cheryl Austin earlier in this section about the stigma she felt as a person with albinism and nystagmus.

We might expect infantile nystagmus in albinism to be disruptive to reading as precise eye movement control plays an important role in skilled reading. I recall being surprised by a participant in one of our early lab studies of low vision and reading who had pronounced nystagmus. For text size that exceeded her critical print size, she read rapidly, matching the speed of normally sighted readers. Kimberly Merrill (2011) and colleagues at the University of Minnesota measured the reading performance of 63 participants with albinism, 29 adults and 34 children. All but one of them had nystagmus. They used the MNREAD test described in Chapter 6 to estimate maximum reading speed, critical print size, and reading acuity. While most of the participants required magnification, their maximum reading speeds were highly functional and near normal (median of 150 words per minute). Another study by Barot et al. (2013) also showed good reading performance by a group of subjects with albinism, with maximum reading speeds being uncorrelated with the extent of nystagmus. The lack of impact of nystagmus on reading speed is surprising. Merrill and colleagues speculated that the eye-movement demands of the reading task might suppress nystagmus.

My best childhood friend, Bob, has albinism. I could spot him from a distance by his white hair. He has been legally blind since birth, with acuity less than 20/200. As kids, we read the same books and played games. We enjoyed sports together, both playing and listening to hockey and baseball on the radio. After seventh grade, we were separated by many miles of Canadian geography, Bob in Saskatchewan and me in Ontario. We kept in touch through high school and college and then lost contact. Decades later, we reconnected and have enjoyed a close friendship at a distance ever since. He has contributed to this book by reviewing and commenting on several chapters. I have met many other people with albinism over the years. They all have low vision but live successful and productive lives.

Congenital cataract

Congenital cataract refers to the lack of clarity and transparency of the crystalline lens in one or both eyes at the time of birth. In the 1940s, it was discovered that rubella (German measles) during the first trimester of a pregnancy could result in congenital cataracts in newborns. Fortunately, the development of a rubella vaccine in the 1960s and its wide adoption has nearly eliminated this cause of congenital cataracts in developed countries. (A vaccine for rubella is combined with vaccinations for mumps and measles in a single MMR shot.)

Congenital cataracts can also have a genetic origin, often following an autosomal dominant pattern of inheritance.

As I discussed in Chapter 3, the development of cataracts in adulthood, if left untreated, results in reduced acuity, problems with glare, and reduced vividness of colors. The treatment for adult-onset cataracts is the removal of the cloudy crystalline lens and its replacement with an artificial intraocular lens (IOL). This procedure usually restores good vision including acuity in the normal range.

Some infants are born with dense congenital cataracts in both eyes, clouding vision from birth. If the cataracts are not removed surgically, normal visual development cannot take place. Permanent low vision occurs if cataract removal is delayed until later childhood or adulthood. The experience of pediatric ophthalmologists and researchers has shown that it is imperative to remove the cataracts in the early weeks of life in order to preserve the development of normal visual acuity.

In 2009, Eileen Birch and colleagues at the Retina Foundation of the Southwest, in Dallas, Texas, reported on the visual acuity of 37 children, tested between ages 5 and 16 years, all born with dense cataracts in both eyes. The children all had cataract surgery, ranging from three days to 31 weeks after birth. The researchers used statistical models to evaluate the impact of the age (in weeks) of cataract removal on long-term acuity. From birth to 14 weeks, average acuity declined by one line of the acuity chart for each three weeks of delay, from an average acuity of 20/30 (6/9) for surgery at one week to 20/80

(6/24) for surgery at 14 weeks. There was no further decline in acuity for cataract surgery from 14 to 31 weeks, with resulting acuities averaging 20/80. This important study had two major conclusions: First, there appears to be a critical period of about 14 weeks during which visual deprivation from dense cataracts can have an impact on long-term visual acuity. Second, within the first 14 weeks of life, the earlier cataracts are removed, the better the prospect for normal or near-normal visual acuity later in life.

It is only in recent decades that we have come to understand the importance of surgical removal of dense congenital cataracts soon after birth. This realization has spared many children from a lifetime of low vision. According to the analysis of data from the Danish registry of children with impaired vision mentioned earlier, in 1980, congenital cataract accounted for 15.6% of cases of childhood vision impairment, but in 2022, only 3.7% of cases.

I've observed the dramatic improvement in the treatment of congenital cataract up close. My friend Michael, born in the early 1960s, and his father were both born with congenital cataracts. Both have had low vision throughout their lives. When Michael and his wife Allison were expecting their first child in the early 1990s, they understood from genetic counseling the possibility that their baby would have congenital cataracts. They made sure to have the baby's eyes examined immediately after birth, and yes, baby Daniel had cataracts in both eyes. Michael was distressed at the prospect that he had passed on low vision to his son. Daniel had cataract surgery on both eyes, one at two weeks of age, and the other at six weeks of age. Subsequent follow-up with Daniel at home involved diligent wearing of glasses, then contact lenses, and ultimately IOL implants. Daniel is now an adult with normal visual acuity. He drives a car, reads regular print, and enjoys healthy vision. A few years later, Daniel's sister Elizabeth was born, also with congenital cataracts. Her cataracts were removed surgically at two weeks of age from both eyes. Elizabeth too has grown up enjoying healthy normal vision. The experience of three generations of this family illustrates the march of progress in our understanding and treatment of eye disease. While my friend Michael has lived a rich and fulfilling life with low vision, we all celebrate the opportunity of his children to live their lives with normal vision.

While surgery soon after birth for congenital cataracts has prevented low vision for children in developed countries, many children in poorer countries with congenital cataracts go untreated and grow up with severe visual impairment. Pawan Sinha in the Department of Brain and Cognitive Sciences at the Massachusetts Institute of Technology realized the plight of many children with untreated congenital cataracts and other eye disorders during a visit to

New Delhi, India, his family home, in 2002. He encountered impoverished blind children on the street and learned that India had more than 400,000 blind children, many of them with congenital cataracts and other treatable conditions. He was inspired to found Project Prakash in collaboration with colleagues from Dr. Shroff's Charity Eye Hospital (Sinha, 2013). Prakash is the Sanskrit word for light. The project has two major goals: to restore sight to children who have treatable forms of blindness and to conduct research on how the brain learns to process visual input following sight deprivation. This project has delivered sight-restoring surgery to many children and adolescents with congenital cataracts, vastly improving their quality of life. As expected from the previous discussion of the need for early cataract surgery, delayed cataract removal does not result in restoration of normal visual acuity and contrast sensitivity, but frequently results in highly functional low vision. In the next chapter, I'll return to an intriguing scientific finding from Project Prakash answering a longstanding philosophical controversy called Molyneux's question.

Retinopathy of prematurity

During the late 19th century and early 20th century, the medical and public health communities made strides in reducing infant mortality. The public became fascinated with the plight of preterm infants. These were infants born before 37 weeks gestational age at high risk of not surviving. Worldwide, about 10% of infants are preterm. Incubators were developed and improved to sustain the lives of preemies. In the early 1900s, preterm babies in incubators were put on public exhibit in many places in the United States including the Wonderland Amusement Park in Minneapolis and Coney Island in New York. At that time, attitudes toward sustaining life in premature infants varied. Some advocates of eugenics believed that preterm infants were weaklings and should not receive special medical care. The story of how many premature infants were nurtured in incubators and exhibited in amusement parks is told in a podcast episode of *99% Invisible*, hosted by Roman Mars (2019), entitled The Infantorium.[4]

In the early 20th century, better practices in hospital nurseries yielded increasing survival rates of premature infants. But, preterm infants often suffered from inadequate blood oxygen levels due to underdeveloped lungs, a condition termed cyanosis because of the bluish tint of the skin from

[4] https://99percentinvisible.org/episode/the-infantorium/.

poorly oxygenated blood. Supplemental oxygen, delivered via newly invented incubators, preserved the lives for many preterm infants.

In the early 1940s, ophthalmologists in Boston identified a new form of eye disease in some premature infants. It was named *retrolental fibroplasia* (RLF, for short), literally meaning scar tissue behind the crystalline lens in the eye. The severe disorder was characterized by complete detachment of the retina. Later, the terminology was changed to *retinopathy of prematurity* (ROP), recognizing the site of the disorder as the retina and its high risk in preterm infants. William Silverman in his 1980 book *Retrolental Fibroplasia: A Modern Parable* described how RLF became an epidemic in the late 1940s and 1950s, accounting for an estimated 7,000 cases of blindness in the United States by 1953. The severe form of the disease often resulted in total blindness. One victim of this epidemic was the musical prodigy Stevie Wonder who was born in Michigan in 1950 and lost his vision to RLF. I grew up in Canada and knew several kids born in the late '40s and early '50s who were blind from RLF.

High concentration of supplemental oxygen was identified in the early 1950s as a likely cause of RLF. Measures were taken to restrict the incubator concentrations of supplemental oxygen delivered to premature infants in order to protect vision. Debate persisted over the dosage and wisdom of reducing supplemental oxygen, given its importance in sustaining life in many preterm infants. Silverman (1980) cited one estimate that the reduction in supplemental oxygen for premature infants may have saved the vision of one infant at the cost of the lives of 16 others. To the present, the appropriate timing and dosage of supplemental oxygen and its impact on retinal development in premature infants remains unclear. In a 2013 review of ROP, led by Ann Hellström, the authors point out that excessive concentrations of oxygen (hyperoxia) immediately after the birth of premature infants may inhibit the healthy growth of retinal blood vessels, but insufficient concentrations of oxygen (hypoxia) in later development may stimulate the release of vascular endothelial growth factor (VEGF) which may promote abnormal vessel development.

Proper development and functioning of the retina relies on blood supply from the retinal vessels. These vessels continue to develop throughout full-term pregnancy. After premature birth, maternal factors in the uterine environment supporting normal development are absent. Vascular development may cease or become abnormal. In typical development, vessels grow outward from the optic disk and cover most of the retina, except for a zone around the fovea. The emergence of ROP has been divided into five stages describing abnormalities in the normal growth of blood vessels across the retina. Stages 1 and 2 refer to deficiencies in the extent of retinal coverage of new vessels. An infant diagnosed with stage 1 or 2 ROP may ultimately achieve normal retinal development and good vision. Stage 3 is associated with the growth of abnormal vessels. They may rupture and develop fibrous scar tissue which can pull on the retina leading to retinal detachment. Stage 4 is characterized by partial retinal detachment and stage 5 by total retinal detachment.

Retinal detachment can lead to vision loss and, in extreme forms, to total blindness. Luka, a friend and former student of mine, was born in the early 1980s with ROP. He was extremely premature (24 weeks of gestational age) with a birth weight of 765 grams (1 pound and 11 ounces). He lost vision entirely to ROP in one eye and has an acuity of about 20/200 in the other eye. Despite his low vision, Luka is an active sportsman, enjoying skateboarding and hunting. As a teenager, he learned to drive a stick shift on rural roads while growing up in Idaho.

In the 1980s, a major clinical trial was undertaken, called the Multicenter Trial of Cryotherapy for Retinopathy of Prematurity. Cryotherapy involves applying an ice-cold probe to the sclera of the eye. The goal of the therapy was to use freezing to repair retinal detachments or to limit or prevent the growth of abnormal blood vessels in infants diagnosed with stage 3 ROP. A 2001 report from the multicenter research team compared the visual outcomes of children at 10 years of age who were diagnosed with ROP as infants and whose eyes were treated with cryotherapy to those of controls who did not receive cryotherapy. At the age of 10 years, roughly a quarter of the treated eyes achieved acuity in the normal range (equal to or better than 20/40). Among the other eyes treated with cryotherapy, substantially fewer were classified as blind (acuity worse than 20/1600) than among the controls. These results show that cryotherapy was successful in preserving vision in a substantial number of eyes with ROP. Despite the therapy, however, a majority of eyes with severe ROP had visual impairment.

Cryotherapy became the dominant treatment for infants with advanced forms of ROP. Kevin, a friend of mine, was born in the late 1950s with ROP (then termed RLF) before the advent of cryotherapy. He was a teacher of the visually impaired (TVI) in the public schools before his retirement. He told me that many of his students with vision impairment due to ROP have better vision than him because they benefited from cryotherapy. More recently, laser ablation therapy has replaced cryotherapy as a means for treating advanced ROP. Both cryotherapy and laser therapy seek to protect central vision at the expense of scarring peripheral retina to treat detachments or neovascularization. There is also research on the effectiveness of injections of anti-VEGF drugs for ROP, similar to the modern drug therapy for wet AMD.

What are the continuing risks to vision of premature birth? The EXPRESS study (Extremely Preterm Infants in Sweden Study) addressed this question (Hellgren et al., 2016). The investigators were able to trace nearly 100% of premature infants in Sweden born in a study period from April 4, 2004, to March 31, 2007. The researchers focused on those born with extreme prematurity, at less than 27 weeks of gestational age. The infants in their study had a median birth weight of 770 grams, almost the same as my friend Luka. Of the 707 live births meeting the study criteria, 494 were alive at one year and 462 at 6.5 years. Of these, 434 participated in the study. 36.6% of these had been diagnosed with mild ROP (stages 1 or 2) and 35.5% with severe ROP (stages 3–5). But, when tested at about the age of 6.5 years, only 8.8% had visual acuity worse than 20/40 (6/12) and just 2% had acuity worse than 20/400 (6/120), the WHO criterion for blindness.

The EXPRESS study tells us that while extremely premature birth is still a risk factor for vision impairment and other vision problems, it is not as dire as it was during the epidemic of the 1940s and 1950s. Advances in medicine now result in the survival of more extremely premature infants, but also better management of ROP. Nevertheless, those infants with the more severe forms of ROP (stages 3–5) are at risk for low vision or blindness.

Data from the Danish registry mentioned earlier show that the impact of ROP has decreased over the years from 11% of children with impaired vision in 1980 to only 1.8% in 2022. While the prevalence of impaired vision due to ROP is declining in high-income countries with good medical care, it is higher in some middle-income countries where survival rates of premature infants are rising but pediatric eye care is less available. In low-income countries where survival rates are much lower for preterm infants, ROP is less prevalent or at least not reported. It is also important to be aware that premature birth is a risk factor for other physical, cognitive, and neurological deficits. This means that some children with vision impairment from ROP also experience these additional deficits.

Cortical visual impairment

Most of the causes of low vision discussed in this chapter and elsewhere in this book are due to disorders of the eye, often referred to as ocular disorders. The eye receives visual information in the form of an optical image on the retina and converts the image data into neural signals sent along the optic nerve to the brain. Visual centers in the brain are responsible for interpreting the visual input coming from the eye. Disorders of visual areas in the brain can result in vision impairment, even when the eye itself is healthy. I discussed the example of hemianopia in Chapter 4 in which vision loss can occur in half of the visual field due to a stroke affecting visual centers in one hemisphere of the brain.

Since the 1980s, there has been a growing realization that many children with early-onset visual impairment have a deficit in the way the brain processes visual information. In education and rehabilitation circles, this form of vision impairment is termed cortical visual impairment (CVI) and refers to a neurological deficit in visual processing beyond the eye. Some vision researchers and neuroscientists refer to CVI as "cerebral visual impairment," noting the deficits in question can be subcortical as well as cortical. An older term, "cortical blindness," is sometimes used to refer to acquired vision impairment associated with brain damage in adults but may be misleading in the pediatric context because most individuals with CVI are not blind but retain some visual function.

In current usage, CVI refers to vision impairment that cannot be explained by ocular disorders. More specifically, Sakki et al. (2018) defined CVI as a "verifiable visual dysfunction which cannot be attributed to disorders of the anterior visual pathways or any potentially co-occurring ocular impairment." In some cases, CVI may coexist with an ocular disorder. For example, some preterm infants diagnosed with ROP may also have neurological deficits consistent with CVI. It is likely that many kids with CVI go undiagnosed because it is difficult for ophthalmologists or optometrists to identify the cause of their vision problems.

CVI is now recognized as a leading cause of childhood vision impairment in developed countries. Kong et al. (2012) obtained diagnostic data for 3,070 students at 16 schools for the blind in the United States. CVI was the most-common diagnosis, affecting 18% (556) of the students. An article by Yahalom et al. (2022) included a summary of the percentages of CVI diagnoses among visually impaired children in studies from several developed countries. The percentages ranged from 48% in a 2004 study in the UK to 7% in studies in Finland in 2004 and Ireland in 2007. This wide variation may be due to differences in geography, sampling procedures, and diagnostic definitions. In aggregate, however, it is clear that CVI is a major cause of childhood visual impairment. It is expected that prevalence estimates of CVI will increase with better diagnosis and with medical advances that enhance the survival of infants with serious neurological problems.

Two important causes of CVI have been identified. Extremely premature infants, those at high risk for ROP, are also at risk for periventricular leukomalacia (PVL). This refers to the damage to the white matter in the brain near the ventricles and can result in the disruption of connectivity between brain areas and disruption of signals sent along the spinal cord for motor control. Infants with CVI resulting from PVL will often have motor disabilities as well as vision impairment.

A second cause of CVI is *hypoxic ischemic encephalopathy* (HIE). This disorder can result from hypoxic ischemic injury at birth. This refers to oxygen deprivation due to asphyxia during a difficult delivery, resulting in reduced blood flow causing damage to the brain. Other causes of CVI include traumatic brain injury from abuse or accidents, some forms of infection, and genetic disorders.

Many children with CVI have additional disabilities including cognitive and motor disorders. Cerebral palsy frequently accompanies CVI. My friend Kevin, the teacher of the visually impaired, had many students with CVI. He told me that he could only recall one student with CVI who had no other disabilities. It is likely that for many children, coexisting disabilities mask CVI, resulting in the lack of appropriate vision rehabilitation.

Children with CVI often show deficits in standard clinical measures of vision, although conducting the tests may be challenging. Acuity, measured with Teller acuity cards or VEPs, is usually below age-matched normal levels and may range from near-normal to total blindness. Visual-field deficits are common, particularly in the lower visual field. Strabismus and refractive error frequently accompany CVI. Higher-level visual, motor, cognitive, and social deficits are typically present as well. The educator Christine Roman-Lantzy, in her 2018 book *Cortical Visual Impairment—An Approach to Assessment and Intervention*, has described in detail 10 visual and behavioral characteristics typically found in CVI. Table 9.1 lists these 10 visual and behavioral characteristics with brief descriptions. These 10 characteristics are present in most children with CVI but with varying degrees of severity. Roman-Lantzy has developed a method for scoring children on these 10 characteristics, based on parental interviews and professional observations of children with CVI. This profile of CVI characteristics, termed the CVI Range, can be used to document changes

Table 9.1 Ten visual and behavioral characteristics of CVI (adapted from Roman-Lantzy [2018]. Cortical visual impairment—An approach to assessment and intervention [2nd ed.]. AFB Press. Chapter 3)

Color preference. Strong preference for a particular bright color such as red or yellow.
Attraction to movement. Captivated by moving objects such as a ceiling fan, TV action, or staring out of the window of a moving car.
Visual latency. Slow visual response to the appearance of a new object in the scene.
Visual-field preferences. Often a preference for noncentral vision. May turn the head to use a particular portion of the peripheral visual field to look at things. Lower visual field is often impaired, impacting mobility.
Difficulty with visual complexity. Simple patterns, such as objects with a single color, are recognized better than multicolored surfaces or objects in cluttered scenes. Difficulty integrating multisensory input such as combined audiovisual stimuli. Difficulty recognizing faces and making eye contact.
Need for light. Gazing at bright lights is common as well as attraction to shiny surfaces.
Difficulty with distance viewing. Distant objects are harder to attend to and recognize, possibly because of confusion with background clutter. A single object held close to the face may be easier to attend to.
Atypical visual reflexes. Delayed or absent blink response when touched on the bridge of the nose. Absent or delayed blink response to an object rapidly approaching the face along the midline.
Difficulty with visual novelty. Unlike typical infants who prefer to look at novel stimuli, those with CVI prefer familiar targets.
Absence of visually guided reach. Failure to spontaneously reach for and touch nearby objects.

over time in a child's condition due to rehabilitation or educational interventions.

The 10 characteristics of CVI affect many aspects of everyday life and reflect the broad impact of CVI on the brain and behavior. Several of the characteristics refer to abnormal attentional focus on simple environmental features such as color, motion, and bright lights. Other characteristics refer to difficulty with complex visual patterns, unfamiliar objects, and multisensory input. Visual-motor actions are impaired as reflected by slow visual response to new objects, difficulty with visual-motor reaching, and reduced visual reflexes to touch or looming stimuli.

My friend Kevin told me about one of his students with CVI. His acuity was evidently quite good. He had a fascination with the color orange and loved orange juice. He could easily spot a bottle of orange drink across the room. But, when he tried to navigate across the room to retrieve the orange drink he would stumble and bump into things in the way. His mobility was poor, perhaps because of a lower visual-field deficit.

Keep in mind that CVI is an umbrella term referring to vision impairment due to a variety of possible neurological issues, manifesting with different symptoms from one person to another. An unusual and interesting case study was described by Katie Lane-Karnas (2023). Her daughter Mae is a "curious, talkative and bright young person" with normal visual acuity. As a child, Mae exhibited some eye-movement difficulties and several types of visual agnosia. In particular, she had difficulty recognizing printed letters and words and struggled with visual reading. At the age of 11, Mae was diagnosed with CVI. Recognizing Mae's difficulty with print reading, Katie introduced her daughter to Braille. Mae immediately took to learning Braille by touch, and she was soon doing her schoolwork and enjoying reading young adult novels in Braille. This is a rare instance in which a person with normal visual acuity has trouble with print reading but reads Braille by touch. It is also an example of how an appropriate intervention for a person with CVI is specific for their type of vision disability.

How can we begin to understand the diverse visual deficits associated with CVI? Behavioral and brain-imaging studies are pointing at some principles that may explain deficits in terms of brain structure. In Chapter 5, I discussed the division of information processing in the visual brain along the ventral and dorsal pathways. The ventral pathway, beginning in the primary visual cortex in the occipital lobe and converging on the temporal lobe, is responsible for object recognition, including faces and words, and is sometimes termed the *what* pathway. The dorsal pathway, beginning in the primary visual cortex and converging on the parietal lobe, plays an important role in space perception and motion perception and is often termed the *where* pathway. The dorsal pathway is also thought to play an important role in visually guided motor behavior such as grasping with the hand and was termed the *how* pathway by Goodale and Milner (1992).

The characteristic problems in CVI with visual-motor control and motion perception imply the possibility of dorsal-stream deficits in the brain. Janette Atkinson from University College London, in her 2017 Davida Teller Award lecture and review article, described mounting evidence for dorsal-stream vulnerability in preterm infants and full-term infants at risk for neurological problems, including those with CVI. A signature marker of dorsal-stream damage is a deficit in global motion perception.

Global motion sensitivity can be tested by asking a subject to look at a display of dots moving in random directions. (Think of a swarm of fireflies moving randomly.) The subject is asked to find a region of the display in which a fraction of the dots move coherently in the same direction. Threshold sensitivity is determined by finding the smallest fraction of coherent dot motion in the region enabling detection. Taylor et al. (2009) tested sensitivity to global motion in two groups of children aged five to nine years. The group born very prematurely (gestational age less than 32 weeks) had much higher thresholds for detecting coherence in global motion than children born at full term.

Christopher Bennett (2020) and colleagues from Massachusetts Eye and Ear, Harvard Medical School, reviewed the growing behavioral and brain-imaging research implicating dorsal-stream damage in CVI. They also found evidence that the ventral stream, primarily involved with object recognition, is affected in CVI. For example, the difficulties with visual complexity and scene clutter, and the lack of interest in novel stimuli, may reflect ventral-stream dysfunction.

While the developing visual brains of infants and young children are vulnerable to disease and deprivation, the young visual brains may also be more amenable to rehabilitation interventions than those of adults. In her book, Roman-Lantzy (2018) emphasized the potential benefits of early interventions at home and at school. Interventions can capitalize on the known visual characteristics of a child. For example, Roman-Lantzy described one child who was unable to learn typical black-on-white printed characters, but when the symbols were outlined in the child's favorite color, red, he was able to learn the characters.

Given that brain plasticity may be the greatest for the youngest children, interventions may be the most effective at the earliest age. Elisa Fazzi (2021) at the University of Brescia, Italy, led an early intervention group that conducted a pilot clinical trial intervention study with infants, with the average age being 5.9 months. Groups of 15 infants with CVI and 15 infants with vision impairment due to ocular disorders (termed PVI for "peripheral visual impairment") participated in a six-month intervention. A comparison group composed of 30 infants (15 with CVI and 15 with PVI) received regular services but not the intervention. The intervention program required adaptations to the home environment such as the preparation of quiet and uncluttered spaces and use of large, colorful, high-contrast targets presented within reach. An important aspect of the intervention was social interaction; caregivers or therapists responded to the infant's attentional focus and interests with relevant activities and with verbal communications through words, nursery rhymes, and songs. The intervention also included training hand–eye coordination through reaching to targets of interest and exercises to improve eye-movement control. The primary outcome measures were visual acuity, contrast sensitivity, and eye-movement measures of fixation, smooth pursuit, and saccade accuracy. Following the six-month intervention program, both the intervention and comparison groups showed improvement in visual acuity and contrast sensitivity, but only the intervention groups exhibited improvements in the eye-movement measurements. The investigators interpreted their findings as promising evidence for the value of early interventions in enhancing the visual capabilities of infants with CVI.

We are still in the early days of understanding CVI, its causes, and strategies for prevention and rehabilitation. A key step is to diagnose CVI early in life and to provide parents and teachers with information about how to maximize the visual and learning environments for the child.

For an informative perspective on the challenges faced by families and children with CVI, I recommend *Kaleidoscope: The Cortical Visual Impairment Podcast.*[5] This podcast is hosted by Jessica Marquardt and describes the challenges faced by her family and other families with a child with CVI. One compelling podcast episode is a direct report from Jessica's daughter Grace about her life experience with CVI.

Optimism

Advances in modern medical science have reduced the prevalence of some forms of childhood low vision, such as congenital cataract, and have reduced the severity of others, such as ROP. Greater understanding has emerged among eye clinicians and rehabilitation specialists about the previously ill-recognized forms of CVI and associated disabilities. Inherited causes of childhood low vision, including albinism and several forms of inherited retinal disease, continue to account for many cases of childhood low vision in developed countries.

Childhood low vision poses challenges for affected kids and their families, but there is every reason to be optimistic about the future for these children. The passage of the Americans with Disabilities Act in 1990 in the United States, the integration of most children with low vision into mainstream classrooms, the realization among eye clinicians and educators of the functional

[5] https://podcasts.apple.com/us/podcast/kaleidoscope-the-cortical-visual-impairment-podcast/id1386780362.

value of even very low vision, and the advent of a wide range of assistive technologies all contribute to enhanced quality of life and career prospects for children with low vision. Of course, parental and family support is critical as well. Parents often play a key role in the education of their children with low vision through interactions with teachers. These exchanges can result in the development of written formal agreements called individualized education plans.

Over the years, I've talked to many young people with low vision or their parents. They ask for my advice about educational programs, career opportunities, and difficulties with social interactions. While there are obviously individual differences in life circumstances, I start with the premise that the sky is the limit. Yes, life with low vision poses challenges, but given motivation and family support, almost anything is possible. My ultimate advice is usually, "Follow your dreams!"

10
Sight Restoration
The Dream

Almost everyone with low vision has thought about recovery of full sight. For most, it is only a dream. For a few, therapies may exist to improve vision. When vision impairment begins at birth or in early childhood, restoration of normal vision later in life is unlikely. I'll describe three famous cases in which vision restoration was attempted through surgery. Modern technologies, including neuroprosthetics and gene therapy, offer some level of improved vision for specific types of eye disorders. The possibility of vision restoration depends on the ability of brain networks to adapt and make sense of modified visual input.

• • • • •

What is sight restoration?

When I was a child attending the school for the blind in Brantford, Ontario, some of the kids with low vision like me would talk about a future when we would get our sight back. I had an expectation that one day, I would have full sight again. We played ball, and I imagined being a major league baseball player. No adults encouraged my vision restoration fantasy, although I suspect that my parents consulted my ophthalmologist hoping to learn about possible sight-restoring cures.

Most people with vision impairment have thought about sight restoration. For some, it may be a distinct possibility. For others, it is a dream. But, what exactly do people mean when they refer to restoring sight?

A popular conception comes from Bible stories about healing of the blind. There are many references in the Bible to blindness, some literal and others metaphorical. The New Testament tells about miracles in which Jesus restored vision to the blind. According to *Matthew chapter 9*:

Low Vision. Gordon E. Legge, Oxford University Press. © Oxford University Press (2026).
DOI: 10.1093/9780198946960.003.0011

> As Jesus went on from there, two blind men followed him, calling out, "Have mercy on us, Son of David!" When he had gone indoors, the blind men came to him, and he asked them, "Do you believe that I am able to do this?" "Yes, Lord," they replied. Then he touched their eyes and said, "According to your faith let it be done to you"; and their sight was restored ...
>
> ***Matthew*** **9: 27-30, New International Version (NIV) of the Bible.**

Modern ophthalmology has treatments that restore normal vision for some eye conditions that cause temporary vision deficits. A common example is cataract surgery. Cataracts occur when the clear crystalline lens in the eye develops opacities that cloud vision. If the cataract is not treated, it eventually results in reduced acuity, glare, and distortion of colors. Cataract surgery involves the removal of the natural crystalline lens and its replacement with a transparent artificial intraocular lens (IOL). In most cases, the loss of vision due to cataracts can be remedied by surgery.

Age-related cataracts are very common. According to the National Eye Institute, more than half of Americans over 80 years either have cataracts or have had surgery to remove cataracts. In developed countries, cataract surgery is usually undertaken before vision impairment becomes severe. Cataract surgery is not as widely available in less-developed countries, and cataracts continue to be a leading cause of vision impairment worldwide. In Chapter 1, I mentioned Nicholas Kristof's 2015 article about the ophthalmologist who was implementing a program of inexpensive cataract surgery in Nepal.

Examples of vision restoration in healthy eyes

Vision restoration can refer to the improvement of some aspect of vision in a person with otherwise healthy sight. I'll briefly mention three examples: the use of eyeglasses, methods for improving color vision, and vision interventions to improve stereoscopic depth perception.

An everyday but supremely important example of vision restoration is the use of eyeglasses (spectacles) or contact lenses to correct for errors of optical focusing in the eyes. Millions of people worldwide wear glasses or contact lenses to correct their myopia (shortsightedness), hyperopia (farsightedness), or astigmatism, collectively referred to as refractive errors. Most people need reading glasses or bifocals by their mid-50s. For many people, misplacing or breaking their glasses results in an immediate and obvious vision deficit. Putting on glasses restores good vision.

An article on the history of glasses by John Dreyfus (1995) traced the first use of glasses to Italy in the late 1200s, with the first manufacture of spectacles occurring in Venice in 1301. Most people in developed countries have access to glasses to correct for refractive errors, providing good acuity at both near and far distances. In the United States, roughly 60% of the population use glasses or contact lenses. But, routine access to glasses is not true worldwide. The Flaxman (2017) article cited in Chapter 1 estimated that more than 50% of acuity reduction in the range of 20/60 to 20/400 worldwide is due to the lack of refractive correction. If people in this category had access to properly prescribed glasses, they could be restored to visual acuity in the normal range.

People with normal acuity but inherited deficits in color vision (see Chapter 3) could benefit from methods for restoring normal trichromatic color vision. An intriguing 2009 article by a team led by Katharine Mancuso at the University of Washington in Seattle described research on a form of gene therapy to enhance color vision in squirrel monkeys. Male squirrel monkeys are dichromatic, lacking the longwave-sensitive L cones present in normal, trichromatic human vision. The researchers surgically delivered genes coding for the L pigment into the photoreceptor layer of the retinas of two male squirrel monkeys. Before the gene therapy, the monkeys were trained on a computer-based test of color vision. Like human dichromats with protanopia, they could not discriminate some reds and greens. But, several weeks after the therapy, they were able to make color distinctions similar to those made by people with normal trichromatic color vision. Despite public interest in gene therapy for human dichromats (those lacking one of the three cone pigments), this therapy is not yet approved for use in humans. The current method for injecting the modified genes into the eye has significant risks including retinal detachment. Later in this chapter, I'll return to gene therapy for restoring vision in inherited retinal diseases.

Several optical methods, involving glasses with color filters, have been proposed to help people with color deficits. One interesting example is the EnChroma lenses intended to enhance color vision for anomalous trichromats. These are individuals (about 6% of males and less than 1% of females) who have three cone pigments but with excessive overlap in the wavelength sensitivity of the middle-wavelength-sensitive (M) and long-wavelength-sensitive (L) cone pigments. This excessive overlap means that people with anomalous trichromacy have difficulty distinguishing among some red and green colors. The EnChroma lenses filter out a narrow band of the overlapping wavelengths, potentially allowing for better discrimination of reds and greens. Online reviews of the effectiveness of these lenses have been mixed. But, John Werner (2020) at the University of California at Davis led a study demonstrating the benefits of these lenses. Seven participants with anomalous trichromacy wore EnChroma lenses several hours a day for two weeks. Several of the participants spontaneously commented that they noticed enhanced visibility of colors in flowers and fall foliage while wearing the lenses. More surprisingly, in careful laboratory tests, even without the glasses, the participants experienced stronger perceptual responses to red/green color contrast, perhaps representing a form of perceptual adaptation facilitated by the lenses. One participant commented, "I now see that my girlfriend's brown hair has hints of red; I now notice it even without wearing the glasses."

Stereoscopic depth perception relies on the slightly different viewpoints of the two eyes in normal binocular vision. In Chapter 4, I pointed out that many people with low vision have poor or no stereo vision because of major differences in vision in their two eyes. Between 5% and 10% of people with normal acuity have stereo deficits as well. A complete absence of stereopsis is called stereoblindness. The traditional view was that stereopsis could not be restored after a critical period ending at about the age of 7. In 2009, in a book called *Fixing My Gaze*, Sue Barry described how she acquired stereoscopic depth perception at 48 years of age for the first time. She did so with the help of vision therapy. A key part of the therapy was devoted to getting her two eyes to properly fuse images. She also had lengthy training sessions in identifying targets in depth. Sue Barry's remarkable recovery of stereo vision motivated wide public interest in methods for restoring or improving stereo vision in adults.

Stereoblindness in adults is often associated with amblyopia. Amblyopia refers to the impairment of vision in one eye due to some form of visual deprivation early in life. There are two major causes of amblyopia—strabismus and anisometropia. Strabismus refers to the misalignment of the two eyes. Often, one eye dominates perception and retains normal acuity while perception is suppressed in the other (amblyopic) eye and acuity is reduced. Anisometropia refers to significantly different refraction in the two eyes. Because the two eyes attempt to focus together, only one eye can be in good focus at a time. When one eye dominates in achieving clear focus, the other eye will be blurred and may become amblyopic. Both types of amblyopia frequently result in deficits or a total loss of stereopsis.

In 2015, Dennis Levi at the University of California at Berkeley and colleagues reviewed the growing research literature on several types of vision interventions to restore stereopsis in adults with the two forms of amblyopia. They found that success in improving or restoring stereopsis was greater in anisometropic amblyopia with more than 50% of subjects showing improvements. By comparison, only 26% of subjects with strabismic amblyopia showed benefits from the interventions. These findings indicate that some degree of restoration of stereopsis is possible in adults. Research is needed to determine what factors are predictive of this improvement.

People with low vision may benefit from these three forms of sight restoration. Of course, many people with low vision improve their vision with glasses. Some people with low vision have the inherited forms of colorblindness and could potentially benefit from methods to improve color vision. Methods for enhancing stereopsis might help those with low vision who have a similar vision status in their two eyes.

Is vision restoration possible after vision loss in early childhood?

The possibility of restoring normal vision seems to depend on prior experience with fully developed normal vision. It is rare to find cases of vision restoration in adulthood following severe early childhood vision loss. There have been a few famous cases in which early-onset cataracts have been removed or corneal transplants have been done that "restore" vision to someone who has been blind or nearly blind for most of their life. Let's look at three well-known cases of sight restoration.

Sidney Bradford

In a famous 1963 report, Richard Gregory and Jean Wallace at the University of Cambridge reported on the case of subject Sidney Bradford (SB). SB had lost most of his vision at the age of 10 months due to an infection that damaged his corneas. In 1959, at the age of 53, SB had separate corneal transplant operations on his two eyes which restored vision in the sense of providing unobstructed optical image formation. Gregory and Wallace evaluated SB's restored vision, based on their tests of his perception, his self-reports, and information from his family and his eye surgeon. They also had access to information from SB's childhood medical records.

Before the corneal transplants, the eye surgeon reported that SB's vision was limited to hand movements only. Gregory and Wallace tested SB with a variety of classical perceptual illusions and drawings of ambiguous figures. He did not see the illusory spatial distortions in the Hering, Zolner, and

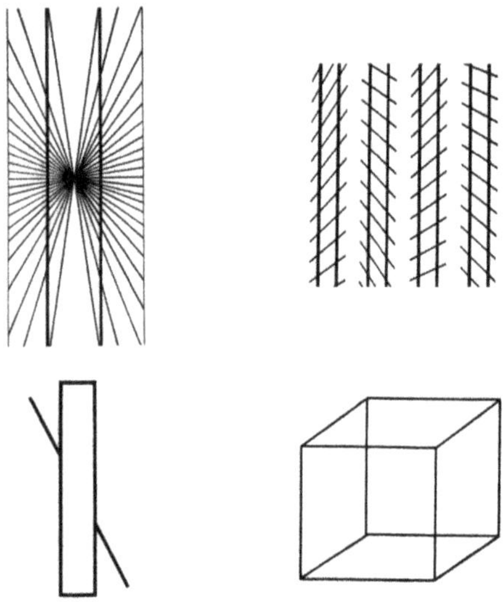

Figure 10.1 Four illusions used by Gregory and Wallace (1963) to test subject SB. A. Hering illusion: The two parallel, vertical straight lines presented in front of the radial spoke pattern appear to bow outward. B. Zolner illusion: The parallel vertical lines do not appear to be parallel in the presence of the superimposed short diagonal crossing lines. C. Poggendorf illusion: The visible sections of a straight slanted line, interrupted by a rectangle, do not appear to be parts of the same straight line. D. Necker cube: The 2-D drawing of a 3-D wire cube has an ambiguous interpretation; either the lower-left or upper-right bounded regions can be seen as the front face of the cube. Adapted from Gregory & Wallace (1963). Recovery from early blindness, a case study. *Experimental Psychology Society Monograph*, *2*, 1–46.

Poggendorf illusions (Figure 10.1). He did not recognize the depth or see perceptual reversals in ambiguous images including the Necker cube.

SB seemed unable to see 3-D perspective in drawings. In contrast, Gregory and Wallace were intrigued by SB's ability to identify the numbers in the Ishihara color test. This revealed that SB had normal color vision. His ability to recognize the numbers visually may have been evidence of the transfer of shape knowledge learned by touch to vision. They observed that SB often learned to recognize objects visually after first touching them.

Gregory and Wallace were surprised that SB was disappointed with his restored vision. When they saw SB six months after their first visit, they reported:

> ... we formed a strong impression that his sight was to him almost entirely disappointing. It enabled him to do a little more, and he had a strong desire to drive a car, but it became clear that the opportunities it afforded him were less than he had

> imagined. We found a still active middle-aged man of fairly high intelligence, but with a laborer's job and unable to read more than a few simple words. His income and status were obviously lower than they would have been if he had not been so handicapped, and these facts were very clear to him. He described the world as rather, drab; he still to a great extent lived the life of a blind man, sometimes not bothering to put on the light at night, and he still made little of the normal visual occupations of the cinema or television.... He certainly relied a great deal on vision, but we've formed the impression that this very reliance cost him his self-respect, for he had been proud of his abilities when the handicap was obvious, but now his previous achievements seemed paltry and his present position almost foolish. He was not a man to talk freely, but was obviously depressed, and we felt that he had lost more than he had gained by recovery of sight.

Virgil

In a 1993 article in the *New Yorker* magazine, the neurologist and essayist Oliver Sacks reported the story of Virgil, a man from Oklahoma who had his vision restored after 45 years of severe vision loss. Virgil's history included severe illness at the age of three which may have resulted in retinal damage, followed later by the formation of dense cataracts at the age of six. Forty-five years later, he had cataract surgery. When the surgical bandage was removed from Virgil's right eye, Sacks reported:

> The dramatic moment stayed vacant, grew longer, sagged. No cry ("I can see!") burst from Virgil's lips. He seemed to be staring blankly, bewildered, without focusing, at the surgeon, who stood before him, still holding the bandages. Only when the surgeon spoke - saying "Well?"- did a look of recognition cross Virgil's face.
>
> Virgil told me later that in this first moment he had no idea what he was seeing. There was light, there was movement, there was color, all mixed up, all meaningless, a blur. Then out of the blur came a voice that said, "Well?" Then, and only then, he said, did he finally realize that this chaos of light and shadow was a face - and, indeed, the face of his surgeon.

Sacks wrote that Virgil was able to recognize colors and movements, but he had difficulty integrating visual features into recognizable objects. He liked large neon signs. He could see the moon. Occasionally, he could see birds but he had no idea of distance. He was able to recognize letters on the eye chart, achieving an acuity of 20/80. But, apparently, this moderately good acuity was not sufficient to support 3-D object recognition and depth perception. Like subject SB, Virgil recognized visual letters, explaining that he had learned their shapes by touch. Similar to Gregory and Wallace, Sacks was impressed by the importance of touch to Virgil in learning to use vision. Referring to Virgil's experience after returning home from the cataract surgery:

> This first month, then, saw a systematic exploration, by sight and touch, of all the smaller things in the house: fruit, vegetables, bottles, cans, cutlery, flowers, the knickknacks on the mantelpiece-turning them round and round, holding them close to him, then at arm's length, trying to synthesize their varying appearances into a sense of unitary objecthood.

Months later, Virgil's restored vision led to fatigue and emotional discontent. Then, his vision began to decline along with his general health. Sacks reported that Virgil's experience with vision restoration, similar to SB's, was ultimately disappointing.

Isn't it amazing that vision restoration after decades of severe vision impairment should lead to unhappiness? Why might vision restoration, even if only partial, be disappointing and emotionally taxing? Gregory and Wallace, and Sacks, speculated on the possible reasons. Might it be due to a change in one's identity and way of life as a person with a vision disability? What about the effort and other challenges in adapting to a new source of sensory input? Might there be disappointment in failing to recover entirely normal vision? Might it be anxiety about meeting the expectations of others? Sudden life changes of any kind, whether positive or negative, can be stressful and emotionally taxing. For anyone contemplating sight-restoring surgery after long-term deprivation, hopes and aspirations should be tempered with a realistic understanding of the range of likely outcomes.

Mike May

A more recent case study was described in dramatic detail in Robert Kurson's (2007) book, *Crashing Through: A True Story of Risk, Adventure, and the Man Who Dared to See.* Mike May had normal vision until the age of three-and-a-half years when a chemical explosion at home caused the loss of one of his eyes and serious corneal damage to the other eye. He retained light perception but no form vision. In 1999, at the age of 46, he had the first of the two surgeries to restore his vision, a transplant of limbal stem cells from a donor. These are cells that grow in the limbus of the eye at the edge of the cornea and are required to replenish corneal cells to sustain clarity. The second surgery was a corneal transplant. Both surgeries were successful. Kurson's book provides many interesting and informative details about Mike's decision to proceed with the surgery and his reactions to the results. What was Mike's vision like following the surgeries? Mike was willing to participate in research to examine his vision status. The research was conducted by a team led by Ione Fine (2003) then at the University of California at San Diego. With the damage to Mike's cornea successfully repaired, his optical image quality should have been good enough to support 20/40 acuity. Mike's accident occurred at three-and-a-half years, an age at which his visual acuity was approaching an adult level. His retinal function appeared to be intact. But, like the previous cases of SB and Virgil, Mike's vision was far from normal. His visual acuity, measured with grating patterns, was low, equivalent to about 20/500. The low acuity measured following the sight-restoring surgery indicated that his pattern vision did not stand still during the years of deprivation but declined. After the surgery, Mike's color and motion perception were quite good. He could recognize simple shapes like squares and circles but had trouble interpreting 3-D shapes. He also had trouble with perception of faces. Similar to the earlier cases of SB and Virgil, he recognized objects visually better after touching them, as if it took some direct multimodal interaction to forge the link.

Using technology not available in the earlier studies, Fine and colleagues tested Mike's vision with brain imaging [functional magnetic resonance imaging (fMRI)]. Dorsal visual areas of Mike's brain, typically responsive to motion, were much more active than ventral pathway areas normally involved with processing faces and objects. Fine and colleagues proposed that Mike's three–and-a-half years of early visual development were sufficient to establish stable color and motion perception but that more complex perceptual functions such as 3-D space perception and face perception were immature and remained incomplete in their development. Mike's visual experience following the long period of deprivation was not effective in re-engaging this development; tests more than ten years later showed no improvement in acuity or visual brain responsiveness (Huber et al., 2015).

Kurson's book describes Mike's very different reaction to sight restoration compared to the disappointment experienced by SB and Virgil. Mike May has a charismatic personality and a forward-looking and intrepid spirit of adventure. Prior to his sight-restoring surgery, he had worked abroad in Ghana, was an analyst for the CIA, and was the founder and CEO for Sendero Group, the company that developed the first widely used GPS apps for blind mobility. He was an accomplished downhill skier with the world speed record for blind skiers (65 miles per hour). He was happily married with a family. As in many of his other life endeavors, he approached the prospect of sight restoration as a challenging adventure. While ultimately not recovering normal vision, Mike has found the adventure fulfilling. He told me that the best part of it was the interesting people that he has met along the way. Unlike SB and Virgil, he did not consider his restored vision to be a disappointment.

What do we conclude from these case studies of sight restoration after many years of vision deprivation? In a 2016 article, Susana Chung and I (Legge and Chung, 2016) reviewed these cases in the context of the larger issue of low vision and brain plasticity. We wrote:

> The conclusion from these case studies is that if experience-dependent visual functions do not develop normally prior to visual deprivation, they will not develop following vision restoration. Some capacities that had matured may also decline through long periods of deprivation, such as visual acuity in the case of Mike May.

It appears that important aspects of visual development slow down and stop in the absence of ongoing visual experience. It is unclear why the restoration of visual input after prolonged visual deprivation cannot trigger the recovery of normal visual functioning. We don't know what biological mechanisms put the brakes on visual development and whether treatment can be found to release the brakes. Persisting questions remain. How many years of normal visual development are required to sustain the potential for full vision restoration after prolonged vision impairment? What level of residual vision (low vision) can sustain the potential for full or partial vision restoration later in life? These questions continue to be important when considering the degree of vision restoration to be expected from retinal implants, gene therapy, or other high-tech methods of sight restoration.

Molyneux's question

Cases of early childhood vision deprivation have been used to address a famous philosophical dilemma known as Molyneux's question and discussed by the philosopher John Locke in his 1689 treatise *An Essay Concerning Human Understanding*. Briefly stated, if a person born blind has learned to identify shapes such as spheres and cubes by touch, would they be able to recognize the same objects by sight if vision were restored? In other words, would knowledge about object shapes learned by touch transfer immediately to restored vision? Locke thought not: "[I] am of the opinion that the blind man, at first, would not be able with certainty to say which was the globe, which the cube ..." In the cases of SB, Virgil, and Mike May, it seems that visual recognition of 3-D objects benefited from combining visual exploration with touch. Visual recognition was not immediate.

Molyneux's question was tested more directly in Project Prakash, introduced in Chapter 9. In a study conducted by Richard Held (2011) and colleagues from MIT, five children from Project Prakash, aged 8–17 years, were tested with visual and tactile stimuli less than 48 hours after receiving sight-restoring surgery. Four had grown up with dense bilateral cataracts and one with dense bilateral corneal opacities. Following the surgery, all of them had sufficient vision to see large, high-contrast 3-D objects with different shapes taken from a children's toy set. Testing consisted of showing the subjects a sample shape (either by touch alone or by vision alone) and then asking them to choose the target from a pair of objects, one being a target and one being a foil. For example, the target might be a rectangle, and the test might require the subject to feel (or view) the rectangle and an oval and choose the one they thought was the target. Sometimes, both the target and test objects were felt by touch, and sometimes, both were viewed with restored vision. In these cases, the subjects performed well, making the correct choice more than 90% of the time. In the critical cross-modal condition, subjects felt the target and then viewed the pair of test objects visually. Would they be able to transfer the shape knowledge acquired by touch to make a correct choice based on vision? Held and colleagues found that performance was very poor in the cross-modal condition, dropping to nearly the guessing level of 50%; the subjects could not use vision to distinguish the target they had touched from a foil. The results answer Molyneux's question: Someone restored to vision after near-total visual deprivation from infancy is not able to immediately transfer knowledge of felt shape to vision. Experience seems to be necessary to connect tactile and visual representations of shape. But, when tested again only a few days later, the subjects did much better in the cross-modal matching task. These findings confirm Locke's supposition that immediate transfer of touch shape knowledge to vision is difficult after long-term vision deprivation, but with relatively brief experience, transfer from touch to vision improves. And indeed, as we saw earlier in the cases of SB, Virgil, and Mike May, transfer of knowledge of touch to vision seems to play a valuable role in enhancing visual understanding of seen objects.

Vision prostheses

Most forms of low vision are due to diseases that affect structures within the eyeball itself, such as the cornea, crystalline lens, and retina. Visual information leaving the eye along the optic nerve is conveyed to the visual areas of the brain in the form of electrical impulses carried by neurons. The brain is responsible for the interpretation of the visual input and conscious perception.

If structures in the eyeball are damaged or diseased so that visual input is blocked, what about bypassing the eyeball and delivering visual input directly to the brain? The concept of neuroprosthetics is to interface technology with the brain or nervous system to enhance or restore human abilities. Could a prosthetic device restore vision to someone who is blind or has low vision?

Cortical implants

By the early 20th century, it was known that visual input from the eyes reaches the occipital lobe at the back of the brain. In 1918, the British neurologist Gordon Morgan Holmes published a map showing how the layout of neural responses in the visual cortex in the occipital lobe corresponds to stimulation across the visual field. The map was based on observations of visual-field loss experienced by soldiers in World War I with penetrating gunshot wounds to the occipital lobes. Holmes observed that the central retina maps to the posterior (back) pole of the occipital lobe and the peripheral retina maps to more anterior (forward) portions.

During the late 19th century and the first half of the 20th century, a few case studies with human patients revealed that electrical stimulation of cortical tissue in the occipital lobe resulted in the perception of visual spots of light, termed phosphenes. Given the knowledge of the mapping from points on the retina to responses in the primary visual cortex (called the retinocortical map) and the observation that localized electrical stimulation of the visual cortex produces a localized percept of light, the idea emerged of designing a visual prosthesis to restore vision to blind people, based on direct electrical stimulation of the visual cortex.

The first major effort to develop and test a working visual prosthesis was undertaken in the 1960s by Giles Brindley, a physiologist at the University of Cambridge. After preliminary testing of the safety and viability of the design in baboons, a prosthetic device was implanted in a 52-year-old nurse with bilateral glaucoma who was nearly totally blind. The results were described by Brindley and Lewin in 1968. A rectangular grid of 80 stimulating electrodes was implanted intracranially to contact the surface of the patient's visual cortex in the occipital lobe of the right hemisphere. The grid-covered surface tissue expected to correspond to a wide region of the visual field.

The electrodes were connected by cable to 80 tiny radio receivers, all embedded within the patient's skull. The radio receivers could be activated wirelessly to selectively initiate electrode stimulation of the corresponding regions of the visual cortex. Thirty-nine of the 80 electrodes produced visual phosphenes. By asking the patient to point at and describe the phosphenes she saw, Brindley and Lewin were able to map the size and layout of the phosphenes in her visual field. The investigators reported:

> ... the phosphene that the patient sees is typically a very small spot of white light, described as "like a star in the sky", or "the size of a grain of sago at arm's length". This is the commonest kind of phosphene, and all phosphenes that are within 10° of the point of regard are of this kind. Phosphenes that lie further from the point of regard are sometimes elongated, the length being from 1 1/2 to 4 times the width. The long axis may be vertical, horizontal, or oblique. The commonest description of such elongated phosphenes is "like a grain of rice at arm's length". One exceptionally long one, 21° from the fixation point, is "like half a matchstick at arm's length".

This experiment demonstrated the plausibility of prosthetic vision. Since the input from the stimulating electrodes was controlled by the researchers and not based on environmental scenes, the prosthetic vision provided to this patient had no functional benefit. Nevertheless, Brindley and Lewin considered their results to be a success. They believed that with a larger grid of electrodes, connected to a camera, functional vision could be achieved. They concluded that:

> Our findings strongly suggest that it will be possible, by improving our prototype, to make a prosthesis that will permit blind patients not only to avoid obstacles when walking, but to read print or handwriting, perhaps at speeds comparable with those habitual among sighted people.

Now, more than 50 years after the Brindley and Lewin publication, the state-of-the-art in prosthetic vision may be approaching the goal of providing vision sufficient to avoid obstacles while walking, but we are still not close to providing vision sufficient to read print at speeds comparable to sighted people.

After 1968, research continued on the development of visual prostheses using direct cortical stimulation, notably by William Dobelle. In 2000, he reported on a cortical implant in a 62-year-old man who had been blind for many years from head trauma. The input to the implant came from a video camera attached to glasses worn by the man. Dobelle described the implant as "the first visual prosthesis providing useful 'artificial vision' to a blind volunteer by connecting a digital video camera, computer, and associated electronics to the visual cortex of his brain." The artificial vision covered a visual field of about 7 degrees wide by 20 degrees high. Within this field, the man could tell the orientation of a large capital E (tumbling E) equivalent in size to a 20/1400 letter. Dobelle was recognized for this accomplishment by the *Guinness Book of World Records* for "the first successful artificial eye."

Progress on the development of visual cortical prostheses (VCPs) has been slow. I recall talking with a young, blind woman in the 1980s who had been told by her ophthalmologist that within five years, she would probably have her sight restored by such a device. Researchers and clinicians need to be cautious in their predictions about the outcomes of unproven treatments and technologies. Challenging barriers in the development of effective VCPs have included safety risks, such as infections or seizures, associated with brain implants, electrical current spread from stimulating electrodes which limits the spatial resolution of the implants, and the nature of the resulting prosthetic vision, limited to coarse shape, motion, and light perception. These issues were reviewed by Lewis and Rosenfeld (2016). A recent VCP, called Orion, is under development by Vivani Medical Inc. and has undergone an early feasibility study with a small number of blind subjects. The promise of this technology remains to be fulfilled.

Retinal implants

In the 1990s, interest in prosthetic vision shifted to the retina. Depending on the nature of the vision condition, it might be possible to take advantage of some residual retinal function. Moreover, surgery for retinal implants is less invasive than that for cortical implants. Interest in retinal implants was also inspired by the success of cochlear implants (CIs) that assist people with severe sensorineural hearing impairment. CIs include a sound processor that sits behind the user's ear. It captures and processes sound and transmits signals to electrodes implanted in the cochlea in the inner ear. These electrodes stimulate auditory nerve fibers. The first CIs were implanted in the 1960s. By the mid-1990s, CI technology enabled many users to understand speech well enough to communicate over the telephone. According to the U.S. National Institutes of Health (NIH), in 2019, there were approximately 737,000 people with CIs worldwide. For a review of the history and design of CIs, see Zeng et al. (2008).

Several types of retinal implants have been developed and tested as vision prosthetics. For a review, see Ayton et al. (2020). The two most-widely tested are the Alpha-IMS, a subretinal implant, and the Argus-II, an epiretinal implant. Both types are intended for people with severe vision loss due to advanced retinal disease affecting the photoreceptor cells (rods and cones), especially retinitis pigmentosa (RP).

Figure 10.2 illustrates the difference between subretinal and epiretinal implants.

Subretinal implants are placed between a patient's retinal pigment epithelium (RPE) and the outer retinal layer containing damaged or dead photoreceptors. The implant contains hundreds of tiny light-sensitive photodiodes (1,500 photodiodes in the Alpha-IMS implant), acting like artificial photoreceptors. Light entering the eye falls on the photodiodes which generate weak electrical signals related to the intensity of the light falling on them. Circuitry is included to amplify the signals which then stimulate the adjacent retinal neurons, initiating a response that is sent to retinal ganglion cells and from there along the optic nerve to the brain. To the extent that retinal cells beyond the photoreceptor layer are healthy, the implant takes advantage of normal retinal processing. No external camera is required but the user has an external battery pack to power the implant. The implant relies on normal image formation by the optics of the eye. The user can scan the environment with normal eye and head movements. The surgery to place the implant beneath the retina is challenging.

Epiretinal implants are placed on the innermost side (vitreous side) of the retina adjacent to the ganglion cell layer. The implant contains an array of electrodes (60 of them in Argus II) that directly stimulate the ganglion cells. The implant receives image data from a camera whose output is processed by a video display unit and then transmitted to the electrode array. The camera is mounted on glasses worn by the user. In order to scan the environment, the user must turn their head to point the camera in the desired direction. This type of implant has the advantage of not needing clarity of the optics of the eye and involves less-risky surgery. This type of retinal implant is most-directly analogous to the CI in the sense that the image capture and signal processing are done by hardware outside the eye.

Both of these types of retinal implants rely on residual retinal functioning and intact optic nerves for conveying visual information to the brain.

To date, these vision prosthetics have succeeded in restoring ultra-low vision to some patients who had no more than light perception. In 2015, Katarina Stingl and colleagues reported on patient findings from a consortium led by the University of Tübingen in Germany. Twenty-nine patients, all

Two Types of Retina Implant

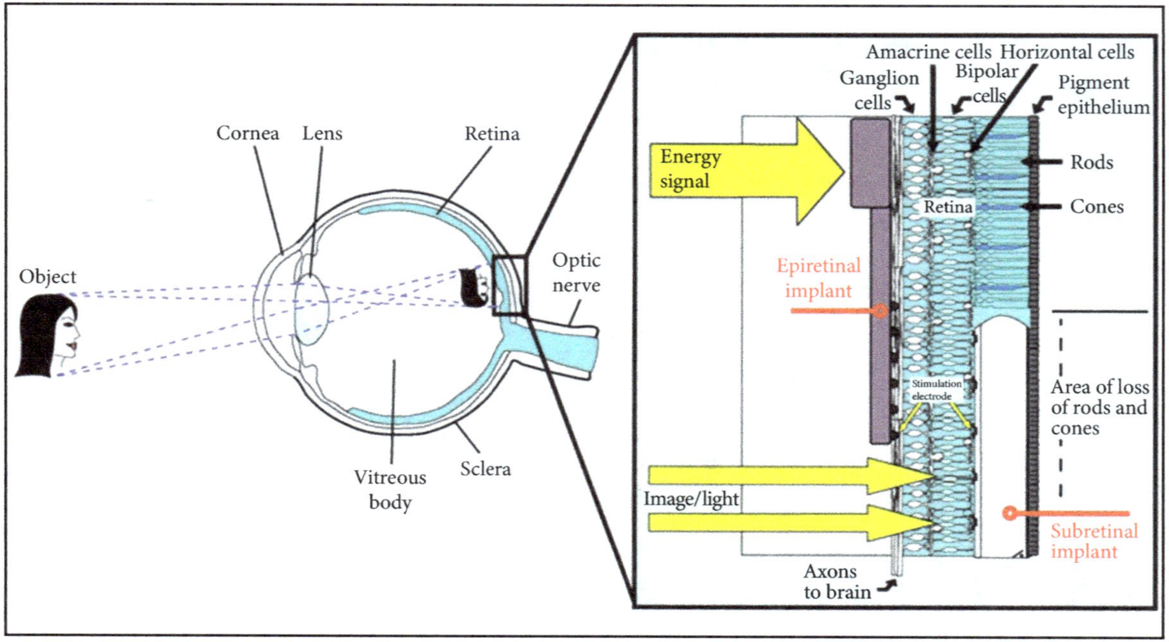

Figure 10.2 The inverted image of a face is projected by the optics of the eye onto the retina and is transformed into neural responses by the photoreceptor cells (rods and cones). A subretinal implant replaces damaged rods and cones with a silicon chip carrying many tiny light-sensitive photodiodes. Light from the image directly activates the photodiodes whose signals are amplified by circuitry that injects currents into the remaining neural cells of the retina. In contrast, an epiretinal implant has no light-sensitive elements but receives input from a camera attached to glasses worn by the user. Electrodes in the epiretinal implant then directly stimulate the axons of ganglion cells that form the optic nerve. Figure adapted from Figure 1 in Zrenner (2002). Will retinal implants restore vision? *Science*, *295*(5557), 1022–1025.

with late-stage forms of hereditary retinal degeneration—25 with RP and four with cone-rod dystrophy—received the Alpha-IMS subretinal implant in one eye. Most of them could localize light sources with the implant, and 13 of them reported useful everyday functions such as vision of "picture frame on the wall, fluorescent tubes, kitchen objects, plates in a good contrast, bottles, cup handle, washbasin, and bottles on shelves."

More than 350 patients have received an Argus II epiretinal implant. The implant contains 60 stimulating electrodes arranged in a 10-by-6 grid. Initial testing with each patient shows how many of the electrodes produce light sensations. The implant covers only 18 by 11 degrees of the visual field. The small field of view means that the user must turn their head to survey the environment. Similar to Alpha-IMS, Argus II yields at best ultra-low vision in recipients.

Efforts to improve the function of retinal implants have focused on enhancing salient environmental features. For example, Lan Yue at the University of Southern California led a team investigating whether color information could be transmitted by retinal implants. Typically, phosphenes produced by retinal implants are thought to be grayscale only, without color. Yue (2021) and colleagues found that five of seven Argus II users reported seeing phosphene colors ranging from yellow to blue when the stimulating electrodes delivered current pulses ranging from low-to-high frequency. But, they did not find a reliable method for encoding red and green colors. (Argus II electrodes deliver stimuli to the retina as brief pulses of current lasting about one millisecond in duration. In the Yue et al. study, the pulse frequency ranged from 6 to 200 pulses per second.)

In another example, Yingchen He (2020) at the University of Minnesota led a team studying the use of a thermal camera for input to Argus II. The camera responded to heat-generating sources, such as human bodies, pets, coffee cups, and ovens, making warm objects stand out against the background. In one experimental test, Argus II users were better at identifying the locations of people in a room with the thermal camera than with a conventional camera sensitive to visible light.

To date, the level of vision provided by retinal implants is very coarse, falling in the ultra-low vision range. It is usually too coarse to be measured with the typical clinical tests of acuity, contrast sensitivity, and visual field described in earlier chapters of this book or by questionnaire methods such as the National Eye Institute Visual Function Questionnaire (NEI-VFQ). How then should the vision provided by retinal implants be evaluated? Prior to approving retinal implants, the U.S. Food and Drug Administration (FDA) asked Second Sight Medical Products, the company that created the Argus

II implant, to develop a method to demonstrate the visual benefits of the implant in real-world contexts. A team led by Duane Geruschat at Johns Hopkins University described the development and initial use of such an assessment instrument in articles published in 2015 and 2016. The method is called the Functional Low-Vision Observer Rated Assessment (FLORA for short). FLORA has three parts: (1) self-report in which subjects respond to a series of open-ended questions about how the implant has affected their everyday lives, such as "Has the system helped you do things you could not do before?"; (2) assessment by an expert rehabilitation specialist of the benefits to a user of the implant for performing 35 daily activities—tasks relevant to orientation and mobility such as locating light sources, windows, doors, or fixtures in the bathroom or social tasks such as spotting movement of people; and (3) a narrative summary report by the expert evaluator. In an initial use of FLORA, 26 subjects who were blind from late-stage RP and who had the Argus II retinal implant were evaluated for an average of three years after the implant surgery. Statistical analysis showed that 24 of the 35 daily tasks in Part 2 of the FLORA were easier to perform with the aid of the implant—for example, finding doorways, crossing a street using the lines of a crosswalk, visually locating a place setting on a dinner table, sorting light from dark laundry, and determining the direction of people walking by. These results from the FLORA showed that the ultra-low vision provided by the implant can be helpful in performing activities of daily living.

What is prosthetic vision like? It is sometimes referred to as "artificial vision" because it differs so much from natural vision. It has been said to resemble a very blurry black-and-white television image. In the case of Argus II, imagine a narrow-field display with 60 grayscale pixels in a 10-by-6 configuration. Such a display could convey coarse information about lighting, shapes, and motion. With proper formatting, it might be capable of delivering information about a small number of adjacent letters.

Imagining visual prosthetics as delivering an image with point-like pixels may be oversimplified. As described by Brindley and Lewin in the quote earlier in this section and by many patients with prosthetic vision, individual stimulating electrodes do not necessarily generate point-like visual phosphenes but sometimes streaks or blobs. Michael Beyeler at the University of California at Santa Barbara led a group that developed software called pulse2percept to simulate prosthetic vision. The software, available as open-source Python computer code, takes into account the response properties of stimulated cells in the retina in creating simulations of prosthetic vision (Beyeler et al., 2017). Figure 10.3 shows two examples of Argus II simulations using this software—a subway platform with pedestrians and a girl jumping into a pool.

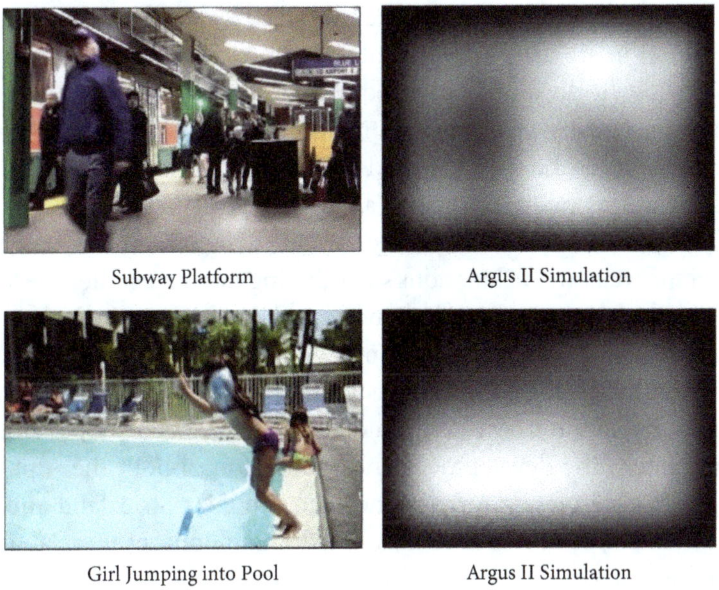

Figure 10.3 Simulations of percepts produced by the Argus II retinal implant for two scenes. Top: A subway platform showing pedestrians and a train. Bottom: A girl about to jump into a swimming pool. The simulations are based on the pulse2percept software and are provided courtesy of Michael Beyeler. See the text for more details.

As expected, the simulated views are low in resolution and do not retain color. People and objects in the scenes are not recognizable in the static images from the simulations. In real life, motion would help in image interpretation: for instance, the motion of the girl jumping into the pool. Michael Beyeler has created motion videos of Argus II simulations of the subway platform and the jumping girl at the pulse2percept[1] website. Beyeler and colleagues have pointed out that image simulations depend on the patterns of phosphenes elicited by individual electrodes. These patterns differ from one implant recipient to another.

How valuable is the ultra-low vision provided by the current generation of retinal implants? In this book, I have emphasized the value of even very low vision. Many recipients of the devices have reported positive benefits. In addition to the functional value in some everyday activities, recipients sometimes describe the pleasure they receive from visual experiences. For example, recipients who have lost sight for many years have reported pleasure at seeing fireworks or lightning again, or Christmas tree lights, or the shapes and movements of their spouses or grandchildren.

[1] https://pulse2percept.readthedocs.io/en/latest/examples/implants/plot_argus.html.

Ross Doerr (2023), a retired attorney, received an Argus II retinal implant in his 60s after many years of nearly total blindness. He has written a memoir describing how he decided to proceed with implant surgery and his experience with prosthetic vision. In reflecting on the potential risks and benefits prior to the surgery, he wrote "I used to be sighted. I know what I'm missing and I want as much of it back as I can get. ... If I pass this up, will I wonder if I blew my last chance for some eyesight?" In the memoir, he described the trials and tribulations surrounding the surgery, how he learned to use his prosthetic vision, and its benefits and limitations. He also described his concerns about cost and insurance. According to a 2023 estimate by http://theophthalmologist.com, the cost of the device, the surgery, and the follow-up rehabilitation services would be about $500,000 per patient.

Unfortunately, the development and production of both the Alpha-IMS and Argus II have ceased. A magazine article by Liza Strickland and Mark Harris, published in February 2022, entitled "their bionic eyes are now obsolete and unsupported,"[2] reported on the sale of Second Sight, the company that developed Argus II. The article provides some examples of how Argus II benefited recipients, and also, how the company's demise left the recipients without adequate technical backup. Ross Doerr has had to deal with this lack of support. Nevertheless, in his memoir, he concluded "Do I have any regrets about getting an Argus II? No, not a single one. I can see something."

The Alpha-IMS and Argus II retinal implants have the goal of restoring vision to individuals with no more than light perception. They were not designed to assist people with useful pattern vision. A newer type of subretinal implant, called Prima, has the goal of assisting people with central-vision loss from the advanced form of dry age-related macular degeneration (AMD) known as geographic atrophy. Prima has the novel goal of providing users with prosthetic central vision simultaneous with their preserved natural peripheral vision. Candidate patients are those who have large central scotomas, that is, no light perception in their central vision. The implant is placed in the subretinal space to substitute for the loss of photoreceptors (rods and cones) in the macula. The implant contains 378 electrodes, responsive to near-infrared light, covering approximately 7 degrees of central vision. When activated, the electrodes produce current pulses that initiate neural activity in retinal neurons, triggering a visual percept. The user wears glasses that contain a camera for capturing image information in the central field, a visual-processing unit, and a tiny projector that produces a focused infrared image on the subretinal chip containing the electrodes. The user has

[2] https://spectrum.ieee.org/bionic-eye-obsolete.

simultaneous access to the prosthetic visual input in central vision and their natural peripheral vision.

Daniel Palanker from Stanford University and his colleagues published the first clinical report on the outcomes of five patients with the Prima implants in 2022. Promising results included evidence that the patients could simultaneously use the prosthetic input for central vision and their natural peripheral vision. The patients achieved acuities averaging 20/500 with a test based on the identification of letters presented one at a time. Like Argus II, reliance on a head-borne camera for image capture means that the user must use head movements to scan the environment. The success of this type of retinal implant will depend on how effectively prosthetic central vision can be combined with natural peripheral vision in reading, mobility, and other everyday activities.

Gene therapy for restoring vision

Inherited retinal diseases (known collectively as IRDs) are important causes of low vision, especially among young people. Variants of more than 270 genes have been identified as contributing to these disorders. (I am using the term *variant* rather than *mutation* because the latter may have a pejorative connotation.)

In principle, if a single gene variant responsible for vision loss can be replaced by a properly functioning gene, it may be possible to restore vision. Modern genetic testing combined with genetic counseling can sometimes pinpoint the gene variant causing an eye disorder and identify potential gene therapies if they exist. Its use in retinal disease is especially promising for three reasons: first, the retina does not have as strong an inflammatory response to foreign biological substances as many other parts of the body; second, it is easier to surgically access the retina than internal organs; and third, gene therapy targets cells in the retina that are present for a lifetime, so only one treatment may be necessary rather than recurring treatments.

Several types of gene therapy are potentially applicable for treating inherited retinal or optic nerve disorders. For a detailed review, see Drag et al. (2023). Replacement of a missing or nonfunctional gene variant with the corresponding functional gene is the only type that has been approved so far for the treatment of a substantial number of patients. I'll describe the use of this form of gene therapy in treating one form of Leber congenital amaurosis (LCA 2). CRISPR-Cas9 is a gene-editing tool with promise for gene therapy. It has been implemented in a proof-of-concept study for LCA 10, demonstrating safety and improvement of vision in some subjects in a small group study (Pierce et al., 2024). You can find a readable description of CRISPR and its history for nonexperts in a book by Kevin Davies (2020).

The German ophthalmologist Theodor Leber described two inherited eye conditions in the 19th century that bear his name—Leber hereditary optic neuropathy (LHON) and Leber congenital amaurosis (LCA). (According to the Merriam-Webster Dictionary, the term *amaurosis* has Greek and Latin origins pertaining to the dimming of sight and refers to vision loss without an identifiable cause.)

LCA is a subtype of RP with onset during infancy, characterized by nystagmus and rapid progression of vision loss. A first symptom is often difficulty seeing at night, sometimes termed nyctalopia, or simply night blindness.

Modern genetics has identified at least 19 gene variants for different types of LCA, designated as LCA 1, LCA 2, etc. Most of these variants have a recessive pattern of inheritance, meaning that a child will be affected only if both parents possess the gene variant.

One variant of the RPE65 gene was associated with LCA 2 in 1997. The functioning version of this gene encodes an enzyme produced by cells in the RPE. This enzyme plays a role in the conversion of light absorbed by the photoreceptors into neural signals. Without healthy RPE65 genes, the photoreceptors, especially the rods, decline in their sensitivity to light and eventually become nonfunctional. Variants of this gene are responsible for the LCA 2 version of Leber congenital amaurosis. Vision deficits usually emerge in early childhood with progression that is likely to lead to total blindness in adulthood.

Feasibility studies on gene therapy for LCA 2 were led by Jean Bennett and Albert Maguire, a married couple at the University of Pennsylvania in Philadelphia. Initial success was demonstrated with dogs. Some members of the Briard breed experienced night blindness but retained functional vision in daylight. It was discovered that the affected dogs had a variant of the RPE65 gene. A study reported in 2001 by Acland and colleagues demonstrated improved light sensitivity in dogs treated with gene therapy to replace the defective RPE65 gene. One of the treated dogs, named Lancelot, became a celebrity, appearing on TV and visiting the United States Congress. Figure 10.4 is a photo of Lancelot which appeared in the journal *Nature Genetics.*

The success of the dog studies motivated the first clinical trials of gene therapy for LCA 2 in humans. Encouraging initial results with human patients were reported separately in 2008 by groups at the University of Pennsylvania and University College London. In 2017, the U.S. FDA approved gene therapy to treat LCA 2. This was the FDA's first approval of a gene therapy for a disease caused by a variant of a single gene.

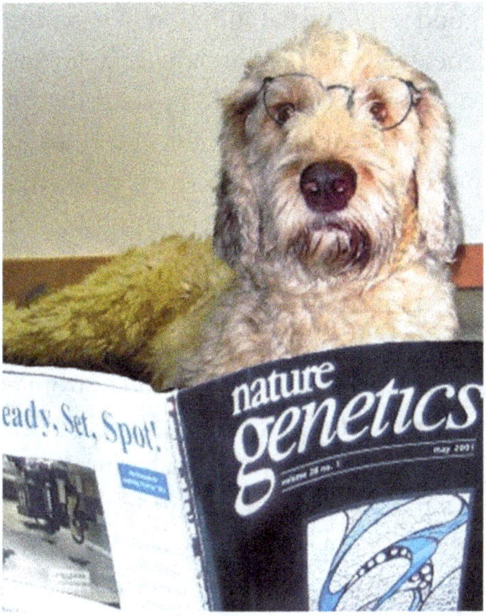

Figure 10.4 A photo of Lancelot, a dog that was treated with gene therapy for a defective RPE65 gene. He is wearing glasses and looking at a copy of *Nature Genetics*. Reproduced from Nature Genetics (2003). Touching base: Mutant of the month. *Nature Genetics, 33*, 119.

The therapy for LCA 2 involves the injection of the drug voretigene neparvovec into the eye, with the brand name Luxturna, manufactured by Spark Therapeutics. The one-time treatment costs \$850,000 for both eyes of a patient.

The gene therapy for LCA 2 requires challenging surgery with patients under general anesthetic. A needle is used to inject tiny droplets under the retina. The droplets contain human-engineered viruses with functioning RPE65 genes. These adeno-associated-viruses (AAVs) are relatively safe and effective at delivering their genetic payload to retinal cells.

How effective is this form of gene therapy for restoring vision in people with LCA 2? A 2017 report by Russell and colleagues described a randomized clinical trial conducted jointly at the Children's Hospital of Philadelphia and the University of Iowa. The results of the trial were presented to the FDA in seeking approval for using Luxturna to treat LCA 2. Evidence was reported for 20 subjects treated with Luxturna and nine controls, all with LCA 2. Ages of the subjects ranged from four to 46 years. Nine of the treated subjects and four of the controls were less than 10 years old. The primary goal of the trial was to determine if the gene therapy would restore visual function in dim lighting.

What would be a good test of visual function in low illumination? Mobility is important at all light levels. The research team developed a new test called the multi-luminance mobility test (MLMT) described in detail by Daniel Chung et al. (2018). This test requires a subject to walk through an obstacle course, following a path defined by black arrows printed on white cloth lying on the floor. The path is constrained to a 5 foot by 10 foot area but can be rearranged for multiple trials. Following a period of dark adaptation, subjects traverse the path on several trials at several low light levels. Calibrated illumination levels in the MLMT include 1, 4, 10, 50, 125, 250, and 400 lux (lx). In Chapter 7, I identified 20–50 lx as being at the bottom end of the photopic (daylight) range for normal vision. The lowest level in MLMT of 1 lx would be in the mesopic range. According to Chung et al., this illumination level would resemble a moonless summer night or an indoor nightlight. The upper end of the MLMT illumination range of 400 lx would be typical for illumination of a letter chart in an eye clinic. A subject's performance in the MLMT test was measured by the time taken to traverse the path and the number of errors (such as bumping into one of the obstacles or veering off the path). A subject passed the test at a given light level if they completed the course within three minutes and with fewer than four errors. The measurement of interest for each subject in the clinical trial was the lowest illumination level for passing the MLMT before and after gene therapy. If the therapy was helpful in restoring vision in dim lighting, we would expect a treated subject to pass the course under lower illumination after treatment. A key outcome measure of the clinical trial was the change in MLMT score at one year after treatment. The results indicated that treated subjects improved by almost two levels on the MLMT. For instance, a patient whose lowest-passing illumination before treatment was 50 lx might have passed at 4 lx following treatment, or another patient might have passed at 125 lx before treatment and 10 lx after treatment. (The mean improvement in the number of illumination levels for the treatment group was 1.8 and for the controls, an insignificant 0.2.) Thirteen of the 20 treated subjects passed the MLMT at the lowest illumination of 1 lx after treatment, but none of the controls passed at this lowest level. These results show that Luxturna enhances light sensitivity, improving mobility in dim lighting for people with LCA 2.

The treated group also exhibited a modest improvement in acuity on the ETDRS chart when tested with typical clinical lighting. The average improvement following gene therapy was between one and two lines on the chart. In another study of 41 patients treated with Luxturna gene therapy at three sites—the Bascom Palmer Eye Institute, Cincinnati Children's Hospital, and Baylor College of Medicine—no persisting improvements in visual acuity were observed following treatment (Sengillo, 2022). This study did not include the MLMT mobility test, but the majority of patients did report improvement in night vision.

What should we make of the vision improvements due to gene therapy with Luxturna? Some dramatic reports in the press have described patients throwing away their white canes and abandoning reading of Braille. There may be wide variability in patient outcomes; some patients may improve much more than others. Improvements in acuity in daylight situations are usually modest. It seems clear that the therapy enhances light sensitivity and is functionally valuable at night and in other dimly lit situations. How valuable is improvement in night vision?

My former PhD student and friend Walter Wu has a different form of RP but also experiences difficulty with night vision. His acuity and limited visual field permit good mobility in daylight; he doesn't need to use a white cane for effective travel. As sunset approaches, his vision becomes more impaired. He slows down in unfamiliar outdoor areas and sometimes uses a cane. He carries a bright flashlight to illuminate ahead at night. His use of a flashlight can be embarrassing; once, in a dimly lit restaurant, he was told not to use it. At home, he has motion-sensitive night lights placed at strategic locations to assist with mobility after dark. He plans visits to parks and other outdoor venues to avoid dimly lit areas at night. Once, he found himself in a large, poorly lit park after sunset without a flashlight. He had trouble seeing his way along the walkway at the ocean's edge. He fell into the water. Fortunately, he was able to scramble back over the retaining wall, avoiding a very serious situation. Walter agrees that enhancing night vision would be helpful to him for mobility. While he has adopted strategies to cope with his greater vision disability at night, therapy to provide better night vision would enable him to travel with more confidence, less anxiety, and less need for planning ahead.

An important issue in evaluating the efficacy of Luxturna treatment is the period of sustained improvement in vision. Reports indicate that the enhancement of light sensitivity is observed within 30 days after the surgery and is sustained for at least one to three years. Patients with LCA 2, if untreated, usually face progressive loss of vision, often ending in total blindness. If gene therapy results in the preservation of vision for years or possibly even a lifetime, its benefits accumulate over time compared with the progressive loss in untreated eyes. So, while the restoration of vision may be limited primarily to improved night vision, the preservation of vision over years may be its greatest benefit.

The price tag of $850,000 for Luxturna is controversial. Who can afford this, and who will pay? Is such a price justifiable for the expected vision improvement? How much is the quality of life enhanced?

Quality of life with a health condition is sometimes quantified as a percentage of the quality of life with full health. In Chapter 1, I described the time-tradeoff (TTO) method for estimating quality of life with AMD. A team led by Scott Johnson at Medicus Economics LLC in Boston conducted a study on the cost of Luxturna treatment for LCA 2 in relation to the expected improvement in quality of life (Johnson et al., 2019). (Some members of the team were affiliated with Spark Therapeutics, the manufacturer of Luxturna.) Box 10.1 provides a brief description of their approach. Their bottom line conclusion was that Luxturna treatment is cost-effective if the visual benefits are sustained over a lifetime.

Box 10.1 Is Luxturna treatment cost-effective?

Suppose a person's quality of life with a given form of vision loss is estimated to be only 60% of their quality of life with full vision. If this condition persists for the rest of their life expectancy, say 50 years, we would say that the number of quality-adjusted life years (QALYs) with the condition is 60% of 50, which is 30 years. Suppose a therapy would result in vision improvement so that the quality of life after the treatment is estimated to be 80%. If sustained across 50 years, the number of QALYs following treatment is 40, a gain of ten QALYs compared to the untreated case. We can also estimate lifetime costs in dollars associated with vision care without the treatment and potential indirect costs such as reduced earning potential, government subsidies, and care-giver costs. If a treatment, such as Luxturna, results in improved vision, we would expect the lifetime of vision-related costs to be less, but the cost of the treatment must be included to assess cost-effectiveness.

Johnson (2019) and colleagues conducted an analysis like this for Luxturna treatment of LCA 2. They developed a model that compared QALYs for LCA 2 patients who did or did not receive Luxturna gene therapy. From their modeling, an average LCA 2 patient receiving gene therapy would enjoy an extra 9.5 QALYs if treatment benefits were sustained throughout their expected lifetime. In computing lifetime costs, the model took several factors into account, including the likely decline in vision of untreated patients, mortality information (life expectancy), direct costs of the therapy, conventional eye care costs, and indirect costs to both groups associated with the impact of impaired vision on educational attainment, work productivity, care-giver costs, and government programs. Using various scenarios for the period and extent of retained vision improvement following gene therapy, they estimated the cost per additional QALY to range from about

$80,000 per year (assuming preservation of vision benefits throughout lifetime) to about $380,000 per year (assuming benefits decline rapidly within a few years). These dollar figures compare with an estimated $150,000 that people might be expected to pay for one extra year of life with full health. Without a doubt, the model estimates contain substantial uncertainty. If the model is reasonably accurate, the cost effectiveness of the Luxturna gene therapy will depend heavily on the number of years of sustained vision improvement.

There continues to be intense research interest in developing gene therapies for other IRDs associated with single gene variants. These are causes of vision loss for which there have been no prior treatments, so gene therapy offers great promise. A review article by Alexis Britten-Jones (2022) and colleagues from the University of Melbourne identified many publications, conference abstracts, and clinical trial registrations regarding clinical studies of retinal and optic nerve disorders associated with 16 distinct gene variants. The authors reviewed reports on safety and outcomes for RPE65-mediated retinal dystrophy (referred to as LCA 2 above), choroideremia, LHON, rod-cone dystrophy, achromatopsia (discussed in Chapter 3), and X-linked retinoschisis. Very few of the reports found improvements in visual acuity, and none as much as three lines (15 letters) on the ETDRS chart. (Three lines are equivalent to an improvement in acuity by a factor of 2, such as an improvement from 20/200 to 20/100 [6/60 to 6/30]). Keep in mind that gene therapy might restore aspects of vision not measured on the acuity chart, such as improved night vision in LCA 2. In some cases, gene therapy may stabilize vision, preventing progressive loss. The major benefit of gene therapy may be preservation of vision rather than restoration of vision.

How do potential recipients of gene therapy for IRDs feel about the pros and cons of the treatment? Britten-Jones (2024) and colleagues conducted an online survey of 496 potential recipients from 35 countries (69% from the U.S.). Ninety percent of the respondents indicated that they would likely accept gene therapy if available to them, but more than half self-reported not having good knowledge of gene therapy. While a majority (63%) understood that one goal of gene therapy was to slow down the vision decline, 53% also thought that a goal was to restore vision back to normal. The authors of the study concluded that education is vital to avoid false expectations and misunderstandings by potential patients.

Before leaving the topic of gene therapy, what about Stargardt disease (SGTD)? Although still quite rare, SGTD is the most-prevalent inherited retinal disorder associated with a single gene, the ABCA4 gene. SGTD is usually first diagnosed in childhood or adolescence. It damages the macula and often leads to central vision loss with visual consequences similar to those discussed in Chapter 5 for AMD. Why hasn't gene therapy been deployed to treat SGTD? One limiting factor is that the ABCA4 gene is too large to be engineered into the viral vectors currently deployed for gene therapy in the eye. Ongoing research is focused on overcoming this limitation.

Brain plasticity and sight restoration

Most low vision results from disorders of the eye or optic nerve. But, most visual information processing and interpretation occur in brain centers and brain networks. In the context of vision restoration, brain plasticity refers to changes in the way the brain processes visual information following the onset of ocular pathology.

Susana Chung and I wrote a review article in 2016 about the role of brain plasticity in understanding low vision and its rehabilitation. We introduced a bridge analogy. Imagine a network of city streets on an island (brain network) and a major bridge (visual pathway) allowing traffic to flow from the mainland (outside world) to the city. In this analogy, the flow of traffic along the city streets represents the flow of neural signals in the brain. Suppose the bridge is damaged so that traffic is reduced or prevented from reaching the city, analogous to eye pathology that reduces visual input to the brain. Although the city streets themselves are unaffected, the traffic patterns in the city would likely change, and the flow of traffic might concentrate more on the use of other bridges from the mainland (other sensory channels). The changing patterns of traffic flow in the city resulting from the bridge closure are analogous to changes in neural information processing in the brain due to reduced visual input from eye pathology.

Pushing the analogy a little further, consider two qualitatively different types of changes that might occur in the city. If the bridge restrictions are long-term, the city engineers might decide on structural changes to the city street map, entirely closing some streets and building new ones to accommodate the modified needs of city traffic. Alternatively, instead of changing the street map, speed limits or other regulations could be introduced so that traffic is reduced along some existing streets and increased along others. The structural changes in the street map are analogous to the formation or pruning of neural connections in the brain network. Changing the controls on existing streets is analogous to changing levels of neural inhibition and excitation within neural networks without changing the network connectivity itself. In a 2010 article, Daphne Bavelier from the University of Rochester and colleagues described these two major categories of brain plasticity—structural changes modifying connectivity within brain networks and changes in the levels of excitation and inhibition within existing neural networks.

Two major issues related to brain plasticity have an impact on the potential for vision restoration—plasticity before and after sensitive periods for visual development and cross-modal reassignment of the visual cortex. First, let's consider sensitive periods and brain plasticity. As I pointed out in Chapter 9 on childhood low vision, the development of normal human vision depends critically on the nature of visual experience after birth. Humans are born with immature vision. Normal visual experience through developmentally sensitive periods is required to achieve healthy adult vision. When the sensitive periods close, biological mechanisms put the "brakes" on further structural modifications. The length of sensitive periods may vary for different aspects of vision, with processing of color and motion developing rapidly and some aspects of object recognition, such as face recognition, maturing much more slowly. Once the sensitive periods have ended, the networks of neural connections remain stable throughout adulthood. For people who experience vision loss as adults, this stability leaves open the possibility of full-vision recovery if a suitable treatment becomes available. For example, full recovery of vision can be expected following surgery for cataracts acquired later in life. On the other hand, if prolonged visual deprivation occurs early in life, as in the cases of SB, Virgil, and Mike May, visual maturation will be incomplete. It appears that once the sensitive periods for visual maturation are past, major structural changes in visual brain networks are no longer possible. By the time SB, Virgil, and Mike May had their vision restored, it was too late for their visual maturation to resume and achieve typical, normal adult levels.

There is research on methods for releasing the brakes on visual maturation to facilitate later sight restoration. In their review, Bavelier and colleagues discussed animal studies with drug therapies aimed at releasing the brakes on structural brain plasticity, but we are not yet close to therapies for humans.

Even if structural changes in visual brain networks are not possible, once the sensitive periods have ended, brain plasticity may take place through alteration of the balance of inhibition and excitation of connections within neural networks. One example, discussed earlier in this chapter, is the research on behavioral interventions to improve stereopsis in amblyopic eyes. In another example, Susana Chung (2011) trained a group of subjects with central-vision loss from AMD on a perceptual reading task. There were six weekly sessions of training, which ultimately yielded an average of 53% improvement in reading speed. Behavioral interventions involving extensive visual practice on a particular task are often called *perceptual learning*, implying that some mechanism in the visual pathway has been modified (possibly through rebalancing of synaptic inhibition and excitation) to perform the visual task more effectively.

A second issue concerns the reassignment of the visual cortex for other cognitive or perceptual functions in the presence of vision deprivation. For people with normal sight, a large proportion of the brain's cortex is devoted to visual processing (at least 30%). What happens to this large portion of the cortex during prolonged visual deprivation? For people born blind, evidence from functional brain-imaging studies has shown that the visual cortex becomes responsive to nonvisual input. In a 1996 report, Norihiro Sadato and colleagues at the NIH used brain imaging (positron emission tomography) to show that the occipital brain area (responsive to visual input in normally sighted subjects) was responsive during Braille reading and other tactile tasks. In a 2015 article, Gabriella Hirsch, Corinna Bauer, and Lotfi Merabet at the Massachusetts Eye and Ear Infirmary in Boston reviewed abundant research showing that the visual areas of the brain in early blind subjects are responsive in tasks involving touch, hearing, smell, and even working memory. This nonvisual responsiveness, termed cross-modal plasticity, may play a role in compensatory functioning in the blind.

Less is known about cortical reorganization in people with low vision. If you read my introduction to this book, you'll know that I had normal vision until the age of six. This is an age by which most but not all visual functions have reached mature levels. When I was six years old, I experienced a life-threatening illness that left me with permanent, severe low vision. How has my visual cortex fared during decades of visual deprivation?

At the age of 56, I participated in a brain-imaging study using fMRI. While in the MRI scanner, I was presented with either coarse visual stimuli (visible within my acuity limit) or tactile patterns (Braille characters and embossed shapes). The study was led by my PhD student Sing-Hang Cheung and described in a 2009 journal article. The results showed that the portion of my primary visual cortex typically responsive to high-acuity central vision in the occipital lobe (posterior portion of area V1) did not respond to the visual stimuli but did respond to the tactile stimuli. The portion of my visual cortex, typically responsive to stimuli in the peripheral visual field (anterior portion of V1), did respond to the visual input. It appears that my brain reorganized so that the region of the visual cortex typically responsive to fine details in central vision has been recruited for tactile functioning. The results showed, at least in my case, that the visual cortex has the capacity to share a portion of its resources with another sensory modality (touch), while retaining a portion for visual processing.

What functional benefit, if any, did I receive from the activation of the visual cortex by touch? Does it enhance my tactile perception? I do rely on touch for Braille reading and numerous daily tasks such as identifying coins. I participated in a follow-up study several years later to address this question. The study was conducted by Edward Silson (2022) and colleagues at the University of York in Yorkshire England. My wife Wendy and I were on vacation in northern England. I devoted a day in the lab at York to testing with fMRI and transcranial magnetic stimulation (TMS). TMS is a noninvasive method of brain stimulation. When applied to the scalp adjacent to a sensory area of cortex, it temporarily disrupts processing in that area. If the region of my visual cortex which responds to touch is important for tactile recognition, we would expect TMS applied to the corresponding region of my occipital lobe to disrupt tactile recognition of Braille characters. When TMS was applied to my somatosensory cortex, I felt a series of pulses delivered to my scalp above my right ear. The TMS caused some slightly unpleasant jaw clenching. As expected, it also made the Braille symbols on my right index finger harder to recognize. But, when TMS pulses were applied to my visual cortex at the back of my head, there was no impact on my ability to feel the Braille symbols.

These results imply that the tactile responsiveness of my visual cortex is not playing a critical role in my ability to recognize Braille characters. It remains uncertain what functional role, if any, the responsiveness of my visual cortex to touch plays.

A study by Samantha Cunningham (2014) and colleagues at the University of Southern California, using fMRI, also found tactile responses in the visual cortex of a group of nine subjects with vision impairment. These subjects had peripheral visual-field loss due to RP. The investigators found a correlation between the regions of visual-field loss and cortical regions responding to tactile stimuli in their subjects.

It remains to be determined if the responsiveness of the visual cortex to tactile or other nonvisual signals in the brains of people with low vision plays a useful functional role. If so, this form of plasticity may pose barriers for any subsequent therapies for sight restoration. We don't yet understand the factors that predispose the visual cortex to become responsive to tactile or other nonvisual stimuli nor the capacity of the visual cortex to re-establish visual responsiveness following sight restoration therapy.

Reflecting on the two major issues concerning brain plasticity and low vision, Susana Chung and I wrote in our 2016 review:

> Visual plasticity has a dual nature when it comes to rehabilitation. Reorganization of visual processing in the presence of low vision, such as cross-modal sharing of visual pathways with tactile or auditory processing, may be of enormous adaptive advantage in the everyday lives of people with low vision. But this reorganization may get in the way of potential sight-restoring therapies or prosthetics later on. On the other hand, decreased plasticity, typical of late-onset low vision from cataract or AMD, may leave the visual pathways more intact and receptive to sight-restoring therapies. The duality of plasticity means that the age of onset of low vision and the number of years of vision impairment will play important roles in determining the potential functional benefits of retinal implants, gene therapy, optogenetics and other innovative treatments for vision loss. Consideration of this duality may help specialists and their low-vision patients/clients decide whether to undertake sight-restoring treatment, devote effort to training with a sensory-substitution device or concentrate on more traditional strategies for adapting to low vision.

Epilogue

Looking Ahead

In this book, I've described what low vision is, how we measure it, and what people with low vision see and do with their eyesight. In recent years, we've seen dramatic growth in society's recognition of the existence of low vision and in our understanding of its diverse characteristics. These advances have made the world a better place for those of us with low vision. What developments might we expect in the near future? Crystal ball gazing is a blurry enterprise, but here are some things I'll be watching for.

• • • • •

Will the prevalence of low vision rise or decline?

With advances in eye and vision research, we might expect the prevalence of low vision and blindness to diminish in coming years. But, most current projections predict an increase in the number of people with low vision in developed countries including the United States. There are two main reasons. First, the proportion of seniors in the population is increasing, and most low vision results from age-related eye diseases. Second, the population as a whole continues to grow.

The worldwide epidemic of myopia (near sightedness) may also have a major impact. The Brian Holden Vision Institute[1] in Australia has reported that the worldwide prevalence of myopia is expected to increase from about 28% (two billion people) in 2010 to about 50% (five billion people) in 2050. It is thought that nearly one billion of the 2050 population will have high myopia (defined as having more than 5 diopters of myopia). In developed countries, myopia can usually be corrected with glasses and is not included in counts of low vision. But, there is growing evidence that high myopia is a risk

[1] https://bhvi.org/.

Low Vision. Gordon E. Legge, Oxford University Press. © Oxford University Press (2026).
DOI: 10.1093/9780198946960.003.0012

factor for several eye conditions, especially myopic macular degeneration, leading to low vision. In a population-based study conducted in the Netherlands, Tideman (2016) and colleagues reported that 39% of people over the age of 75 years with high myopia were visually impaired, compared with only 3.8% of those with milder levels of myopia. In short, as the worldwide prevalence of myopia rises, so too will the prevalence of high myopia, with a corresponding increase in the number of people with low vision. There is ongoing research into the causes of the rising prevalence of myopia, possible preventative measures such as increased daylight exposure for children, and, ultimately, ways to reduce the risk of high myopia and corresponding vision impairment.

Meanwhile, efforts will continue to eradicate or treat preventable causes of blindness and low vision, with a focus on less developed countries. For example, in 2024, the World Health Organization declared the total elimination of the blinding disease trachoma in Pakistan, the 19th country where the disease has been eliminated. Accomplishments like this will contribute to lower prevalence of impaired vision worldwide.

New ways to measure low vision

In Part I of this book, I described the common clinical tests for measuring low vision—acuity, contrast sensitivity, and visual-field perimetry. These methods are used primarily to diagnose and follow the progression of eye disease and to evaluate the outcomes of treatments. These tests have also been used as indirect measures of everyday visual functioning by people with low vision. We will continue to see updated and improved versions of these tests, some with applications to low vision, and new digital versions of the tests for use on the web or in mobile applications. In addition, two different approaches for assessing visual function have been emerging in the past couple of decades and are likely to be used more frequently with direct impact on low-vision rehabilitation.

First, performance measures are being designed for more direct evaluation of vision in important everyday tasks. These include tests of reading (my own development of the MNREAD test, described in Chapter 6, is an example), mobility, face perception, and even driving. The implementation of such tests in virtual reality or other digital formats is likely to increase.

A second approach involves self-reports from low-vision participants about difficulties they experience in daily life. Visual function questionnaires ask participants to rate their difficulty in performing a wide range of tasks. Psychometric methods are then employed to use the responses to estimate a quantity called a person's *visual ability.* Think of visual ability as an overall estimate of how well the person is able to use vision in accomplishing a wide range of daily activities. Robert Massof and colleagues at Johns Hopkins University have introduced a psychometric method, item response theory (IRT), into vision science to estimate a person's visual ability across a range of tasks and to estimate the visual difficulty of those tasks. In a 2007 paper, Massof and colleagues described the development and use of the Activity Inventory consisting of 459 questions about visual difficulty covering four visual domains—reading, mobility, visual-motor activities, and information gathering. Data from 1,880 low-vision participants revealed that underlying visual ability splits into at least two dimensions; visual ability for reading is different from visual ability for orientation and mobility. I anticipate more applications of visual function questionnaires. In Chapter 2, I described the development of a questionnaire for people with low vision to relate their measured acuity on the eye chart (such as 20/100) to their ability to accomplish a wide range of everyday visual tasks (Wu et al., 2024). Another application is the assessment of multisensory function. Xiong (2024) and colleagues developed a questionnaire in which participants rated both their auditory and visual abilities in locating everyday audiovisual objects such as people talking and cars moving. The study included participants with vision and/or hearing impairment and assessed their spatial localization abilities in both sensory modalities. A questionnaire of this type could be useful in evaluating spatial orientation and mobility of people with dual-sensory impairment.

What about advances in high tech?

I see at least three ways in which artificial intelligence (AI) will have an impact on low vision. First, there is already burgeoning research on using AI to diagnose eye disease early from large databases of retinal images and other ocular measures. Early and improved diagnosis may lead to lower incidence and severity of eye conditions leading to low vision.

Second, AI may become useful in planning rehabilitation strategies for low vision, either directly by providing information to low-vision consumers or by guiding rehab specialists. If you have low vision, imagine describing your condition to AI, answering its questions in a conversational format, and receiving its suggestions for assistive tech or strategies to overcome your specific everyday problems.

Third, AI is rapidly being incorporated into assistive technology for people with vision impairment. There are already apps that provide detailed and fairly reliable descriptions of pictures and photos. Mostly, they provide descriptions of single, static images. But, as technology advances, it is likely that AI agents will be able to provide a running commentary to a visually impaired user of streaming video from their phone or smart glasses. Imagine an app that describes what's ahead as you walk down the street or what can be viewed out of the window of a car, bus, train, or airplane. It remains to be seen if AI agents will ultimately replace the value of remote human assistance offered by services such as Aira and Be My Eyes. Some users may prefer the social contact and common sense of humans to even very clever AI agents.

People have asked me if companies can use AI to safely navigate autonomous vehicles at auto speeds safely, why can't we provide people who are blind or who have low vision with effortless mobility? There are two major barriers. First, autonomous vehicles rely on numerous cameras and other sensors. Will it be possible to package a similar array of technology into a practical, wearable, and cost-effective system for pedestrians with impaired vision? Maybe so, with miniaturization and lower prices. Second, there is the interface problem. For human mobility, the sensor data need to be converted to accurate, timely, real-time information for the user, potentially in a visual display but more likely in speech, audio, or tactile formats. Perhaps, an array of wearable sensors could feed a real-time AI agent who would in turn provide descriptive information to guide a visually impaired person along a busy street or across a traffic intersection.

I will continue to watch for efforts to make autonomous vehicles accessible for visually impaired users, first as rideshare vehicles and ultimately as personally owned vehicles.

Let's not forget about the future of high-tech vision aids. There continues to be interest in developing cost-effective head-mounted video magnifiers to help with reading and mobility. As I briefly reviewed in Chapter 6, there are still design challenges ahead related to cost, appearance, ergonomics, and range of magnification. The CCTV and its portable electronic offspring have been a big success for people with low vision. It remains to be seen if head-mounted descendants will have similar success. Modern mainstream technology may provide options for use in low vision such as the Apple Vision Pro and the Meta Smart Glasses. And, there is still room and opportunity for creative optical designs, such as the Peli prisms for hemianopia discussed in Chapter 4 or improved bioptic telescopes for driving (Chapter 8).

What about advances in technology for vision restoration?

There is already extensive research on gene therapies for inherited retinal diseases with initial success in treating Leber congenital amaurosis

(Chapter 10). Almost certainly, treatments will emerge for other single-gene disorders. Depending how early in the disease process these treatments can be delivered, they may be particularly important in forestalling decline of vision or even in improving vision. And perhaps, the impact will be the greatest if these treatments are safe for children early in life.

What about the potential of vision prostheses? Will Brindley and Lewin's (1968) optimistic prediction come to pass that direct cortical stimulation will restore vision adequate for effective visual mobility and effortless reading (Chapter 10)? We are still a long way from achieving these goals. Given the sophisticated processing of visual signals by the retinal and cortical neural networks, it will be a heavy lift to simply stimulate cortical cells with processed video from a camera and expect high-quality transfer of visual information. I remain skeptical but hopeful. Progress may depend on methods to target specific cell types in the retina or visual cortex with patterns of electrical stimulation customized for those cells. To date, prosthetics have provided only very low vision, sometimes termed ultra-low vision. What is the ceiling? How good can prosthetic vision be? Time will tell.

In 2024, there was an exciting report of a whole-eye transplant (Ceradini et al., 2024). The patient had lost an eye in a serious injury from a high-voltage electrical accident. While aspects of the complex surgery were successful, including sustained blood flow to the retina, the patient experienced no recovery of vision. Will it be possible to replace an entirely blind eye with a seeing eye? In a 2024 commentary, Bradley and Woog identified significant issues concerning the likelihood of restoring vision through such complex surgery. I remain skeptical that a whole eye can be transplanted and vision restored. But, who would have thought heart transplants would be possible when they were first proposed in the early 20th century?

Here's a thought experiment. Suppose you are a person with severe low vision like me or someone who is totally blind. To function well in our visuocentric (ableist) world, would you prefer to invest your time, energy, and money in surgery to restore coarse low vision from a prosthetic system? Or would you prefer to invest your effort in learning nonvisual rehabilitation strategies including the use of AI apps on your smartphone to help with mobility and reading text? I'm fairly certain in saying that in order to read hard-copy text on a page or sign, the phone app will be more effective than the vision prosthesis, at least in the foreseeable future. But, of course, it need not be an either/or choice. A person who chooses prosthesis can also make use of apps that describe scenes in speech or Braille.

What can we expect to learn from brain imaging about low vision?

There have been many brain-imaging studies of how the visual pathways adapt to blindness, but less is known about how the brain adapts to low vision. Big questions remain. Answers will almost certainly depend on the age of onset of vision impairment and its interaction with sensitive periods for visual development. If visual areas of the brain have reorganized in response to early visual deprivation, can normal visual function be restored later on and at what cost? In my own case with the onset of vision impairment at six years, a portion of my visual cortex is unresponsive to visual input but responsive to touch (discussed in Chapter 10). What is the functional benefit, if any, of this cortical reorganization?

If normal adult vision is in place before the onset of low vision, can we rely on reviving normal brain processing years later if future research permits normal visual input to be restored? How long can this dormant functionality last—for years or decades?

For those considering vision restoration through prosthetics, can tests be developed to assess the surviving integrity of visual processing in the brain?

Brain imaging will clearly continue to help us understand the structural and functional consequences of vision loss due to brain lesions found in cortical visual impairment (CVI).

What are the future prospects for education and employment of people with low vision?

In my own education and academic career, I've crossed over from the visuocentric world of hard-copy text, chalkboard diagrams, and slide projectors to the era of screen magnification, text-to-speech, web accessibility guidelines, and growing awareness of accessibility issues in classrooms and the workplace. In the United States, the Americans with Disabilities Act (ADA) has had a profoundly positive influence. In April 2024, the U.S. Federal government published a Final Rule from the ADA requiring public educational institutions to make web content and mobile apps readily accessible for students with disabilities. Although still challenging, especially in science, technology, engineering, and mathematics (STEM) fields, it has become more feasible today for students with low vision to keep pace with peers in school and compete for quality jobs. With the growing use of graphics and data charts in many fields including STEM, more needs to be done to enhance accessibility of figures of all kinds for people with impaired vision. Advances in optical character recognition and its implementation in text-to-speech, beginning with the pioneering work of Ray Kurzweil in the 1970s and 1980s, has made most text readily accessible to people with impaired vision. I look forward to a day when maps, data figures, and other forms of graphics are as readily accessible to people with impaired vision as most text is now.

Teachers and professors who routinely incorporate accessible practices in their classrooms are engaging in inclusive design. Making PowerPoint files available to students in advance and clearly verbalizing key points of graphics in classroom presentations benefits all students and especially those with impaired vision.

The increasing societal recognition of the potential of people with low vision means an increased need for rehabilitation programs. Even in wealthy countries, we need wider availability of rehabilitation information and services. This is especially true in small communities and rural areas. Telerehabilitation is likely to play an increasing role, in which people with low vision access occupational therapy and other forms of rehabilitation over the internet. A study led by Ava Bittner (2024) at the University of California at Los Angeles showed that follow-up training with reading magnifiers at home over a video link was as effective as similar in-office instruction by optometrists.

Enhancement of environmental accessibility and lifestyle improvements

Society has a growing realization and responsibility, embodied in the ADA, to make public life more accessible for people with impaired vision in all realms. In Chapter 7, I described the concept of visual accessibility in architectural design. The goal is to provide architects and designers with tools to make hazards and other key features of built spaces highly visible, taking variations in lighting and viewpoint into account. Visual accessibility is a goal in public spaces of all kinds, including clinics, hospitals, shopping centers, community centers, senior residences, and apartment buildings. Accessible design for low vision can be incorporated into other realms, such as websites, computer apps, classrooms, and public transportation. I look forward to creative designs and approaches. And, of course, accessibility must go beyond visual design to include nonvisual accessibility for people who are blind or have severe low vision.

At the individual level, we are learning more about how lifestyle changes can enhance quality of life for people with low vision. In Chapter 7, I talked about how lighting, contrast, and other factors can enhance accessibility at home. Exercise programs may be developed and shown to improve safe mobility and reduce falls and injuries by seniors with impaired vision.

We already know that nutritional supplements can slow down progression of AMD (Chapter 5). Research by Emily Chew (2020) and colleagues at the U.S. National Eye Institute has shown that a healthy diet can also be good for vision. The American Academy of Ophthalmology recommends the Mediterranean Diet: Healthy Eating for Healthier Eyes.[2]

• • • • •

I am composing these closing remarks in the early days of 2025. By the time you read this book, there will be progress on the topics I've touched on, and new ideas will have emerged. For those of us with low vision and for professionals who are engaged in research or rehabilitation to improve the quality of life for people with low vision, the future is bright. I'm excited to see what comes next.

[2] https://www.aao.org/eye-health/news/mediterranean-diet-healthy-eating-healthier-eyes

APPENDIX

Structures of the Eye

This appendix includes a brief overview of the structures of the eye and the neural connections of the eyes to the visual cortex in the brain.

• • • • •

Anatomy of the eye

Many books and online resources provide more detailed descriptions. The presentation here is intended to give you sufficient background to understand the anatomical references made in this book. Internet searches will provide you with lots of additional information about any of the anatomical terms mentioned below.

Figure A1 is a drawing of the major structures of the eye, with an accompanying blow-up showing key components of the retina. We pay special attention to the retina because much of low vision results from retinal disorders.

The schematic eye in the drawing is looking at a cartoon figure of a carrot. Light rays from the carrot are brought to focus by the optics of the eye (cornea and crystalline lens) to form a small, inverted image of the carrot on the retina.

The human eye is approximately spherical (hence the term "eye ball"), with a diameter of about 24 mm (nearly one inch). The eyeball contains three concentric layers—sclera, choroid, and retina—with additional important interior structures.

The *sclera,* the "white of the eye," is a tough, fibrous outer, protective layer of the eye, covering about 80% of the surface area. It forms a boundary with the cornea at the front of the eye. The border between the sclera and the cornea (where the white of the eye meets the clear portion) is called the *limbus.* The sclera has a hole at the back for the optic nerve to leave the eye.

The *cornea* is the transparent front surface of the eye. The front surface of the cornea is the major refracting surface in the eye. The eye as a whole has a refractive power of about 60 diopters. The front surface of the cornea contributes about 42 diopters. At its center, the cornea is very nearly spherical. Away from the center, the cornea flattens slightly. This flattening helps improve optical image quality by reducing spherical aberration in the eye. The cornea's major role in vision is to bend incoming light rays to focus on the retina.

When light leaves the cornea, it passes through the *aqueous humor.* This is a dilute, watery solution (similar to salt water) that lies between the cornea and the crystalline lens. It is produced by the ciliary body and is maintained under pressure and helps retain the shape of the eye. Eye shape (especially the distance between cornea and retina) is optically important for creating focused images on the retina.

The *choroid* is a layer of the eyeball that lies between the retina and the sclera. It contains blood vessels that provide metabolic support to the retina and other structures of the eye.

The *iris* is the forward portion of the choroid. Variations in its pigment molecules (melanin) determine eye color—blue, green, brown, and occasionally other colors. Distinctive individual variations in pigmentation texture have been exploited for biometric recognition systems. (John Daugman, a fellow graduate student of mine at Harvard University, developed and patented the first algorithms to do iris recognition.)

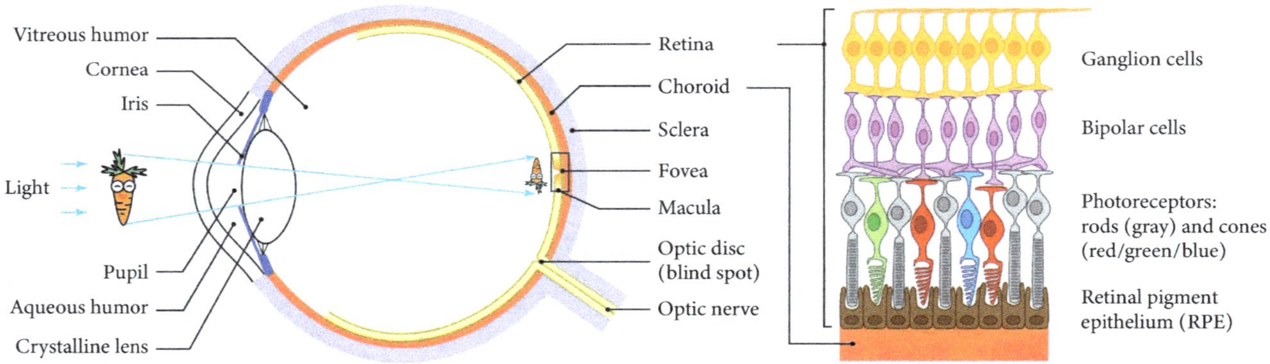

Figure A1 A schematic diagram of the human eye. An eye is facing to the left, viewing a cartoon carrot wearing glasses. Blue lines depict light rays from the carrot entering the eye. The rays are refracted by the cornea and lens to form an inverted and left-right reversed image of the carrot on the retina. Important structures are color-coded for ease of identification: sclera (light purple), choroid (orange), iris (dark blue), retina (light yellow) containing the macula (darker yellow), and retinal pigment epithelium (brown). A blow-up of the retina is shown at the right, including rods (gray), three types of cones (red, green, and blue), bipolar cells (purple), and ganglion cells (dark yellow).

The *pupil* is an opening at the center of the iris. The size of the pupil is variable and is controlled by two muscles working in opposition, sphincter to narrow pupil size and dilator to widen it. The pupil acts as an aperture of variable size. It plays a role like the F-stop on a camera. Generally, pupil size decreases with increasing light intensity. Pupil diameter ranges from a minimum of two millimeters to eight millimeters. Wider pupils allow more light to enter the eye creating brighter retinal images. The range of pupil size decreases with age so that older people experience less pupil dilation in dim illumination.

The *crystalline lens* is a transparent structure without blood vessels or nerves. It is convex on both its front and back surfaces (biconvex) and plays a role in bringing light to focus on the retina. The shape of the crystalline lens is controlled by the ciliary muscle. The variation in shape gives the eye adjustable refractive power, permitting focus on objects at different distances. As an object approaches the eye, the lens must exert more refractive power (by becoming more convex) to keep the object in focus on the retina. The increase in dioptric power of the lens is termed *visual accommodation*. As people get older, the ability of the crystalline lens to change shape declines, resulting in a reduced ability to change focus. This is why older people need reading glasses or bifocals.

The *vitreous humor* is a jelly-like substance that fills the posterior chamber between the crystalline lens and the retina. Sometimes, people notice stable dark spots in their vision when they view a uniform field such as the sky. The spots move when the eyes move. These *floaters* are usually due to shadows cast on the retina from clumping of microscopic fibers within the vitreous. They are usually harmless, but a sudden onset of many floaters might be a symptom of a retinal disorder.

The *retina* is a third layer of the eye, lying inside the choroid and extending only part way around the eyeball. Light-sensitive responses from the retina provide the input to vision. Any damage to the retina is likely to have an adverse impact on visual perception. The retina in each eye has an area of about 10 cm^2 (1.5 $inch^2$), slightly larger than the area of a postage stamp. The retina has a thickness of only 0.3 mm (1/100 inch) and is even thinner in the foveal region.

There are several layers of cells in the retina. The photoreceptors (rods and cones) are the cells that absorb light and initiate neural responses. They are located on the choroidal side of the retina. Light must pass through transparent layers of the retina in order to reach the photoreceptors. There are about 90 million rods and about five million cones in each eye (Lamb, 2016). The cones are responsible for daylight vision (photopic vision) and the rods for night vision (scotopic vision). People with normal color vision have cones with three types of pigments sensitive to different bands of visible light—long-wavelength-sensitive (L) cones absorb medium and long wavelengths (yellow-red light), medium-wavelength-sensitive (M) cones absorb medium wavelengths (green-yellow light), and the short-wavelength-sensitive (S) cones absorb short wavelengths (blue light). Abnormalities in the wavelength-sensitivity profiles of one or more of the cone pigments, or a total absence of a pigment, account for several forms of inherited color-vision deficits.

The *macula* is a region at the center of the retina with a high concentration of cones. At the center of the macula is a small depression in the retina called the *fovea*. The foveal depression has a diameter of about 1.5 mm. It is the region of densest concentration of cones. The central 0.5 mm of the fovea is rod-free. This rod-free region is estimated to contain about 34,000 cones. The fovea, with its dense packing of cones, is the region of highest visual acuity.

When photoreceptors absorb light, they generate electrical signals which are passed through the retina, first to *bipolar* cells and from the bipolars to *ganglion* cells. Other cells in the retinal network (amacrine cells and horizontal cells) make lateral connections within the retina.

The *retinal pigment epithelium* (RPE) is a layer of light-absorbing cells that lies adjacent to the photoreceptors. The tips of the photoreceptors (outer segments) containing light-absorbing pigment molecules are embedded in the RPE. The RPE plays a biologically active role in supporting photoreceptor function. Disease in the RPE underlies macular degeneration. Read more about macular degeneration in Chapter 5.

The *optic nerve* in each eye is a bundle of neuron fibers that carries information from the retina to the optic chiasm and onward to visual centers in the brain. The neural information includes the signals used in visual perception as well as signals controlling pupil size, visual accommodation, and circadian rhythms. The optic nerve in each eye has approximately one million nerve fibers, composed of the axons of the retinal ganglion cells.

The *optic disc* is a gap in the retina where the optic nerve leaves the eye. It corresponds to the naturally occurring *blind spot* in the visual field. It is offset from the fovea in the nasal side of the retina. Because of the laws of optical image formation, this means that the blind spot occurs in the peripheral visual field in each eye on the side toward the temple. More about the blind spot in Chapter 4.

Neural connections from the two eyes to the two hemispheres of the brain

Figure A2 illustrates how the eyes are connected to the primary visual cortex in the left and right hemispheres of the brain. In the two panels, the eyes are looking at a fixation point ahead. The visual axes (dotted gray lines) show that an image of the fixation point is formed on the fovea in each retina. The two panels show the resulting patterns of projections for targets in the left and right visual fields (Panel A) and for a target on the midline (Panel B).

Half of the optic nerve fibers from each eye project to the opposite (contralateral) hemisphere, crossing at the *optic chiasm*. The remaining nerve fibers project to the hemisphere on the same side (ipsilateral hemisphere). The optic nerve axons form synapses on neurons in a structure in the thalamus called the *lateral geniculate nucleus* (LGN). Axons from the LGN neurons form the *optic radiation* and make synapses on neurons in the *primary visual cortex*, also known as *area V1*, in the left and right hemispheres.

Let's examine the interesting arrangement of connections along the retinocortical pathway that underlies binocular vision. In Panel A, there is a red stop sign in the right visual field and a blue parking sign in the left visual field. Light rays from the blue parking sign in the left visual field create an image on the nasal (toward the nose) side of the retina in the left eye and the temporal (toward the temple) side of the retina in the right eye. Neural signals from the nasal retina in the left eye are routed to the right hemisphere, indicated by the blue lines in the drawing. Neural signals from the temporal retina in the right eye also project to the right hemisphere. In short, visual signals produced by a target in the left visual field are routed through the two eyes to the primary visual cortex in the right hemisphere. The opposite pattern holds for the red stop sign in the right visual field; neural information about this target is routed to the primary visual cortex in the left hemisphere. This arrangement means that the left visual field of both eyes is represented in the right hemisphere and the right visual field of both eyes is represented in the left hemisphere.

This pattern of projection enables information about a single object entering both eyes to converge on binocular neurons in the visual cortex of one hemisphere (either right or left). Binocular neurons are responsive to the corresponding input from the two eyes. These binocular neurons provide the basis for stereoscopic depth perception.

People sometimes mistakenly think that the eyes, like the hands and feet, project to the contralateral hemispheres—left eye to the right hemisphere and right eye to the left hemisphere. But, as we've just seen, it's the right visual field, not the right eye, that projects to the left hemisphere, and vice versa.

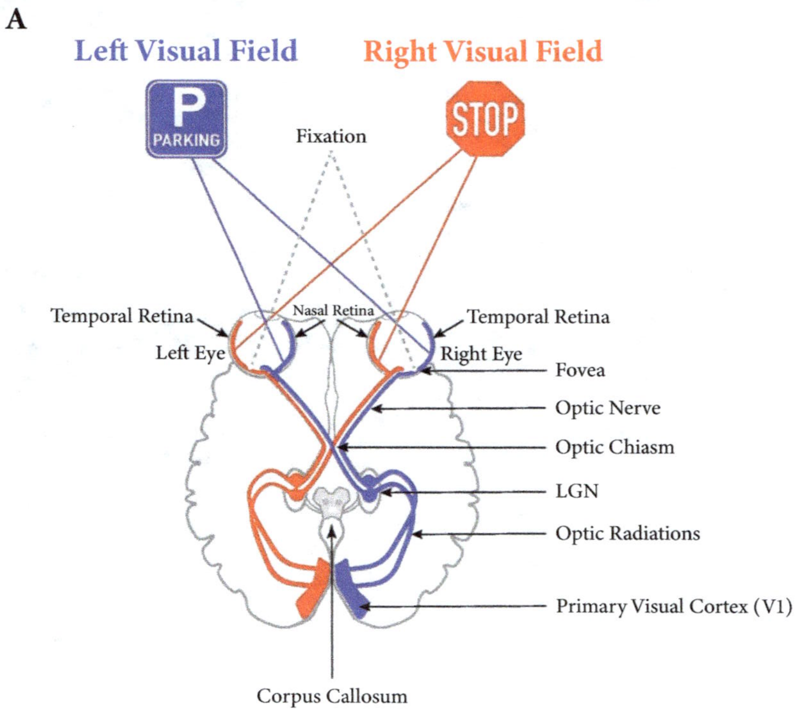

Figure A2 Schematic diagrams of the connections from the two eyes to the visual cortex in the left and right hemispheres of the brain. Viewed from above, the two eyes are looking at a fixation point on the midline ahead. Panel A illustrates the patterns of projection for a target in the left visual field (blue parking sign) and a target in the right visual field (red stop sign). Blue and red lines show how light rays from these targets form images on nasal and temporal retina in the two eyes, and how the pathways carry neural signals from the eyes to the brain. The diagram shows how the optic nerve fibers divide at the optic chiasm and project to the lateral geniculate nucleus (LGN) on both sides. Neurons from the LGN pass along the optic radiation to the primary visual cortex (area V1). A large bundle of nerve fibers called the corpus callosum allows for communication between the left and right hemispheres. Panel B illustrates the pattern of projection for a target on the midline (green exit sign) nearer to the observer than the point of fixation.

Panel B illustrates a different pattern of projection for targets lying on or near the midline between the two visual axes. These are targets that lie in opposite hemi-fields in the two eyes. For example, the green exit sign in Panel B is in the right visual field of the left eye and the left visual field of the right eye. The corresponding images are formed on temporal retina in both eyes with neural signals routed to visual cortex in ipsilateral hemispheres on opposite sides. This would seem to pose a problem for binocular vision since neural signals from the two eyes project to different hemispheres. Similarly, when objects lie between the visual axes, farther away than the fixation point, their images are formed on nasal retina in both eyes, with neural projections to the opposite hemispheres. Both of these cases seem to be problematic for stereoscopic depth perception because signals from the two eyes end up in different hemispheres. But, it is well-known that stereopsis is very good for judging the depth of objects on or near the midline. How do we resolve this seeming paradox?

The *corpus callosum* is a large bundle of fibers connecting the two hemispheres permitting interhemispheric communication. It is known that the corpus callosum carries visual information between the two hemispheres. It is possible that visual information about objects on or near the midline is brought back together via the corpus callosum. In a 1970 study, Donald Mitchell and Colin Blakemore, then at the University of California at Berkeley, evaluated stereoscopic depth perception in a split-brain patient. This was a patient whose corpus callosum was cut to prevent epileptic seizures from propagating from one hemisphere to the other. This patient was able to make stereo depth judgments for targets in the left and right peripheral fields but was unable to make stereo depth judgments along the midline. This interesting result provides evidence that an intact corpus callosum is required for stereoscopic depth perception for targets lying on or near the midline.

References

Acland, G. M., Aguirre, G. D., Ray, J., Zhang, Q., Aleman, T. S., Cideciyan, A. V., Pearce-Kelling, S. E., Anand, V., Zeng, Y., Maguire, A. M., Jacobson, S. G., Hauswirth, W. W., & Bennett, J. (2001). Gene therapy restores vision in a canine model of childhood blindness. *Nature Genetics, 28*, 92–95. https://doi.org/10.1038/ng0501-92

Adkisson, J. (n.d.). LostEye. http://LostEye.com

Alexander, M. S., Lajoie, K., Neima, D. R., Strath, R. A., Robinovitch, S. N., & Marigold, D. S. (2014a). Effect of ambient light and age-related macular degeneration on precision walking. *Optometry & Vision Science, 91*(8), 990–999. https://doi.org/10.1097/OPX.0000000000000316

Alexander, M. S., Lajoie, K., Neima, D. R., Strath, R. A., Robinovitch, S. N., & Marigold, D. S. (2014b). Effects of age-related macular degeneration and ambient light on curb negotiation. *Optometry & Vision Science, 91*(8), 975–989. https://doi.org/10.1097/OPX.0000000000000286

American Academy of Ophthalmology. (2024, April 3). *Mediterranean diet: healthy eating for healthier eyes.* https://www.aao.org/eye-health/news/mediterranean-diet-healthy-eating-healthier-eyes

American Council of the Blind (2011, July 12). *Best practices and guidelines for large print documents used by the low vision community.* https://www.acb.org/large-print-guidelines

American Foundation for the Blind (AFB) (n.d.). *CCTVs/Video Magnifiers.* https://www.afb.org/blindness-and-low-vision/using-technology/assistive-technology-products/video-magnifiers

American Foundation for the Blind (AFB). (n.d.). Statistics about children and youth with vision loss. https://www.afb.org/research-and-initiatives/statistics/statistics-blind-children

American Printing House (APH). (2023). *The low vision history timeline.* https://aphconnectcenter.org/wp-content/uploads/sites/5/2023-Low-Vision-History-Timeline.pdf

Arditi, A. (1988). The volume visual-field: A basis for functional perimetry. *Clinical Vision Sciences, 3*(3), 173–183.

Arditi, A. (1999). *Making text legible: Designing for people with partial sight.* Lighthouse International. https://accessible-techcomm.org/wp-content/uploads/making_text_legible.pdf

Arditi, A. (2005). Improving the design of the letter contrast sensitivity test. *Investigative Ophthalmology and Visual Science, 46*(6), 2225–2229. https://doi.org/10.1167/iovs.04-1198

Arditi, A. (2017). Rethinking ADA signage standards for low-vision accessibility. *Journal of Vision, 17*(5), 8. https://doi.org/10.1167/17.5.8

Arditi, A. (n.d.). *Effective color contrast: Designing for people with partial sight and color deficiencies.* Lighthouse International. https://pages.mtu.edu/~nilufer/classes/cs3611/interesting-stuff/designing-with-colors-1/color_contrast.htm

Arunkumar, R., Calvo, C. M., Conrady, C. D., & Bernstein, P. S. (2018). What do we know about the macular pigment in AMD: The past, the present, and the future. *Eye, 32*, 992–1004. https://doi.org/10.1038/s41433-018-0044-0

Ashmead, D., & Wall, R. (2002). Low frequency sound as a navigational tool for people with visual impairments. *Journal of Low Frequency Noise, Vibration and Active Control, 21*(4), 199–205. https://doi.org/10.1260/026309202321834645

Atilgan, N., Xiong, Y. -Z., & Legge, G. E. (2020). Reconciling print-size and display-size constraints on reading. *Proceedings of the National Academy of Sciences, 117*(48), 30276–30284. https://doi.org/10.1073/pnas.2007514117

Atkinson, J. (2017). The Davida Teller Award Lecture, 2016: Visual brain development: A review of "Dorsal Stream Vulnerability"—motion, mathematics, amblyopia, actions, and attention. *Journal of Vision, 17*(3), 26. https://doi.org/10.1167/17.3.26

Audio Description Project. (n.d.). https://adp.acb.org/index.html

Austin, C. L. (2018). Step toward acceptance: My journey as a woman with albinism and implications for practice. *Journal of Visual Impairment & Blindness, 112*(6), 713–715. https://doi.org/10.1177/0145482X1811200606

Authié, C. N., Berthoz, A., Sahel, J. -A., & Safran, A. B. (2017). Adaptive gaze strategies for locomotion with constricted visual field. *Frontiers in Human Neuroscience, 11*, 387. https://doi.org/10.3389/fnhum.2017.00387

Ayton, L. N., Barnes, N., Dagnelie, G., Fujikado, T., Goetz, G., Hornig, R., Jones, B. W., Muqit, M. M. K., Rathbun, D. L., Stingl, K., Weiland, J. D., & Petoe, M. A. (2020). An update on retinal prostheses. *Clinical Neurophysiology, 131*(6), 1383–1398. https://doi.org/10.1016/j.clinph.2019.11.029

Bailey, I. L., & Lovie, J. E. (1976). New design principles for visual acuity letter charts. *American Journal of Optometry and Physiological Optics, 53*(11), 740–745. https://doi.org/10.1097/00006324-197611000-00006

Bailey, I. L., Jackson, A. J., Minto, H., Greer, R. B., & Chu, M. A. (2012). The Berkeley Rudimentary Vision Test. *Optometry and Vision Science, 89*(9), 1257–1264. https://doi.org/10.1097/OPX.0b013e318264e85a

Barot, N., McLean, R. J., Gottlob, I., & Proudlock, F. A. (2013). Reading performance in infantile nystagmus. *Ophthalmology, 120*(6), 1232–1238. https://doi.org/10.1016/j.ophtha.2012.11.032

Barraga, N. C. (1964). *Increased visual behavior in low vision children.* American Foundation for the Blind.

Barry, S. R., & Sacks, O. (2009). *Fixing my gaze: A scientist's journey into seeing in three dimensions.* Basic Books.

Bavelier, D., Levi, D. M., Li, R. W., Dan, Y., & Hensch, T. K. (2010). Removing brakes on adult brain plasticity: From molecular to behavioral interventions. *Journal of Neuroscience, 30*(45), 14964–14971. https://doi.org/10.1523/JNEUROSCI.4812-10.2010

Beckmann, P. J., & Legge, G. E. (1996). Psychophysics of reading. XIV. The page-navigation problem in using magnifiers. *Vision Research, 36*(22), 3723–3733. https://doi.org/10.1016/0042-6989(96)00084-3

Bennett, C. R., Bauer, C. M., Bailin, E. S., & Merabet, L. B. (2020). Neuroplasticity in cerebral visual impairment (CVI): Assessing functional vision and the neurophysiological correlates of dorsal stream dysfunction. *Neuroscience & Biobehavioral Reviews, 108*, 171–181. https://doi.org/10.1016/j.neubiorev.2019.10.011

Bernard, J. B., & Chung, S. T. L. (2018). Visual acuity is not the best at the preferred retinal locus in people with macular disease. *Optometry and Vision Science, 95*(9), 829–836. https://doi.org/10.1097/opx.0000000000001229

Bernard, J. -B., Aguilar, C., & Castet, E. (2016). A new font, specifically designed for peripheral vision, improves peripheral letter and word recognition, but not eye-mediated reading performance. *PLoS ONE*, 11(4), e0152506. https://doi.org/10.1371/journal.pone.0152506

Beyeler, M. (2024, January 29) *Simulating Argus II.* Pulse2percept. https://pulse2percept.readthedocs.io/en/latest/examples/implants/plot_argus.html

Beyeler, M., Boynton, G. M., Fine, I., & Rokem, A. (2017). pulse2percept: A Python-based simulation framework for bionic vision. *Proceedings of the 16th Python in Science Conference (SciPy)*, 81–88. https://doi.org/10.1101/148015

Beyeler, M., Nanduri, D., Weiland, J. D., Rokem, A., Boynton, G. M., & Fine, I. (2019). A model of ganglion axon pathways accounts for percepts elicited by retinal implants. *Scientific Reports*, *9*(1), 9199. https://doi.org/10.1038/s41598-019-45416-4

Birch, E. E., Cheng, C., Stager, D. R., Jr., Weakley, D. R., Jr., & Stager, D. R., Sr. (2009). The critical period for surgical treatment of dense congenital bilateral cataracts. *Journal of the American Association for Pediatric Ophthalmology and Strabismus*, *13*(1), 67–71. https://doi.org/10.1016/j.jaapos.2008.07.010

Bittner, A. K., Kaminski, J. E., Yoshinaga, P. D., Shepherd, J. D., Chan, T. L., Malkin, A. G., Deemer, A., Gobeille, M., Thoene, S. J., Rossi, A., & Ross, N. C., for the BeST-AID Study Team. (2024). Outcomes of telerehabilitation versus in-office training with magnification devices for low vision: A randomized controlled trial. *Translational Vision Science & Technology*, *13*(1), 6. https://doi.org/10.1167/tvst.13.1.6

Blackmore-Wright, S., Georgeson, M. A., & Anderson, S. J. (2013). Enhanced text spacing improves reading performance in individuals with macular disease. *PLoS ONE*, 8(11), e80325. https://doi.org/10.1371/journal.pone.0080325

Blake, R. (1988). Cat spatial vision. *Trends in Neurosciences*, *11*(2), 78–83. https://doi.org/10.1016/0166-2236(88)90169-5

Bochsler, T. M., Legge, G. E., Gage, R., & Kallie C. S. (2013). Recognition of ramps and steps by people with low vision. *Investigative Ophthalmology & Visual Science*, *54*(1), 288–294. https://doi.org/10.1167/iovs.12-10461

Boucart, M., Despretz, P., Hladiuk, K., & Desmettre, T. (2008). Does context or color improve object recognition in patients with low vision? *Visual Neuroscience*, *25*(5-6), 685–691. https://doi.org/10.1017/S0952523808080826

Bouma, H. (1970). Interaction effects in parafoveal letter recognition. *Nature*, *226*, 177–178. https://doi.org/10.1038/226177a0

Bourne, R., Steinmetz, J. D., Flaxman, S., Briant, P. S., Taylor, H. R., Resnikoff, S., Casson, R. J., Abdoli, A., Abu-Gharbieh, E., Afshin, A., Ahmadieh, H., Akalu, Y., Alamneh, A. A., Alemayehu, W., Alfaar, A. S., Alipour, V., Anbesu, E. W., Androudi, S., Arabloo, J … . Vos, T. (2021). Trends in prevalence of blindness and distance and near vision impairment over 30 years: An analysis for the Global Burden of Disease Study. *The Lancet Global Health* *9*(2), e130–e143. https://doi.org/10.1016/S2214-109X(20)30425-3

Bowers, A. R., Keeney, K., & Peli, E. (2014). Randomized crossover clinical trial of real and sham peripheral prism glasses for hemianopia. *JAMA Ophthalmology*, *132*(2), 214–222. https://doi.org/10.1001/jamaophthalmol.2013.5636

Bowers, A. R., Meek, C., & Stewart, N. (2001). Illumination and reading performance in age-related macular degeneration. *Clinical & Experimental Optometry*, 84(3), 139–147. https://doi.org/10.1111/j.1444-0938.2001.tb04957.x

Bradley, E. A., & Woog, J. J. (2024). Whole eye transplant—the journey begins. *JAMA Ophthalmology*, *142*(10), 897–899. https://doi.org/10.1001/jamaophthalmol.2024.3670

Brady, F. B. (2004). *A singular view: The art of seeing with one eye* (6th ed.). Frank B Brady.

Braille Institute of America. (n.d.). Braille Challenge. https://brailleinstitute.org/braille-challenge/

Brian Holden Vision Institute. (n.d.). https://bhvi.org

Brindley, G. S., & Lewin, W. S. (1968). The sensations produced by electrical stimulation of the visual cortex. *The Journal of Physiology*, *196*(2), 479–493. https://doi.org/10.1113/jphysiol.1968.sp008519

Britten-Jones, A. C., Jin, R., Gocuk, S. A., Cichello, E., O'Hare, F., Hickey, D. G., Edwards, T. L., & Ayton, L. N. (2022). The safety and efficacy of gene therapy treatment for monogenic retinal and optic nerve diseases: A systematic review. *Genetics in Medicine, 24(*3), 521–534. https://doi.org/10.1016/j.gim.2021.10.013

Britten-Jones, A. C., McGuinness, M. B., Chen, F. K., Grigg, J. R., Mack, H. G., & Ayton, L. N. (2024). A multinational survey of potential participant perspectives on ocular gene therapy. *Gene Therapy, 31*, 314–323. https://doi.org/10.1038/s41434-024-00450-4

Bronstad, P. M., Albu, A., Bowers, A. R., Goldstein, R., & Peli, E. (2015). Driving with central visual field loss II: How scotomas above or below the preferred retinal locus (PRL) affect hazard detection in a driving simulator. *PLoS One, 10*(9), e0136517. https://doi.org/10.1371/journal.pone.0136517

Bronstad, P. M., Bowers, A. R., Albu, A., Goldstein, R., & Peli, E. (2013). Driving with central field loss I: Effect of central scotomas on responses to hazards. *JAMA Ophthalmology, 131*(3), 303–309. https://doi.org/10.1001/jamaophthalmol.2013.1443

Brown, A. M., Opoku, F. O., & Stenger, M. R. (2018). Neonatal contrast sensitivity and visual acuity: Basic psychophysics. *Translational Vision Science & Technology, 7*(3), 18. https://doi.org/10.1167/tvst.7.3.18

Bruni, F. (2022). *The beauty of dusk: On vision lost and found.* Simon & Schuster.

Bullimore, M. A., Bailey, I. L., & Wacker, R. T. (1991). Face recognition in age-related maculopathy. *Investigative Ophthalmology & Visual Science, 32*(7), 2020–2029.

Calabrèse, A., Bernard, J. -B., Hoffart, L., Faure, G., Barouch, F., Conrath, J., & Castet, E. (2010). Small effect of interline spacing on maximal reading speed in low-vision patients with central field loss irrespective of scotoma size. *Investigative Ophthalmology & Visual Science,* 51(2), 1247–1254. https://doi.org/10.1167/iovs.09-3682

Campbell, A. J., Robertson, M. C., Grow, S. J. L., Kerse, N. M., Sanderson, G. F., Jacobs, R. J., Sharp, D. M., & Hale, L. A. (2005). Randomised controlled trial of prevention of falls in people aged ≥75 with severe visual impairment: The VIP trial. *BMJ, 331*(7520), 817. https://doi.org/10.1136/bmj.38601.447731.55

Caves, E. M., Brandley, N. C., & Johnsen, S. (2018). Visual acuity and the evolution of signals. *Trends in Ecology & Evolution, 33*(5), 358–372. https://doi.org/10.1016/j.tree.2018.03.001

Ceradini, D. J., Tran, D. L., Dedania, V. S., Gelb, B. E., Cohen, O. D., Flores, R. L., Levin, J. P., Saadeh, P. B., Staffenberg, D. A., Youss, Z. B., Filipiak, P., Baete, S. H., & Rodriguez, E. D. (2024). Combined whole eye and face transplant: Microsurgical strategy and 1-year clinical course. *Jama, 332*(18), 1551–1558. https://doi.org/10.1001/jama.2024.12601

Chan, T., Friedman, D. S., Bradley, C., & Massof, R. (2018). Estimates of incidence and prevalence of visual impairment, low vision, and blindness in the United States. *JAMA Ophthalmology, 136*(1), 12–19. https://doi.org/10.1001/jamaophthalmol.2017.4655

Cheong, A. M. Y., Legge, G. E., Lawrence, M., Cheung, S. -H., & Ruff, M. (2008). Relationship between visual span and reading performance in age-related macular degeneration. *Vision Research, 48*(4), 577–588. https://doi.org/10.1016/j.visres.2007.11.022

Cheung, S. -H., & Legge, G. E. (2005). Functional and cortical adaptations to central vision loss. *Visual Neuroscience, 22*(2), 187–201. https://doi.org/10.1017/S0952523805222071

Cheung, S. H., Fang, F., He, S., & Legge, G. E. (2009). Retinotopically specific reorganization of visual cortex for tactile pattern recognition. *Current Biology, 19*(7), 596–601. https://doi.org/10.1016/j.cub.2009.02.063

Chew, E. Y. (2020). Age-related macular degeneration: Nutrition, genes and deep learning-The LXXVI Edward Jackson Memorial Lecture. *American Journal of Ophthalmology, 217*, 335–347. https://doi.org/10.1016/j.ajo.2020.05.042

Chung, D. C., McCague, S., Yu, Z. -F., Thill, S., DiStefano-Pappas, J., Bennett, J., Cross, D., Marshall, K., Wellman, J., & High, K. A. (2018). Novel mobility test to assess functional vision in patients with inherited retinal dystrophies. *Clinical & Experimental Ophthalmology, 46*(3), 247–259. https://doi.org/10.1111/ceo.13022

Chung, S. T. L. (2013). Cortical reorganization after long-term adaptation to retinal lesions in humans. *Journal of Neuroscience*, *33*(46), 18080–18086. https://doi.org/10.1523/JNEUROSCI.2764-13.2013

Chung, S. T. L. (2011). Improving reading speed for people with central vision loss through perceptual learning. *Investigative Ophthalmology & Visual Science*, *52*(2), 1164–1170. https://doi.org/10.1167/iovs.10-6034

Chung, S. T. L., & Bernard, J. -B. (2018). Bolder print does not increase reading speed in people with central vision loss. *Vision Research*, *153*, 98–104. https://doi.org/10.1016/j.visres.2018.10.012

Chung, S. T. L., Jarvis, S. H., Woo, S. Y., Hanson, K., & Jose, R. T. (2008). Reading speed does not benefit from increased line spacing in AMD patients. *Optometry & Vision Science*, *85*(9), 827–833. https://doi.org/10.1097/OPX.0b013e31818527ea

Chung, S. T. L., Mansfield, J. S., & Legge, G. E. (1998). Psychophysics of reading. XVIII. The effect of print size on reading speed in normal peripheral vision. *Vision Research*, *38*(19), 2949–2962. https://doi.org/10.1016/S0042-6989(98)00072-8

Colenbrander, A. (2002). *Visual standards: Aspects and ranges of vision loss with emphasis on population surveys.* Report prepared for the International Council of Ophthalmology at the 29th International Congress of Ophthalmology Meeting. https://www.researchgate.net/publication/248343777_Visual_Standards_aspects_and_ranges_of_vision_loss_with_emphasis_on_population_surveys

Colón-Emeric, C. S., McDermott, C. L., Lee, D. S., & Berry, S. D. (2024). Risk assessment and prevention of falls in older community-dwelling adults: A review. *JAMA*. https://doi.org/10.1001/jama.2024.1416

Costela, F. M., Sheldon, S. S., Walker, B., & Woods, R. L. (2018). People with hemianopia report difficulty with TV, computer, cinema use, and photography. *Optometry and Vision Science*, *95*(5), 428–434. https://doi.org/10.1097/OPX.0000000000001215

Cowey, A. (2010). The blindsight saga. *Experimental Brain Research*, *200*(1), 3–24. https://doi.org/10.1007/s00221-009-1914-2

Crabb, D. P., Smith, N. D., Glen, F. C., Burton, R., & Garway-Heath, D. F. (2013). How does glaucoma look?: Patient perception of visual field loss. *Ophthalmology*, *120*(6), 1120–1126. https://doi.org/10.1016/j.ophtha.2012.11.043

Creem-Regehr, S. H., Barhorst-Cates, E. M., Tarampi, R. M., Rand, K. M., & Legge, G. E. (2021). How can basic research on spatial cognition enhance the visual accessibility of architecture for people with low vision? *Cognitive Research: Principles and Implications* 6(1), 3. https://doi.org/10.1186/s41235-020-00265-y

Crossland, M., & Rubin, G. (2007). The Amsler chart: Absence of evidence is not evidence of absence. *British Journal of Ophthalmology*, *91*(3), 391–393. https://doi.org/10.1136/bjo.2006.095315

Crossland, M. D. (2024). *Vision impairment: Science, art and lived experience.* UCL Press.

Crossland, M. D., Culham, L. E., & Rubin, G. S. (2004). Fixation stability and reading speed in patients with newly developed macular disease. *Ophthalmic & Physiological Optics*, *24*(4), 327–333. https://doi.org/10.1111/j.1475-1313.2004.00213.x

Crossland, M. D., Macedo, A. F., & Rubin, G. S. (2010). Electronic books as low vision aids. *British Journal of Ophthalmology*, *94*(8), 1109. https://doi.org/10.1136/bjo.2009.170167

Cryotherapy for Retinopathy of Prematurity Cooperative Group. (2001). Multicenter trial of cryotherapy for retinopathy of prematurity: Ophthalmological outcomes at 10 years. *Archives of Ophthalmology*, *119*(8), 1110–1118. https://doi.org/10.1001/archopht.119.8.1110

Cunningham, S. I., Weiland, J. D., Bao, P., Lopez-Jaime, G. R., & Tjan, B. S. (2014). Correlation of vision loss with tactile-evoked V1 responses in retinitis pigmentosa. *Vision Research, 111, Part B*, 197–207. https://doi.org/10.1016/j.visres.2014.10.015

Curcio, C. A., Owsley, C., & Jackson, G. R. (2000). Spare the rods, save the cones in aging and age-related maculopathy. *Investigative Ophthalmology & Visual Science, 41*(8), 2015–2018.

Davies, K. (2020) *Editing Humanity: The CRISPR Revolution and the New Era of Genome Editing*. Pegasus Books.

Dearen, J. (2018, April 13). *Driverless cars give hope to blind – Are automakers onboard?* Associated Press. https://apnews.com/article/02cf7e83ead84493be10ad0dec745151

DeCarlo, D. K., Scilley, K., Wells, J., & Owsley, C. (2003). Driving habits and health-related quality of life in patients with age-related maculopathy. *Optometry and Vision Science, 80*(3), 207–213. https://doi.org/10.1097/00006324-200303000-00010

Deffler, R. A., Xu, J., Bittner, A. K., Bowers, A. R., Hassan, S. E., Ross, N., Cooley, S. -S. L., Doubt, A., Davidorf, F. H., & Dougherty, B. E., for the RADARS Study Group (2022). Use and perceptions of advanced driver assistance systems by older drivers with and without age-related macular degeneration. *Translational Vision Science & Technology, 11*(3), 22. https://doi.org/10.1167/tvst.11.3.22

Delahunt, P. B., Webster, M. A., Ma, L., & Werner, J. S. (2004). Long-term renormalization of chromatic mechanisms following cataract surgery. *Visual Neuroscience, 21*(3), 301–307. https://doi.org/10.1017/s0952523804213025

Dobelle, W. H. (2000). Artificial vision for the blind by connecting a television camera to the visual cortex. *ASAIO Journal, 46*(1), 3–9.

Doerr, R. A. (2023, January 19). *One of the last new argonauts: A review of the Argus II artificial retinal implant*. Top Tech Tidbits. https://www.toptechtidbits.com/138.html

Drag, S., Dotiwala, F., & Upadhyay, A. K. (2023). Gene therapy for retinal degenerative diseases: Progress, challenges, and future directions. *Investigative Ophthalmology & Visual Science, 64*(7), 39. https://doi.org/10.1167/iovs.64.7.39

Dreyfus, J. (1995). The invention of spectacles and the advent of printing. In *Into print: Selected writings on printing history, typography, and book production*. David R. Godine Publishing.

E, J. Y., Li, T., McInally, L., Thomson, K., Shahani, U., Gray, L., Howe, T. E., & Skelton, D. A. (2020). Environmental and behavioural interventions for reducing physical activity limitation and preventing falls in older people with visual impairment. *Cochrane Database of Systematic Reviews 2020*(9). https://doi.org/10.1002/14651858.CD009233.pub3

Elliott, D. B., & Bullimore, M. A. (1993). Assessing the reliability, discriminative ability, and validity of disability glare tests. *Investigative Ophthalmology & Visual Science, 34*(1), 108–119.

Enoch, J., McDonald, L., Jones, L., Jones, P. R., & Crabb, D. P. (2019). Evaluating whether sight is the most valued sense. *JAMA Ophthalmology, 137*(11), 1317–1320. https://doi.org/10.1001/jamaophthalmol.2019.3537

Eperjesi, F., Fowler, C. W. & Evans, B. J. W. (2002). Do tinted lenses or filters improve visual performance in low vision? A review of the literature. *Ophthalmic and Physiological Optics, 22*(1), 68–77. https://doi.org/10.1046/j.1475-1313.2002.00004.x

Eye Diseases Prevalence Research Group. (2004). Causes and prevalence of visual impairment among adults in the United States. *Archives of Ophthalmology, 122*(4), 477–485. https://doi.org/10.1001/archopht.122.4.477

Eye Diseases Prevalence Research Group. (2004). Prevalence of open-angle glaucoma among adults in the United States. *Archives of Ophthalmology, 122*(4), 532–538. https://doi.org/10.1001/archopht.122.4.532

Faye, E. (1976). *Clinical low vision*. Little, Brown.

Fazzi, E., Micheletti, S., Calza, S., Merabet, L., Rossi, A., Galli, J., & Early Visual Intervention Study Group. (2021). Early visual training and environmental adaptation for infants with visual impairment. *Developmental Medicine & Child Neurology*, *63*(10), 1180–1193. https://doi.org/10.1111/dmcn.14865

Ferris, F. L., III, Kassoff, A., Bresnick, G. H., & Bailey, I. (1982). New visual acuity charts for clinical research. *American Journal of Ophthalmology*, *94*(1), 91–96. https://doi.org/10.1016/0002-9394(82)90197-0

Fine, I., Wade, A. R., Brewer, A. A., May, M. G., Goodman, D. F., Boynton, G. M., Wandell, B. A., & MacLeod, D. I. A. (2003). Long-term deprivation affects visual perception and cortex. *Nature Neuroscience*, *6*(9), 915–916. https://doi.org/10.1038/nn1102

Fink, P. D. S., Doore, S. A., Lin, X., Maring, M., Zhao, P., Nygaard, A., Beals, G., Corey, R. R., Perry, R. J., Freund, K., Dimitrov, V., & Giudice, N. A. (2023). The Autonomous Vehicle Assistant (AVA): Emerging technology design supporting blind and visually impaired travelers in autonomous transportation. *International Journal of Human-Computer Studies*, *179*, 103125. https://doi.org/10.1016/j.ijhcs.2023.103125

Flaxman, A. D., Wittenborn, J. S., Robalik, T., Gulia, R., Gerzoff, R. B., Lundeen, E. A., Saaddine, J., & Rein, D. B., for the Vision and Eye Health Surveillance System Study Group (2021). Prevalence of visual acuity loss or blindness in the US: A bayesian meta-analysis. *JAMA Ophthalmology*, *139*(7), 717–723. https://doi.org/10.1001/jamaophthalmol.2021.0527

Flaxman, S. R., Bourne, R. R. A., Resnikoff, S., Ackland, P., Braithwaite, T., Cicinelli, M. V., Das, A., Jonas, J. B., Keeffe, J., Kempen, J. H., Leasher, J., Limburg, H., Naidoo, K., Pesudovs, K., Silvester, A., Stevens, G. A., Tahhan, N., Wong, T. Y., Taylor, H. R., and the Vision Loss Expert Group of the Global Burden of Disease Study (2017). Global causes of blindness and distance vision impairment 1990–2020: A systematic review and meta-analysis. *The Lancet Global Health*, *5*(12), e1221–e1234. https://doi.org/10.1016/S2214-109X(17)30393-5

Fletcher, D. C., & Schuchard, R. A. (1997). Preferred retinal loci relationship to macular scotomas in a low-vision population. *Ophthalmology*, *104*(4), 632–638. https://doi.org/10.1016/S0161-6420(97)30260-7

Fletcher, D. C., Schuchard, R. A., & Renninger, L. W. (2012). Patient awareness of binocular central scotoma in age-related macular degeneration. *Optometry & Vision Science*, *89*(9), 1395–1398. https://doi.org/10.1097/OPX.0b013e318264cc77

Franklin, A., Lund, P., Bradbury-Jones, C., & Taylor, J. (2018). Children with albinism in African regions: Their rights to 'being' and 'doing.' *BMC International Health and Human Rights*, *18*(1), 2. https://doi.org/10.1186/s12914-018-0144-8

Freedman, A., Achtemeier, J., Baek, Y., & Legge, G. E. (2019). Gaze behavior during navigation with reduced acuity. *Experimental Eye Research*, *183*, 20–28. https://doi.org/10.1016/j.exer.2018.11.002

Genensky, S. M. (1969). Some comments on a closed-circuit TV system for the visually handicapped. *Optometry & Vision Science*, 46(7), 519–524.

Genensky, S. M. (2001). One man's story: Samuel M. Genensky. *The Braille Forum*, *39*(9). https://www.acb.org/sites/default/files/BF0301.TXT

Geruschat, D. R., Flax, M., Tanna, N., Bianchi, M, Fisher, A., Goldschmidt, M., Fisher, L., Dagnelie, G., Deremeik, J., Smith, A., Anaflous, F., & Dorn, J. (2015). FLORA: Phase I development of a functional vision assessment for prosthetic vision users. *Clinical and Experimental Optometry*, *98*(4), 342–347. https://doi.org/10.1111/cxo.12242

Geruschat, D. R., Richards, T. P., Arditi, A., da Cruz, L., Dagnelie, G., Dorn, J. D., Duncan, J. L., Ho, A. C., Olmos de Koo, L. C., Sahel, J. -A., Stanga, P. E., Thumann, G., & Wang, V. (2016). An analysis of observer-rated functional vision in patients implanted with the Argus II Retinal Prosthesis System at three years. *Clinical and Experimental Optometry*, 99(3), 227–232. https://doi.org/10.1111/cxo.12359

Goodale, M. A., & Milner, D. (1992). Separate visual pathways for perception and action. *Trends in Neuroscience, 15*(1), 20–25. https://doi.org/10.1016/0166-2236(92)90344-8

Google. (2012, March 28). Self-Driving Car Test: Steve Mahan (Audio Described) [Video]. YouTube. https://www.youtube.com/watch?v=peDy2st2XpQ

Granquist, C., Wu, Y. -H., Gage, R., Crossland, M. D., & Legge, G. E. (2018). How people with low vision achieve magnification in digital reading. *Optometry and Vision Science, 95*(9), 711–719. https://doi.org/10.1097/OPX.0000000000001261

Granville, W. C. (1990). Colors do look different after a lens implant! *Color Research & Application, 15*(1), 59–62. https://doi.org/10.1002/col.5080150110

Gregory, R. L., & Wallace, J. G. (1963). Recovery from early blindness, a case study. *Experimental Psychology Society Monograph, No. 2*, 1–46.

Guo, X., Swenor, B. K., & Goldstein, J. E. (2020). Association of visual acuity improvement with uncorrected refractive error in patients new to low vision clinics. *JAMA Ophthalmology, 138*(7), 765–771. https://doi.org/10.1001/jamaophthalmol.2020.1677

Guth, D. (2008). Why does training reduce blind pedestrians' veering? In J. J. Rieser, D. H. Ashmead, F. F. Ebner and A. L. Corn (Eds.), *Blindness and Brain Plasticity in Navigation and Object Perception* (pp. 353–365). Taylor & Francis Group.

Hansen, T., Pracejus, L., & Gegenfurtner, K. R. (2009). Color perception in the intermediate periphery of the visual field. *Journal of Vision, 9*(4), 26. https://doi.org/10.1167/9.4.26

Hassan, S. E. (2012). Are normally sighted, visually impaired, and blind pedestrians accurate and reliable at making street crossing decisions? *Investigative Ophthalmology & Visual Science, 53*(6), 2593–2600. https://doi.org/10.1167/iovs.11-9340

Hassan, S. E., Hicks, J. C., Lei, H., & Turano, K. A. (2007). What is the minimum field of view required for efficient navigation? *Vision Research, 47*(16), 2115–2123. https://doi.org/10.1016/j.visres.2007.03.012

He, Y., Sun, S. Y., Roy, A., Caspi, A., & Montezuma, S. R. (2020). Improved mobility performance with an artificial vision therapy system using a thermal sensor. *Journal of Neural Engineering, 17*(4), 045011. https://doi.org/10.1088/1741-2552/aba4fb

Held, R., Ostrovsky, Y., de Gelder, B., Gandhi, T., Ganesh, S., Mathur, U., & Sinha, P. (2011). The newly sighted fail to match seen with felt. *Nature Neuroscience, 14*(5), 551–553. https://doi.org/10.1038/nn.2795

Hellgren, K. M., Tornqvist, K., Jakobsson, P. G., Lundgren, P., Carlsson, B., Källén, K., Serenius, F., Hellström, A., & Holmström, G. (2016). Ophthalmologic outcome of extremely preterm infants at 6.5 years of age: Extremely preterm infants in Sweden study (EXPRESS). *JAMA Ophthalmology, 134*(5), 555–562. https://doi.org/10.1001/jamaophthalmol.2016.0391

Hellström, A., Smith, L. E. H., & Dammann, O. (2013). Retinopathy of prematurity. *The Lancet, 382*(9902), 1445–1457. https://doi.org/10.1016/S0140-6736(13)60178-6

Hemianopsia.net. (n.d.). http://www.hemianopsia.net/visual-fields-in-brain-injury/

Hirsch, G. V., Bauer, C. M., & Merabet, L. B. (2015). Using structural and functional brain imaging to uncover how the brain adapts to blindness. *Annals of Neuroscience and Psychology, 2*(5).

Holmes, G. (1918). Disturbances of vision by cerebral lesions. *The British Journal of Ophthalmology, 2*(7), 353–384. https://doi.org/10.1136%2Fbjo.2.7.353

Hood, D. C., Raza, A. S., de Moraes, C. G. V., Johnson, C. A., Liebmann, J. M., & Ritch, R. (2012). The nature of macular damage in glaucoma as revealed by averaging optical coherence tomography data. *Translational Vision Science & Technology, 1*(1), 3. https://doi.org/10.1167/tvst.1.1.3

Horton, J. C. (2005). Vision restoration therapy: Confounded by eye movements. *British Journal of Ophthalmology, 89*(7), 792–794. https://doi.org/10.1136/bjo.2005.072967

Huber, E., Webster, J. M., Brewer, A. A., MacLeod, D. I. A., Wandell, B. A., Boynton, G. M., Wade, A. R., & Fine, I. (2015). A lack of experience-dependent plasticity after more than a decade of recovered sight. *Psychological Science, 26*(4), 393–401. https://doi.org/10.1177/0956797614563957

Hull, J. M. (1990). *Touching the rock: An experience of blindness.* Pantheon Books.

Huss, C., & Corn, A. (2004). Low vision driving with bioptics: An overview. *Journal of Visual Impairment & Blindness, 98*(10), 641–653. https://doi.org/10.1177/0145482x0409801008

International Agency for the Prevention of Blindness. (n.d.). *The Vision Atlas.* https://www.iapb.org/learn/vision-atlas/#main

Jacobs, A. (2018, May 5). A simple way to improve a billion lives: Eyeglasses. *The New York Times.* https://www.nytimes.com/2018/05/05/health/glasses-developing-world-global-health.html

Jacobs, A. (2024, April 4). Glasses improve income, not just eyesight. *The New York Times.* https://www.nytimes.com/2024/04/04/health/eyeglasses-income-bangladesh.html

Jauregui, R., Huryn, L. A., & Brooks, B. P. (2018). Comprehensive review of the genetics of albinism. *Journal of Visual Impairment & Blindness, 112*(6), 683–700. https://doi.org/10.1177%2F0145482X1811200604

Jin, H., Zhou, Y., Stagg, B. C., & Ehrlich, J. R. (2024). Association between vision impairment and increased prevalence of falls in older US adults. *Journal of the American Geriatrics Society.* https://doi.org/10.1111/jgs.18879

Johnson, C. A. (2008). Occupational psychophysics to establish vision requirements. *Optometry & Vision Science, 85*(10), 910–923. https://doi.org/10.1097/OPX.0b013e3181888953

Johnson, C. A., Wall, M., & Thompson, H. S. (2011). A history of perimetry and visual field testing. *Optometry and Vision Science, 88*(1), E8–15. https://doi.org/10.1097/OPX.0b013e3182004c3b

Johnson, S., Buessing, M., O'Connell, T., Pitluck, S., & Ciulla, T. A. (2019). Cost-effectiveness of voretigene neparvovec-rzyl vs standard care for RPE65-mediated inherited retinal disease. *JAMA Ophthalmology, 137*(10), 1115–1123. https://doi.org/10.1001/jamaophthalmol.2019.2512

Jones, R. K., & Lee, D. N. (1981). Why two eyes are better than one: The two views of binocular vision. *Journal of Experimental Psychology: Human Perception and Performance, 7*(1), 30–40. https://psycnet.apa.org/doi/10.1037/0096-1523.7.1.30

Kallie, C. S., Schrater, P. R., & Legge, G. E. (2007). Variability in stepping direction explains the veering behavior of blind walkers. *Journal of Experimental Psychology: Human Perception and Performance, 33*(1), 183–200. https://doi.org/10.1037/0096-1523.33.1.183

Kanwisher, N. (2010). Functional specificity in the human brain: A window into the functional architecture of the mind. *Proceedings of the National Academy of Sciences, 107*(25), 11163–11170. https://doi.org/10.1073/pnas.1005062107

Keller, H. (1905) *The Story of My Life.* Parts I & II by Helen Keller, (1880–1968); Part III from the letters and reports of Anne Mansfield Sullivan (ca.1867–1936); Edited by John Albert Macy. Doubleday, Page & Company.

Kessel, L., Jensen, H., Larsen, A. -C., Rosenberg, T., & Rothe Nissen, K. (2024). Temporal changes in incidence, prevalence and causes of childhood visual impairment – Learnings from 45 years with the National Danish Registry of Children with Visual Impairment. *Acta Ophthalmologica.* https://doi.org/10.1111/aos.16700

Khan, J. C., Thurlby, D. A., Shahid, H., Clayton, D. G., Yates, J. R. W., Bradley, M., Moore, A. T., & Bird, A. C. for the Genetic Factors in AMD Study. (2006). Smoking and age related macular degeneration: The number of pack years of cigarette smoking is a major determinant of risk for both geographic atrophy and choroidal neovascularization. *British Journal of Ophthalmology, 90*(1), 75–80. https://doi.org/10.1136/bjo.2005.073643

Kim, L. A., & D'Amore, P. A. (2012). A brief history of anti-VEGF for the treatment of ocular angiogenesis. *The American Journal of Pathology*, *181*(2), 376–379. https://doi.org/10.1016/j.ajpath.2012.06.006

Kish, D. (2015, March 31). *How I use sonar to navigate the world* [Video]. TED. https://www.ted.com/talks/daniel_kish_how_i_use_sonar_to_navigate_the_world?subtitle=en

Klemen, J., Hoffmann, M. B., & Chambers, C. D. (2012). Cortical plasticity in the face of congenitally altered input into V1. *Cortex*, *48*(10), 1362–1365. https://doi.org/10.1016/j.cortex.2012.03.012

Kong, L., Fry, M., Al-Samarraie, M., Gilbert, C., & Steinkuller, P. G. (2012). An update on progress and the changing epidemiology of causes of childhood blindness worldwide. *Journal of American Association for Pediatric Ophthalmology and Strabismus*, *16*(6), 501–507. https://doi.org/10.1016/j.jaapos.2012.09.004

Kristof, N. (2015, November 7). In five minutes he lets the blind see. *The New York Times*. https://www.nytimes.com/2015/11/08/opinion/sunday/in-5-minutes-he-lets-the-blind-see.html

Kromberg, J. G. R., Flynn, K. A., & Kerr, R. A. (2023). Determining a worldwide prevalence of oculocutaneous albinism: A systematic review. *Investigative Ophthalmology & Visual Science*, *64*(10), 14. https://doi.org/10.1167/iovs.64.10.14

Kuborn, A. M., & Hassan, S. E. (2024). The impact of vision loss on attitudes toward autonomous vehicles: A vision-centric analysis. *Optometry and Vision Science*, *101*(6), 424–434. https://doi.org/10.1097/OPX.0000000000002145

Kumin, M. (2013, February 2). Seeing things. *The New York Times*. https://www.nytimes.com/2013/02/03/opinion/sunday/seeing-things.html

Kurson, R. (2007). *Crashing through: A true story of risk, adventure, and the man who dared to see*. Random House.

Kuyk, T., Elliot, J. L., & Fuhr, P. S. W. (1998). Visual correlates of mobility in real world settings in older adults with low vision. *Optometry and Vision Science*, *75*, 538–547. https://doi.org/10.1097/00006324-199807000-00023

Kuyk, T., Elliott, J. L., Biehl, J., & Fuhr, P. S. (1996). Environmental variables and mobility performance in adults with low vision. *Journal of the American Optometric Association*, *67*(7), 403–409.

Kwon, M., Huisingh, C., Rhodes, L. A., McGwin, G., Wood, J. M., & Owsley, C. (2016). Association between glaucoma and at–fault motor vehicle collision involvement among older drivers: A population-based study. *Ophthalmology*, *123*(1), 109–116. https://doi.org/10.1016/j.ophtha.2015.08.043

Kwon, M., Liu, R., Patel, B. N., & Girkin, C. (2017). Slow reading in glaucoma: Is it due to the shrinking visual span in central vision? *Investigative Ophthalmology & Visual Science*, *58*(13), 5810–5818. https://doi.org/10.1167/iovs.17-22560

Kwon, M., Nandy, A. S., & Tjan, B. S. (2013). Rapid and persistent adaptability of human oculomotor control in response to simulated central vision loss. *Current Biology*, *23*(17), 1663–1669. https://doi.org/10.1016/j.cub.2013.06.056

Lamb, T. D. (2016). Why rods and cones? *Eye*, *30*(2), 179–185. https://doi.org/10.1038/eye.2015.236

Lane-Karnas, K. (2023). A case study on cerebral visual impairment, reading and braille. *Journal of Visual Impairment & Blindness*, *117*(6), 498–504. https://doi.org/10.1177/0145482X231218069

Latham, K., Subhi, H., & Shaw, E. (2023). Further validation of comfortable print size as a parameter for clinical low-vision assessment. *Translational Vision Science & Technology*, *12*(6), 18. https://doi.org/10.1167/tvst.12.6.18

Legge, G. E., & Chung, S. T. L. (2016). Low vision and plasticity: Implications for rehabilitation. *Annual Review of Vision Science, 2*, 321–343. https://doi.org/10.1146/annurev-vision-111815-114344

Legge, G. E. (2007). *Psychophysics of Reading in Normal and Low Vision*. CRC Press.

Legge, G. E., & Bigelow, C. A. (2011). Does print size matter for reading? A review of findings from vision science and typography. *Journal of Vision, 11*(5), 8. https://doi.org/10.1167/11.5.8

Legge, G. E., Granquist, C., Baek, Y., & Gage, R. (2016). Indoor spatial updating with impaired vision. *Investigative Ophthalmology & Visual Science, 57*(15), 6757–6765. https://doi.org/10.1167/iovs.16-20226

Legge, G. E., Madison, C., & Mansfield, J. S. (1999). Measuring Braille reading speed with the MNREAD test. *Visual Impairment Research, 1*, 131–145. https://doi.org/10.1076/vimr.1.3.131.4438

Legge, G. E., Mansfield, J. S., & Chung, S. T. L. (2001). Psychophysics of reading. XX. Linking letter recognition to reading speed in central and peripheral vision. *Vision Research, 41*(6), 725–734. https://doi.org/10.1016/S0042-6989(00)00295-9

Legge, G. E., Mullen, K. T., Woo, G. C., & Campbell, F. W. (1987). Tolerance to visual defocus. *Journal of the Optical Society of America A, 4*(5), 851–863. https://doi.org/10.1364/JOSAA.4.000851

Legge, G. E., Parish, D. H., Luebker, A., & Wurm, L. H. (1990). Psychophysics of reading. XI. Comparing color contrast and luminance contrast. *Journal of the Optical Society of America A, 7*(10), 2002–2010.

Legge, G. E., Ross, J. A., Isenberg, L. M., & LaMay, J. M. (1992). Psychophysics of reading XI. Clinical predictors of low-vision reading speed. *Investigative Ophthalmology & Visual Science, 33*(3), 677–687.

Legge, G. E., Rubin, G. S., & Luebker, A. (1987). Psychophysics of reading. V. The role of contrast in normal vision. *Vision Research, 27*(7), 1165–1177.

Legge, G. E., Rubin, G. S., & Schleske, M. M. (1986). Contrast-polarity effects in low-vision reading. In G. C. Woo (Ed.), *Low vision: Principles and applications* (pp. 288–307). Springer-Verlag.

Legge, G. E., Yu, D., Kallie, C. S., Bochsler, T. M., & Gage, R. (2010). Visual accessibility of ramps and steps. *Journal of Vision, 10*(11), 8. https://doi.org/10.1167/10.11.8

Lei, Q., Gage, R., Kersten, D., & Legge, G. E. (2024). The effect of illumination on the visibility of steps and ramps for people with low vision. *Optometry & Vision Science, 101*(6), 399–407. https://doi.org/10.1097/OPX.0000000000002146

Leland, A. (2023). *The country of the blind: A memoir at the end of sight*. Penguin Publishing Group.

Lettvin, J. Y., Maturana, H. R., McCullock, W. S., & Pitts, W. H. (1959). What the frog's eye tells the frog's brain. *Proceedings of the Institute of Radio Engineers, 47*(11), 1940–1951. https://doi.org/10.1109/JRPROC.1959.287207

Levi, D. M., Knill, D. C, & Bavelier, D. (2015). Stereopsis and amblyopia: A mini-review. *Vision Research 114*, 17–30. https://doi.org/10.1016/j.visres.2015.01.002

Lewis, P. M., & Rosenfeld, J. V. (2016). Electrical stimulation of the brain and the development of cortical visual prostheses: An historical perspective. *Brain Research, 1630*, 208–224. https://doi.org/10.1016/j.brainres.2015.08.038

Logan, A. J., Gordon, G. E., & Loffler, G. (2020). The effect of age-related macular degeneration on components of face perception. *Investigative Ophthalmology & Visual Science, 61*(6), 38. https://doi.org/10.1167/iovs.61.6.38

Lord, S. R., & Dayhew, J. (2001). Visual risk factors for falls in older people. *Journal of the American Geriatrics Society, 49*(5), 508–515. https://doi.org/10.1046/j.1532-5415.2001.49107.x

Lovie-Kitchin, J., & Feigl, B. (2005). Assessment of age-related maculopathy using subjective vision tests. *Clinical and Experimental Optometry, 88*(5), 292–303. https://doi.org/10.1111/j.1444-0938.2005.tb06713.x

Ludt, R., & Goodrich, G. L. (2002). Change in visual perceptual detection distances for low vision travelers as a result of dynamic visual assessment and training. *Journal of Visual Impairment & Blindness, 96*(1), 7–15. https://doi.org/10.1177/0145482X0209600103

Luo, G., Vargas-Martin, F., & Peli, E. (2008). The role of peripheral vision in saccade planning: Learning from people with tunnel vision. *Journal of Vision, 8*(14), 25–25. https://doi.org/10.1167/8.14.25

Lusseyran, J. (1998). *And there was light: Autobiography of Jacques Lusseyran, blind hero of the French resistance.* Parabola Books.

Mahoney, R. (2014). *For the benefit of those who see: Dispatches from the world of the blind.* Little, Brown and Company.

Mancuso, K., Hauswirth, W. W., Li, Q., Connor, T. B., Kuchenbecker, J. A., Mauck, M. C., Neitz, J., & Neitz, M. (2009). Gene therapy for red-green colour blindness in adult primates. *Nature, 461*, 784–787. https://doi.org/10.1038/nature08401

Marmor, D. J., & Marmor, M. F. (2010). Simulating vision with and without macular disease. *Archives of Ophthalmology, 128*(1), 117–125. https://doi.org/10.1001/archophthalmol.2009.366

Marmor, M. F. (2000). A brief history of macular grids: From Thomas Reid to Edvard Munch and Marc Amsler. *Survey of Ophthalmology, 44*(4), 343–353. https://doi.org/10.1016/S0039-6257(99)00113-7

Marmor, M. F. (2006). Ophthalmology and art: Simulation of Monet's cataracts and Degas' retinal disease. *Archives of Ophthalmology, 124*(12), 1764–1769. https://doi.org/10.1001/archopht.124.12.1764

Marquardt, J (Host). Kaleidoscope: The Cortical Visual Impairment Podcast. https://podcasts.apple.com/us/podcast/kaleidoscope-the-cortical-visual-impairment-podcast/id1386780362

Mars, R. (host). (2019, December 3). The Infantorium (381) [Audio podcast episode]. In 99 Percent Invisible. https://99percentinvisible.org/episode/the-infantorium/

Martelli, M., Majaj, N. J, & Pelli, D. G. (2005). Are faces processed like words? A diagnostic test for recognition by parts. *Journal of Vision, 5*(1), 58–70. https://doi.org/10.1167/5.1.6

Massof, R. W., Ahmadian, L., Grover, L. L., Deremeik, J. T., Goldstein, J. E., Rainey, C., Epstein, C., & Barnett, G. D. (2007). The Activity Inventory: An adaptive visual function questionnaire. *Optometry and Vision Science, 84*(8), 763–774. https://doi.org/10.1097/OPX.0b013e3181339efd

Mayer, D. L., Beiser, A. S., Warner, A. F., Pratt, E. M., Raye, K. N., & Lang, J. M. (1995). Monocular acuity norms for the Teller Acuity Cards between ages one month and four years. *Investigative Ophthalmology & Visual Science, 36*(3), 671–685.

McDonnall, M. C., & Sui, Z. (2019). Employment and unemployment rates of people who are blind or visually impaired: Estimates from multiple sources. *Journal of Visual Impairment & Blindness, 113*(6), 481–492. https://doi.org/10.1177/0145482x19887620

McGuinness, M. B., Le, J., Mitchell, P., Gopinath, B., Cerin, E., Saksens, N. T. M., Schick, T., Hoyng, C. B., Guymer, R. H., & Finger, R. P. (2017). Physical activity and age-related macular degeneration: A systematic literature review and meta-analysis. *American Journal of Ophthalmology, 180*, 29–38. https://doi.org/10.1016/j.ajo.2017.05.016

McLean, R. J., Windridge, K. C., & Gottlob, I. (2012). Living with nystagmus: A qualitative study. *British Journal of Ophthalmology, 96*(7), 981–986. https://doi.org/10.1136/bjophthalmol-2011-301183

McLuhan, M. (1962). *The Gutenberg Galaxy: The making of typographic man.* University of Toronto Press.

Mellor, C. M. (2006). *Louis Braille: A Touch of Genius.* National Braille Press.

Merrill, K., Hogue, K., Downes, S., Holleschau, A. M., Kutzbach, B. R., MacDonald, J. T., & Summers, C. G. (2011). Reading acuity in albinism: Evaluation with MNREAD charts. *Journal of American Association for Pediatric Ophthalmology and Strabismus, 15*(1), 29–32. https://doi.org/10.1016/j.jaapos.2010.12.005

Miller, A., Crossland, M. D., Macnaughton, J., & Latham, K. (2023). Are wearable electronic vision enhancement systems (wEVES) beneficial for people with age-related macular degeneration? A scoping review. *Ophthalmic and Physiological Optics 43*(4), 680–701. https://doi.org/10.1111/opo.13117

Miller, P. E., & Murphy, C. J. (1995). Vision in dogs. *Journal of the American Veterinary Medical Association, 207*(12), 1623–1634.

Minhas, R., Jaiswal, A., Chan, S., Trevisan, J., Paramasivam, A., & Spruyt-Rocks, R. (2022). Prevalence of individuals with deafblindness and age-related dual-sensory loss. *Journal of Visual Impairment & Blindness 116*(1), 36–47. https://doi.org/10.1177/0145482X211072541

Mitchell, D. E., & Blakemore, C. (1970). Binocular depth perception and the corpus callosum. *Vision Research, 10*(1), 49–54. https://doi.org/10.1016/0042-6989(70)90061-1

Moharrer, M., Wang, S., Dougherty, B. E., Cybis, W., Ott, B. R., Davis, J. D., & Luo, G. (2020). Evaluation of the driving safety of visually impaired bioptic drivers based on critical events in naturalistic driving. *Translational Vision Science & Technology, 9*(8), 14. https://doi.org/10.1167/tvst.9.8.14

Moore, L. W., Constantino, R.E., & Allen, M. (2000). Severe visual impairment in older women. *Western Journal of Nursing Research, 22*(5), 571–595. https://doi.org/10.1177/01939450022044601

Moreland, B. L., Kakara, R., Haddad, Y. K., Shakya, I., & Bergen, G. (2021). A descriptive analysis of location of older adult falls that resulted in emergency department visits in the United States, 2015. *American Journal of Lifestyle Medicine, 15*(6), 590–597. https://doi.org/10.1177/1559827620942187

MyReadingDisplay. (n.d.). *My Reading Display.* https://myreadingdisplay.umn.edu/

National Eye Institute. (n.d.). *Eye conditions and diseases.* https://www.nei.nih.gov/learn-about-eye-health/eye-conditions-and-diseases

National Eye Institute. Eye disease simulations. Available from https://nei.nih.gov/health/examples

National Institute of Building Sciences (NIBS). 2015. *Design Guidelines for the Visual Environment.* https://nibs.org/design-guidelines-for-the-visual-environment/

National Organization for Albinism and Hypopigmentation. (n.d.) Information bulletin - What do you call me? https://www.albinism.org/information-bulletin-what-do-you-call-me/#main

Nature Genetics (2003). Touching base: Mutant of the month. *Nature Genetics, 33*, 119. https://www.nature.com/articles/ng0203-119

Nordby, K. (1990). Vision in a complete achromat: A personal account. In R. F. Hess, L. T. Sharpe, & K. Nordby (Eds.), *Night vision: Basic, clinical and applied aspects* (pp. 290–315). Cambridge University Press. http://consc.net/misc/achromat.html

Owsley, C. & McGwin, G., Jr. (2010). Vision and driving. *Vision Research, 50*(23), 2348–2361. https://doi.org/10.1016/j.visres.2010.05.021

Owsley, C. (2011). Aging and vision. *Vision Research, 51*(13), 1610–1622. https://doi.org/10.1016/j.visres.2010.10.020

Owsley, C., Ball, K., McGwin, G., Jr., Sloane, M. E., Roenker, D. L., White, M. F., & Overley, E. T. (1998). Visual processing impairment and risk of motor vehicle crash among older adults. *JAMA, 279*(14), 1083–1088. https://doi.org/10.1001/jama.279.14.1083

Owsley, C., McGwin, G., Jr., Scilley, K., & Kallies, K. (2006). Development of a questionnaire to assess vision problems under low luminance in age-related maculopathy. *Investigative Ophthalmology & Visual Science, 47*(2), 528–535. https://doi.org/10.1167/iovs.05-1222

Owsley, C., McGwin, G., Jr., Sloane, M., Wells, J., Stalvey, B. T., & Gauthreaux, S. (2002). Impact of cataract surgery on motor vehicle crash involvement by older adults. *JAMA, 288*(7), 841–849. https://doi.org/10.1001/jama.288.7.841

Palanker, D., Le Mer, Y., Mohand-Said, S., & Sahel, J. A. (2022). Simultaneous perception of prosthetic and natural vision in AMD patients. *Nature Communications, 13*(1), 513. https://doi.org/10.1038/s41467-022-28125-x

Pang, L. (2016). Hallucinations experienced by visually impaired: Charles Bonnet Syndrome. *Optometry and Vision Science, 93*(12), 1466–1478. https://doi.org/10.1097/opx.0000000000000959

Pelli, D. G., Palomares, M., & Majaj, N. J. (2004). Crowding is unlike ordinary masking: Distinguishing feature detection and integration. *Journal of Vision, 4*(12), 1136–1169. https://doi.org/10.1167/4.12.12

Pelli, D. G., Robson, J. G., & Wilkins, A. J. (1988). The design of a new letter chart for measuring contrast sensitivity. *Clinical Vision Sciences, 2*(3), 187–199.

Perales, E., Martínez-Verdú, F. M., Linhares, J. M. M., & Nascimento, S. M. C. (2010). Number of discernible colors for color-deficient observers estimated from the MacAdam limits. *Journal of the Optical Society of America A, 27*(10), 2106–2114. https://doi.org/10.1364/JOSAA.27.002106

Pierce, E. A., Aleman, T. S., Jayasundera, K. T., Ashimatey, B. S., Kim, K., Rashid, A., Jaskolka, M. C., & Pennesi, M. E. (2024). Gene editing for CEP290-associated retinal degeneration. *The New England Journal of Medicine, 390*(21), 1972–1984. https://doi.org/10.1056/NEJMoa2309915

Polyak, S. L. (1957). *The vertebrate visual system.* University of Chicago Press.

Porcheron, A., Mauger, E., Soppelsa, F., Liu, Y., Ge, L., Pascalis, O., Russell, R., & Morizot, F. (2017). Facial contrast is a cross-cultural cue for perceiving age. *Frontiers in Psychology, 8*, 1208. https://doi.org/10.3389/fpsyg.2017.01208

Prosopagnosia Research Center. (n.d.). Faceblind. https://www.faceblind.org/

Racette L., Fischer, M., Bebie, H., Holló, G., Johnson, C. A., & Matsumoto, C. (2019). Visual field digest: A guide to perimetry and the Octopus Perimeter (8th ed.). Haag-Streit AG. https://haag-streit.com/2%20Products/Speciality%20diagnostics/Perimetry/Category%20assets/Books/HS_perimetry_br_xxx_visual_field_digest_8th_en.pdf

Radner, W. (2017). Reading charts in ophthalmology. *Graefe's Archive for Clinical and Experimental Ophthalmology, 255*(8), 1465–1482. https://doi.org/10.1007/s00417-017-3659-0

Ramulu, P. (2009). Glaucoma and disability: Which tasks are affected, and at what stage of disease? *Current Opinion in Ophthalmology, 20*(2), 92–98. https://doi.org/10.1097/ICU.0b013e32832401a9

Ravin, J. G. (1999). Sesquicentennial of the ophthalmoscope. *Archives of Ophthalmology, 117*(12), 1634–1638. https://doi.org/10.1001/archopht.117.12.1634

Reid, V. M., Dunn, K., Young, R. J., Amu, J., Donovan, T., & Reissland, N. (2017). The human fetus preferentially engages with face-like visual stimuli. *Current Biology, 27*(12), 1825–1828. https://doi.org/10.1016/j.cub.2017.05.044

Reinhard, J., Schreiber, A., Schiefer, U., Kasten, E., Sabel, B. A., Kenkel, S., Vonthein, R., & Trauzettel-Klosinski, S. (2005). Does visual restitution training change absolute homonymous visual field defects? A fundus controlled study. *British Journal of Ophthalmology*, *89*(1), 30–35. https://doi.org/10.1136/bjo.2003.040543

Reymond, L., & Wolfe, J. (1981). Behavioural determination of the contrast sensitivity function of the eagle Aquila audax. *Vision Research*, *21*(2), 263–271. https://doi.org/10.1016/0042-6989(81)90120-6

Robinson, J. L., Liu, Y., & Chen, Q. (2021). Licensure and driving status among visually impaired persons. *Optometry and Vision Science*, *98*(12), 1334–1339. https://doi.org/10.1097/OPX.0000000000001812

Roman-Lantzy, C. (2018). *Cortical visual impairment – An approach to assessment and intervention* (2nd ed.). AFB Press.

Rosenfeld, P. J., Brown, D. M., Heier, J. S., Boyer, D. S., Kaiser, P. K., Chung, C. Y., & Kim, R. Y., for the MARINA Study Group. (2006). Ranibizumab for neovascular age-related macular degeneration. *The New England Journal of Medicine*, *355*(14), 1419–1431. https://doi.org/10.1056/NEJMoa054481

Rubin, G. S. (2013). Measuring reading performance. *Vision Research*, *90*, 43–51. https://doi.org/10.1016/j.visres.2013.02.015

Runyan, M. [Vision Loss Resources] (2014, February 21). *Marla Runyan at Vision Loss Resources, Part 1 of 2* [Video]. Youtube. https://www.youtube.com/watch?v=zlBuyRoyDMg

Russell, S., Bennett, J., Wellman, J. A., Chung, D. C., Yu, Z. -F., Tillman, A., Wittes, J., Pappas, J., Elci, O., McCague, S., Cross, D., Marshall, K. A., Walshire, J., Kehoe, T. L., Reichert, H., Davis, M., Raffini, L., George, L. A., Hudson, F. P., Dingfield, L., ... Maguire, A. M. (2017). Efficacy and safety of voretigene neparvovec (AAV2-hRPE65v2) in patients with RPE65-mediated inherited retinal dystrophy: A randomised, controlled, open-label, phase 3 trial. *The Lancet*, *390*(10097), 849–860. https://doi.org/10.1016/S0140-6736(17)31868-8

Russell-Minda, E., Jutai, J. W., Strong, J. G., Campbell, K. A., Gold, D., Pretty, L., & Wilmot, L. (2007). The legibility of typefaces for readers with low vision: A research review. *Journal of Visual Impairment & Blindness*, *101*(7), 402–415. https://doi.org/10.1177/0145482X0710100703

Sacks, O. (1993, May). To see and not see. *The New Yorker*, 59–73.

Sacks, O. (1996). The island of the colorblind. Vintage Books.

Sacks, O. (2010). *The mind's eye.* Alfred A. Knopf.

Sadato, N., Pascual-Leone, A., Grafman, J., Ibanez, V., Deiber, M. -P., Dold, G., & Hallett, M. (1996). Activation of the primary visual cortex by Braille reading in blind subjects. *Nature*, *380*, 526–528. https://doi.org/10.1038/380526a0

Sakki, H. E. A., Dale, N. J., Sargent, J., Perez-Roche, T., & Bowman, R. (2018). Is there consensus in defining childhood cerebral visual impairment? A systematic review of terminology and definitions. *British Journal of Ophthalmology*, *102*(4), 424–432. https://doi.org/10.1136/bjophthalmol-2017-310694

Sandberg, M. A., & Gaudio, A. R. (2006). Reading speed of patients with advanced retinitis pigmentosa or choroideremia. *Retina*, *26*(1), 80–88. https://doi.org/10.1097/00006982-200601000-00013

Sehrin, F., Jin, L., Naher, K., Das, N. C., Chan, V. F., Li, D. F., Berson, S., Gudwin, E., Clarke, M., Stephan, T., & Congdon, N. (2024). The effect on income of providing near vision correction to workers in Bangladesh: The THRIVE (Tradespeople and Hand-workers Rural Initiative for a Vision-enhanced Economy) randomized controlled trial. *PLoS One*, *19*(4), e0296115. https://doi.org/10.1371/journal.pone.0296115

Seiple, W., Overbury, O., Rosenthal, B., Arango, T., Odom, J. V., & Morse, A. R. (2018). Effects of lighting on reading speed as a function of letter size. *American Journal of Occupational Therapy, 72*(2), 7202345020. https://doi.org/10.5014/ajot.2018.021873

Sengillo, J. D., Gregori, N. Z., Sisk, R. A., Weng, C. Y., Berrocal, A. M., Davis, J. L., Mendoza-Santiesteban, C. E., Zheng, D. D., Feuer, W. J., & Lam, B. L. (2022). Visual acuity, retinal morphology, and patients' perceptions after voretigene neparovec-rzyl therapy for RPE65-associated retinal disease. *Ophthalmology Retina, 6*(4), 273–283. https://doi.org/10.1016/j.oret.2021.11.005

Silson, E. H., Gouws, A. D., Legge, G. E., & Morland, A. B. (2022). In a case of longstanding low vision regions of visual cortex that respond to tactile stimulation of the finger with Braille characters are not causally involved in the discrimination of those same Braille characters. *Cortex, 155*, 277–286. https://doi.org/10.1016/j.cortex.2022.07.012

Silverman, W. A. (1980). Retrolental fibroplasia: A modern parable. Grune & Stratton.

Sinha, P. (2013). Once blind and now they see. *Scientific American Magazine, 309*(1), 48–55. https://www.scientificamerican.com/article/blind-kids-gain-vision-late-childhood-while-giving-lesson-in-brain-science/

Solomon, A. (2012) *Far from the tree: Parents, children and the search for identity*. Scribner.

Srinivasan, M. V. (2011). Honeybees as a model for the study of visually guided flight, navigation, and biologically inspired robotics. *Physiological Reviews, 91*(2), 413–460. https://doi.org/10.1152/physrev.00005.2010

Stein, J. D., Brown, M. M., Brown, G. C., Hollands, H., & Sharma, S. (2003). Quality of life with macular degeneration: Perceptions of patients, clinicians, and community members. *British Journal of Ophthalmology, 87*(1), 8–12. https://doi.org/10.1136/bjo.87.1.8

Steinkuller, P. G. (2010). Legal vision requirements for drivers in the United States. *AMA Journal of Ethics*, 938–940. https://doi.org/10.1001/virtualmentor.2010.12.12.hlaw1-1012

Stingl, K., Bartz-Schmidt, K. U., Besch, D., Chee, C. K., Cottriall, C. L., Gekeler, F., Groppe, M., Jackson, T. L., MacLaren, R. E., Koitschev, A., Kusnyerik, A., Neffendorf, J., Nemeth, J., Naeem, M. A. N., Peters, T., Ramsden, J. D., Sachs, H., Simpson, A., Singh, M. S., Wilhelm, B., ... & Zrenner, E. (2015). Subretinal visual implant Alpha IMS—Clinical trial interim report. *Vision Research, 111*(Part B), 149–160. https://doi.org/10.1016/j.visres.2015.03.001

Strasburger, H., Rentschler, I., & Jüttner, M. (2011). Peripheral vision and pattern recognition: A review. *Journal of Vision, 11*(5), 13. https://doi.org/10.1167/11.5.13

Strickland, E., & Harris, M. (2022, February 15). Their bionic eyes are now obsolete and unsupported. *IEEE Spectrum*. https://spectrum.ieee.org/bionic-eye-obsolete

Strong, P. (n.d.). *The history of the white cane*. The New Jersey Council of the Blind. https://www.njcounciloftheblind.org/brochures/history_of_white_cane.htm

Summers, C. G. (2009). Albinism: Classification, clinical characteristics, and recent findings. *Optometry & Vision Science, 86*(6), 659–662. https://doi.org/10.1097/OPX.0b013e3181a5254c

Swain, T. A., McGwin, G., Wood, J. M., & Owsley, C. (2021). Motion perception as a risk factor for motor vehicle collision involvement in drivers ≥ 70 years. *Accident Analysis & Prevention, 151*, 105956. https://doi.org/10.1016/j.aap.2020.105956

Switzer, J. V. (2003). *Disabled rights: American disability policy and the fight for equality*. Georgetown University Press.

Tarampi, M. R., Creem-Regehr, S. H., & Thompson, W. B. (2010). Intact spatial updating with severely degraded vision. *Attention, Perception & Psychophysics, 72*(1), 23–27. https://doi.org/10.3758/APP.72.1.23

Tarita-Nistor, L., Brent, M. H., Steinbach, M. J., Markowitz, S. N., & Gonzalez, E. G. (2014). Reading training with threshold stimuli in people with central vision loss: A feasibility study. *Optometry & Vision Science, 91*(1), 86–96. https://doi.org/10.1097/OPX.0000000000000108

Tarita-Nistor, L., Lam, D., Brent, M. H., Steinbach, M. J., & Gonzalez, E. G. (2013). Courier: A better font for reading with age-related macular degeneration. *Canadian Journal of Ophthalmology*, *48*(1), 56–62. https://doi.org/10.1016/j.jcjo.2012.09.017

Tarita-Nistor, L., Sverdlichenko, I., & Mandelcorn, M. S. (2023). What is a preferred retinal locus? *Annual Review of Vision Science*, *9*, 201–220. https://doi.org/10.1146/annurev-vision-111022-123909

Taylor, D. J., Edwards, L. A., Binns, A. M., & Crabb, D. P. (2018). Seeing it differently: Self-reported description of vision loss in dry age-related macular degeneration. *Ophthalmic and Physiological Optics*, *38*(1), 98–105. https://doi.org/10.1111/opo.12419

Taylor, N. M., Jakobson, L. S., Maurer, D., & Lewis, T. L. (2009). Differential vulnerability of global motion, global form, and biological motion processing in full-term and preterm children. *Neuropsychologia*, *47*(13), 2766–2778. https://doi.org/10.1016/j.neuropsychologia.2009.06.001

Tefft, B. C. (2017). Rates of motor vehicle crashes, injuries and deaths in relation to driver age, United States, 2014-2015. Washington, D.C., AAA Foundation for Traffic Safety.

Teller, D. Y. (1997). First glances: The vision of infants. The Friedenwald Lecture. *Investigative Ophthalmology & Visual Science*, *38*(11), 2183–2203.

Teng, S., Puri, A., & Whitney, D. (2012). Ultrafine spatial acuity of blind expert human echolocators. *Experimental Brain Research*, *216*(4), 483–488. https://doi.org/10.1007/s00221-011-2951-1

Thompson, W. B., Shakespeare, R. A., Liu, S., Kersten, D. J., Creem-Regehr, S., & Legge, G. E. (2021). Evaluating the visibility of architectural features for people with low vision: A quantitative approach. *LEUKOS: The Journal of the Illuminating Engineering Society*, *18*(2), 154–172 https://doi.org/10.1080/15502724.2021.1890115

Tideman, J. W. L., Snabel, M. C. C., Tedja, M. S., van Rijn, G. A., Wong, K. T., Kuijpers, R. W. A. M., Vingerling, J. R., Hofman, A., Buitendijk, G. H. S., Keunen, J. E. E., Boon, C. J. F., Geerards, A. J. M., Luyten, G. P. M., Verhoeven, V. J. M, & Klaver, C. C. W. (2016). Association of axial length with risk of uncorrectable visual impairment for Europeans with myopia. *JAMA Ophthalmology*, *134*(12), 1355–1363. https://doi.org/10.1001/jamaophthalmol.2016.4009

Tinker, M. A. (1963). *Legibility of print*. Iowa State University Press.

Tong, J., Huang, J., Khou, V., Martin, J., Kalloniatis, M., & Ly, A. (2021). Topical review: Assessment of binocular sensory processes in low vision. *Optometry and Vision Science*, *98*(4), 310–325. https://doi.org/10.1097/opx.0000000000001672

Traquair, H. M. (1927). *An introduction to clinical perimetry* (1st ed.). Henry Kimpton.

Tsang, J. Y., Wright, A., Carr, M. J., Dickinson, C., Harper, R. A., Kontopantelis, E., Van Staa, T., Munford, L., Blakeman, T., & Ashcroft, D. M. (2023). Risk of falls and fractures in individuals with cataract, age-related macular degeneration, or glaucoma. *JAMA Ophthalmology*, *142*(2), 96–106. https://doi.org/10.1001/jamaophthalmol.2023.5858

Tyler, C. W. (2015). Peripheral color demo. *i-Perception*, *6*(6), 1–5. https://doi.org/10.1177%2F2041669515613671

van der Aa, H. P. A., Garcia-Piña, F., van Nispen, R. M. A., Hoogland, J., Roberts, C., & Seiple, W. (2024). Performance on clinical outcomes, activities of daily living and user experience on head-mounted displays for people with vision impairment. *Ophthalmic and Physiological Optics*, *44*(5), 840–853. https://doi.org/10.1111/opo.13329

Venugopal, D., Wood, J. M., Black, A. A., & Bentley, S. A. (2023). Effect of low luminance on face recognition in adults with central and peripheral vision loss. *Ophthalmic and Physiological Optics*, *43*(6), 1344–1355. https://doi.org/10.1111/opo.13198

Verghese, P., Vullings, C., & Shanidze, N. (2021). Eye movements in macular degeneration. *Annual Review of Vision Science*, *7*, 773–791. https://doi.org/10.1146/annurev-vision-100119-125555

Wang, S., Moharrer, M., Baliutaviciute, V., Dougherty, B. E., Cybis, W., Bowers, A. R., & Luo, G. (2020). Bioptic telescope use in naturalistic driving by people with visual impairment. *Translational Vision Science & Technology*, *9*(4), 11. https://doi.org/10.1167/tvst.9.4.11

Weale, R. A. (1963). *The Aging Eye*. Hoeber Medical Division, Harper & Row.

Weiskrantz, L., Warrington, E. K., Sanders, M. D., & Marshall, J. (1974). Visual capacity in the hemianopic field following a restricted occipital ablation. *Brain*, *97*(1), 709–728.

Wells-Gray, E. M., Choi, S. S., Bries, A., & Doble, N. (2016). Variation in rod and cone density from the fovea to the mid-periphery in healthy human retinas using adaptive optics scanning laser ophthalmoscopy. *Eye*, *30*(8), 1135–1143. https://doi.org/10.1038/eye.2016.107

Werner, J. S., Marsh-Armstrong, B., & Knoblauch, K. (2020). Adaptive changes in color vision from long-term filter usage in anomalous but not normal trichromacy. *Current Biology*, *30*(15), 3011–3015. https://doi.org/10.1016/j.cub.2020.05.054

West, S. K., Munoz, B., Rubin, G. S., Schein, O. D., Bandeen-Roche, K., Zeger, S., German, P. S., & Fried, L. P. (1997). Function and visual impairment in a population-based study of older adults. The SEE project. Salisbury Eye Evaluation. *Investigative Ophthalmology & Visual Science*, *38*(1), 72–82.

West, S. K., Rubin, G. S., Broman, A. T., Munoz, B., Bandeen-Roche, K., & Turano, K. (2002). How does visual impairment affect performance on tasks of everyday life? The SEE Project. *Archives of Ophthalmology*, *120*(6), 774–780. https://doi.org/10.1001/archopht.120.6.774

White, U. E., Black, A. A., Wood, J. M., & Delbaere, K. (2015). Fear of falling in vision impairment. *Optometry & Vision Science*, *92*(6), 730–735. http://doi.org/10.1097/OPX.0000000000000596

Whittaker, S. G., & Lovie-Kitchin, J. (1993). Visual requirements for reading. *Optometry & Vision Science*, *70*(1), 54–65.

Wiecek, E., Lashkari, K., Dakin, S. C., & Bex, P. (2015a). Metamorphopsia and interocular suppression in monocular and binocular maculopathy. *Acta Ophthalmologica*, *93*(4), e318–e320. https://doi.org/10.1111/aos.12559

Wiecek, E., Lashkari, K., Dakin, S. C., & Bex, P. (2015b). Novel quantitative assessment of metamorphopsia in maculopathy. *Investigative Ophthalmology & Visual Science*, *56*(1), 494–504. https://doi.org/10.1167/iovs.14-15394.

Wilkinson, M. E., & McGehee, D. V. (2019). Auditory global positioning system and advanced driver assistance systems: A safer alternative to bioptic telescopes for drivers who are visually impaired? *Optometry and Vision Science*, *96*(2), 130–132. https://doi.org/10.1097/OPX.0000000000001326

Windsor, R. L., Ford, C. A., & Windsor, L. K. (2022). *State laws for bioptic driving by state*. Bioptic Driving USA. http://www.biopticdrivingusa.com/state-laws/

Witkop, C. J., Jr., Nance, W. E., Rawls, R. F., & White, J. G. (1970). Autosomal recessive oculocutaneous albinism in man. Evidence for genetic heterogeneity. *American Journal of Human Genetics*, *22*(1), 55–74.

Wolffsohn, J. S., Palmer, E., Rubinstein, M., & Eperjesi, F. (2012). Effect of light-emitting diode colour temperature on magnifier reading performance of the visually impaired. *Clinical and Experimental Optometry*, *95*(5), 510–514. https://doi.org/10.1111/j.1444-0938.2011.00702.x

Wood, J. M., Black, A. A., Mallon, K., Kwan, A. S., & Owsley, C. (2018). Effects of age-related macular degeneration on driving performance. *Investigative Ophthalmology & Visual Science*, *59*(1), 273–279. https://doi.org/10.1167/iovs.17-22751

Wood, J. M., Black, A. A. Anstey, K. J., & Horswill, M. S. (2021). Hazard perception in older drivers with eye disease. *Translational Vision Science & Technology*, *10*(1), 31. https://doi.org/10.1167/tvst.10.1.31

Wood, J. M., Lacherez, P., Black, A. A., Cole, M. H., Boon, M. Y., & Kerr, G. K. (2011). Risk of falls, injurious falls, and other injuries resulting from visual impairment among older adults with age-related macular degeneration. *Investigative Ophthalmology & Visual Science, 52*(8), 5088–5092. https://doi.org/10.1167/iovs.10-6644

Wood, J. M., McGwin, G., Elgin, J., Searcey, K., & Owsley, C. (2013). Characteristics of on-road driving performance of persons with central vision loss who use bioptic telescopes. *Investigative Ophthalmology & Visual Science, 54*(5), 3790–3797. https://doi.org/10.1167/iovs.12-11485

World Health Organization (WHO). (2019). *World report on vision*. https://www.who.int/publications/i/item/9789241516570

Wu, Y. -H., Granquist, C., Gage, R., Crossland, M. D., & Legge, G. E. (2020). Online survey of digital reading by adults with low vision. *Optometry & Vision Science, 97*(4), 249–256. https://doi.org/10.1097/OPX.0000000000001503

Wu, Y. -H., Yu, D., Goldstein, J. Kwon, M., Gobeille, M., Watson, E., Waked, L., Gage, R., & Legge, G. E. (2024). Estimating visual acuity without an acuity chart. *Translational Vision Science & Technology, 13*(9), 20. https://doi.org/10.1167/tvst.13.9.20

Wurm, L. H., Legge, G. E., Isenberg, L. M., & Luebker, A. (1993). Color improves object recognition in normal and low vision. *Journal of Experimental Psychology: Human Perception and Performance, 19*(4), 899–911. https://doi.org/10.1037/0096-1523.19.4.899

Wyszecki, G., & Stiles, W. S. (1982). *Color science: Concepts and methods, quantitative data and formulae*. John Wiley & Sons.

Xiong, Y., Nemargut, J. P., Bradley, C., Wittich, W., & Legge, G. E. (2024). Development and validation of a questionnaire for assessing visual and auditory abilities in dual sensory impairment. *Scientific Reports, 14*, 7911. https://doi.org/10.1038/s41598-024-58363-6

Xiong, Y. -Z., Kwon, M., Bittner, A. K., Virgili, G., Giacomelli, G., & Legge, G. E. (2020). Relationship between acuity and contrast sensitivity: Differences due to eye disease. *Investigative Ophthalmology and Visual Science, 61*(6), 40. https://doi.org/10.1167/iovs.61.6.40

Xiong, Y. -Z., Liu, R., Kwon, M., Bittner, A. K., Owsley, C., & Legge, G. E. (2021). A unified rule for binocular contrast summation applies to normal vision and common eye diseases. *Investigative Ophthalmology & Visual Science, 62*(13), 6. https://doi.org/10.1167/iovs.62.13.6

Xiong, Y. -Z., Lorsung, E. A., Mansfield, J. S., Bigelow, C., & Legge, G. E. (2018). Fonts designed for macular degeneration: Impact on reading. *Investigative Ophthalmology & Visual Science, 59*(10), 4182–4189. https://doi.org/10.1167/iovs.18-24334

Xu, J., Kendrick, K., & Bowers, A. R. (2022). Experiences of a driver with vision impairment when using a Tesla car. *Optometry and Vision Science, 99*(4), 417–421. https://doi.org/10.1097/OPX.0000000000001876

Xu, J., Kendrick, K., & Bowers, A. R. (2023). Letter to the editor: Update on experiences of a driver with vision impairment when using a Tesla car—Full self-driving (beta) in city driving. *Optometry and Vision Science, 100*(6), 351–353. https://doi.org/10.1097/OPX.0000000000002023

Yahalom, C., Braun, R., Patal, R., Saadeh, I., Blumenfeld, A., Macarov, M., & Hendler, K. (2022). Childhood visual impairment and blindness: 5-year data from a tertiary low vision center in Israel. *Eye, 36*, 2052–2056. https://doi.org/10.1038/s41433-021-01743-3

Yu, D., Chung, S. T. L., & Bailey, I. L. (2024). Conspicuity of staircase configuration: Effects of markings and contrast. *Ophthalmic and Physiological Optics, 44*(5), 854–866. https://doi.org/10.1111/opo.13333

Yue, L., Castillo, J., Calle Gonzalez, A., Neitz, J., & Humayun, M. S. (2021). Restoring color perception to the blind: An electrical stimulation strategy of retina in patients with end-stage retinitis pigmentosa. *Ophthalmology, 128*(3), 453–462. https://doi.org/10.1016/j.ophtha.2020.08.019

Zeng, F. G., Rebscher, S., Harrison, W., Sun, X., & Feng, H. (2008). Cochlear implants: System design, integration, and evaluation. *IEEE Reviews in Biomedical Engineering, 1*, 115–142. https://doi.org/10.1109/RBME.2008.2008250

Zhang, X., Bullard, K. M., Cotch, M. F., Wilson, M. R., Rovner, B. W., McGwin, G., Owsley, C., Barker, L., Crews, J. E., & Saaddine, J. B. (2013). Association between depression and functional vision loss in persons 20 years of age or older in the United States, NHANES 2005-2008. *JAMA Ophthalmology, 131*(5), 573–581. https://doi.org/10.1001/jamaophthalmol.2013.2597

Zrenner, E. (2002). Will retinal implants restore vision? *Science, 295*(5557), 1022–1025. https://doi.org/10.1126/science.1067996

Author Index

For the benefit of digital users, indexed terms that span two pages (e.g., 52–53) may, on occasion, appear on only one of those pages.

Subject Index

For the benefit of digital users, indexed terms that span two pages (e.g., 52–53) may, on occasion, appear on only one of those pages.

Tables, figures, and boxes are indicated by an italic *t*, *f*, or *b*.

The manufacturer's authorised representative in the EU for product safety is Oxford University Press España S.A. of el Parque Empresarial San Fernando de Henares, Avenida de Castilla, 2 – 28830 Madrid (www.oup.es/en or product.safety@oup.com). OUP España S.A. also acts as importer into Spain of products made by the manufacturer.

www.ingramcontent.com/pod-product-compliance
Lightning Source LLC
LaVergne TN
LVHW011633200926
848484LV00014B/2586/J
* 9 7 8 0 1 9 8 9 4 6 9 3 9 *